Platinum and Other Heavy Metal Compounds in Cancer Chemotherapy

Andrea Bonetti • Roberto Leone
Franco M. Muggia • Stephen B. Howell
Editors

Platinum and Other Heavy Metal Compounds in Cancer Chemotherapy

Molecular Mechanisms and Clinical Applications

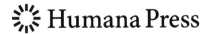 Humana Press

Editors
Andrea Bonetti
Department of Oncology
Mater Salutis Hospital
Legnago
Italy
andrea.bonetti@aulsslegnago.it

Roberto Leone
University of Verona
Institute of Pharmacology
Verona, Italy
rleone@sfm.univr.it

Franco M. Muggia
Division of Medical Oncology
New York University School of Medicine
    and the NYU Cancer Institute
New York, NY, USA
france.muggia@nyumc.org

Stephen B. Howell
Department of Medicine
    and the Moores Cancer Center
University of California, San Diego
La Jolla, CA
USA
showell@ucsd.edu

ISBN: 978-1-60327-458-6   e-ISBN: 978-1-60327-459-3
DOI: 10.1007/978-1-60327-459-3

Library of Congress Control Number: 2008939849

This book is dedicated to the memory of Lloyd R. Kelland, Ph.D., a generous and thoughtful colleague whose careful investigating of the mechanisms by which the platinum-containing drugs kill tumor cells provided valuable insights into how to improve their use in the management of cancer.

Preface

Cisplatin, the first member of the family of platinum-containing chemotherapeutic agents, was discovered by Barnett Rosenberg in 1965 and approved by the FDA for marketing in 1978. After 30 years of use in the clinic, cisplatin remains a central element of many treatment regimens. Cisplatin is still an irreplaceable component of a regimen that produces high cure rates in even advanced nonseminomatous germ-cell cancers, and is widely used in the treatment of ovarian cancers and other gynecologic cancers, head and neck, and numerous other tumor types. The development of carboplatin has reduced some of the adverse events associated with cisplatin treatment, and the introduction of the DACH platinum compound oxaliplatin has broadened the spectrum of activity of the platinums to include gastro-intestinal cancers, especially colorectal cancer. The clinical importance of this family of drugs continues to drive investigation into how these drugs work and how to improve their efficacy and reduce their toxicity.

The papers in this volume were presented in Verona, Italy, during the tenth International Symposium on Platinum Coordination Compounds in Cancer Chemotherapy. The symposium was jointly organized by the Department of Oncology of the Mater Salutis Hospital – Azienda Sanitaria Locale 21 of the Veneto Region – and by the Department of Medicine and Public Health, Section of Pharmacology, the University of Verona. They reflect the vitality of this field and the increasing use of new molecular and cell biologic, genetic, and biochemical tools to identify approaches to further improve their use.

Legnago, Italy   Andrea Bonetti
La Jolla, California, USA   Stephen B. Howell
Verona, Italy   Roberto Leone
New York, New York, USA   Franco M. Muggia

Contents

Contributors

Brooke J. Andrews
Department of Medicine, Indiana University School of Medicine,
Indianapolis, IN, USA;
Biomedical Science Graduate Program, Wright State University, Dayton,
OH, USA

Daniela Antonucci
Department of Biotechnology and Environmental Science, University of Salento,
Lecce, Italy

Lea Baer
Department of Radiation Oncology, New York University School of Medicine,
New York, NY, USA;
NYU Cancer Institute, New York, NY, USA

Giacomo Baldi
Division of Medical Oncology, Azienda USL 6, Istituto Toscano Tumori,
Livorno, Italy

Enzo Banelli
Department of Radiation Oncology, University "Sapienza," Rome, Italy

Philip Beale
Sydney Cancer Centre, Concord Repatriation General Hospital, Concord,
Australia

Michele Benedetti
Department of Biotechnology and Environmental Science, University of Salento,
Lecce, Italy

Valentina Benedetti
Department of Experimental Oncology, Fondazione IRCCS Istituto Nazionale
Tumori, Milan, Italy;
Department of Experimental Oncology and Laboratories, Preclinical
Chemotherapy and Pharmacology Unit, Istituto Nazionale per lo Studio e la Cura
dei Tumori, Milan, Italy

Alberta Bergamo
Callerio Foundation Onlus, Trieste, Italy

Roberta Bertani
Department of Chemical Processes of Engineering, University of Padova,
Padova, Italy

Debadeep Bhattacharyya
Department of Biochemistry and Biophysics, School of Medicine,
University of North Carolina, Chapel Hill, NC, USA

Andrea Bonetti
Department of Oncology, Mater Salutis Hospital, Legnago, Italy

Ovidio Bussolati
Unit of General and Clinical Pathology, Department of Experimental Medicine,
University of Parma, Parma, Italy

Sharon Campbell
Department of Biochemistry and Biophysics, School of Medicine,
University of North Carolina, Chapel Hill, NC, USA

Guido Cavaletti
Department of Neurosciences and Biomedical Technologies, University of Milan
"Bicocca," Monza, Italy

Stephen G. Chaney
Department of Biochemistry and Biophysics, School of Medicine,
Lineberger Comprehensive Cancer Center, University of North Carolina,
Chapel Hill, NC, USA

Etienne Chatelut
EA3035, Institut Claudius Regaud, Toulouse, France
Paul Sabatier University, University of Toulouse, Toulouse, France

Christine Chevreau
EA3035, Institut Claudius-Regaud, Toulouse, France

Giuliano Ciarimboli
Universitätsklinikum Münster, Medizinische Klinik und Poliklinik D,
Experimentelle Nephrologie, Münster, Germany

Giovanni Codacci-Pisanelli
Department of Experimental Medicine and Pathology, University "Sapienza,"
Rome, Italy

Samanta Cupini
Division of Medical Oncology, Azienda USL 6, Istituto Toscano Tumori,
Livorno, Italy

Esteban Cvitkovic
AAIOncology, Kremlin-Bicêtre, France

Ross Davey
Bill Walsh Cancer Research Laboratories, Department of Medical Oncology,
Royal North Shore Hospital, Sydney, Australia;
The University of Sydney, Lidcombe, NSW, Australia

Anton I.P.M. de Kroon
Biochemistry of Membranes, Bijvoet Institute and Institute of Biomembranes,
Utrecht University, Utrecht, The Netherlands

Angelo De Milito
Department of Therapeutic Research and Medicines Evaluation, Unit of Antitumor
Drugs, Drug Resistance and Experimental Therapeutic, Istituto Superiore
di Sanità, Rome, Italy

Shanta Dhar
Department of Chemistry, Massachusetts Institute of Technology, Cambridge,
MA, USA

Francesco Dionisi
Department of Radiation Oncology, University "Sapienza," Rome, Italy

Nikolay V. Dokholyan
Department of Biochemistry and Biophysics, School of Medicine, Lineberger
Comprehensive Cancer Center, University of North Carolina, Chapel Hill, NC,
USA

Fabrizio Drudi
Department of Oncology and Oncohematology, Infermi Hospital, Rimini, Italy

Cosimo Ducani
Department of Biotechnology and Environmental Science, University of Salento,
Lecce, Italy

Stefano Fais
Department of Therapeutic Research and Medicines Evaluation, Unit of Antitumor
Drugs, Drug Resistance and Experimental Therapeutic, Istituto Superiore
di Sanità, Rome, Italy

Sandrine Faivre
RayLab and Department of Medical Oncology, Beaujon University Hospital,
Clichy, France

Alfredo Falcone
Division of Medical Oncology, Azienda USL 6, Istituto Toscano Tumori,
Livorno, Italy;
Department of Oncology, Transplantations and New Technologies in Medicine,
University of Pisa, Italy

Francesco P. Fanizzi
Department of Biotechnology and Environmental Science, University of Salento,
Lecce, Italy

Manuela Fantini
Department of Oncology and Oncohematology, Infermi Hospital, Rimini, Italy

Gwenaël Ferron
Department of Surgical Oncology, Institut Claudius Regaud, Toulouse, France

Antonio T. Fojo
Experimental Therapeutics Section, Medical Oncology Branch, Center for Cancer
Research, National Cancer Institute, National Institutes of Health, Bethesda, MD,
USA

Lorenzo Fornaro
Division of Medical Oncology, Azienda USL 6, Istituto Toscano Tumori, Livorno,
Italy

Silvia C. Formenti
Department of Radiation Oncology, New York University School of Medicine,
New York, NY, USA;
NYU Cancer Institute, New York, NY, USA

Renata Franchi-Gazzola
Unit of General and Clinical Pathology, Department of Experimental Medicine,
University of Parma, Parma, Italy

Lara Furini
Department of Oncology, Mater Salutis Hospital, Legnago, Italy

Elisabetta Gabano
Department of Environmental and Life Sciences, University of Piemonte
Orientale "A. Avogadro," Alessandria, Italy

Valentina Gandin
Department of Pharmaceutical Sciences, University of Padova, Padova, Italy

Marzia B. Gariboldi
Department of Structural and Functional Biology, University of Insubria,
Busto Arsizio, Italy;

Laura Gatti
Department of Experimental Oncology, Fondazione IRCCS Istituto Nazionale
Tumori, Milan, Italy;
Department of Experimental Oncology and Laboratories, Preclinical
Chemotherapy and Pharmacology Unit, Istituto Nazionale per lo Studio e la Cura
dei Tumori, Milan, Italy

Amélie Gesson-Paute
Department of Surgical Oncology, Institut Claudius Regaud, Toulouse, France

Aïda Ghoul
RayLab and Department of Medical Oncology, Beaujon University Hospital,
Clichy, France

Giuseppe Giaccone
Medical Oncology Branch, National Cancer Institute, National Institutes
of Health, Bethesda, MD, USA

Lorenzo Gianni
Department of Oncology and Oncohematology, Infermi Hospital, Rimini, Italy

Alessandra Gilardini
Department of Neurosciences and Biomedical Technologies, University of Milan
"Bicocca," Monza, Italy

Laurence Gladieff
Department of Medical Oncology, Institut Claudius Regaud, Toulouse, France

Michael M. Gottesman
Laboratory of Cell Biology, National Cancer Institute, National Institutes
of Health, Bethesda, MD, USA

Ying Guo
Department of Biochemistry, School of Medicine, Morgantown, WV, USA
Mary Babb Randolph Cancer Center, Robert C. Byrd Health Sciences Center,
West Virginia University, Morgantown, WV, USA

Martin Gutierrez
Medical Oncology Branch, National Cancer Institute, National Institutes
of Health, Bethesda, MD, USA

Matthew D. Hall
Laboratory of Cell Biology, National Cancer Institute, National Institutes
of Health, Bethesda, MD, USA

Irene H.L. Hamelers
Biochemistry of Membranes, Bijvoet Institute and Institute of Biomembranes,
Utrecht University, Utrecht, The Netherlands

Qi He
Department of Biochemistry, School of Medicine, Morgantown, WV, USA;
Mary Babb Randolph Cancer Center, Robert C. Byrd Health Sciences Center,
West Virginia University, Morgantown, WV, USA

Paul J. Hoskins
British Columbia Cancer Agency, Vancouver, BC, Canada

Stephen B. Howell
Department of Medicine and the Moores Cancer Center, University of California,
San Diego, La Jolla, CA, USA

Fazlul Huq
Discipline of Biomedical Sciences, Cumberland Campus, The University of
Sydney, Lidcombe, NSW, Australia

Manuela Imola
Department of Oncology and Oncohematology, Infermi Hospital, Rimini, Italy

Claudio Isella
Division of Molecular Oncology, Institute for Cancer Research and Treatment,
Candiolo, Torino, Italy

Ulrich Jaehde
Department of Clinical Pharmacy, Institute of Pharmacy, University of Bonn,
Bonn, Germany

Dirk Jäger
National Center for Tumor Diseases, Department of Medical Oncology,
University of Heidelberg, Heidelberg, Germany

Ganna V. Kalayda
Department of Clinical Pharmacy, Institute of Pharmacy, University of Bonn,
Bonn, Germany

Maurizio Lanfranchi
Department of General and Inorganic, Analytical, and Physical Chemistry,
University of Parma, Parma, Italy

Cinzia Lanzi
Department of Experimental Oncology, Fondazione IRCCS Istituto Nazionale
Tumori, Milan, Italy;
Department of Experimental Oncology and Laboratories, Preclinical
Chemotherapy and Pharmacology Unit, Istituto Nazionale per lo Studio e la Cura
dei Tumori, Milan, Italy

Armelle Laurand
Institut Bergonié, Université Victor Segalen, Bordeaux, France

Michele Laus
Department of Environmental and Life Sciences, University of Piemonte
Orientale "A. Avogadro," Alessandria, Italy

Valérie Le Morvan
Institut Bergonié, Université Victor Segalen, Bordeaux, France

Xiaobing Liang
Department of Biochemistry, School of Medicine, Morgantown, WV, USA;
Mary Babb Randolph Cancer Center, Robert C. Byrd Health Sciences Center,
West Virginia University, Morgantown, WV, USA

Xing-Jie Liang
Laboratory of Cell Biology, National Cancer Institute, National Institutes
of Health, Bethesda, MD, USA;
Division of Nanomedicine and Nanobiology, National Center of Nanoscience
and Technology of China, Zhongguancun, Beijing, China

Stephen J. Lippard
Department of Chemistry, Massachusetts Institute of Technology, Cambridge,
MA, USA

François Lokiec
Rene Huguenin Cancer Center, Saint-Cloud, France

Florian Lordick
National Center for Tumor Diseases, Department of Medical Oncology,
University of Heidelberg, Heidelberg, Germany

Fotios Loupakis
Division of Medical Oncology, Azienda USL 6, Istituto Toscano Tumori,
Livorno, Italy;
Department of Oncology, Transplantations and New Technologies in Medicine,
University of Pisa, Italy

Francesca Luciani
Department of Therapeutic Research and Medicines Evaluation, Unit of Antitumor
Drugs, Drug Resistance and Experimental Therapeutic, Istituto Superiore
di Sanità, Rome, Italy

Maurizio Marangolo
Department of Oncology, Santa Maria Delle Croci Hospital, Ravenna, Italy

Luciano Marchiò
Department of General and Inorganic, Analytical, and Physical Chemistry,
University of Parma, Parma, Italy

Cristina Marzano
Department of Pharmaceutical Sciences, University of Padova, Padova, Italy

Gianluca Masi
Division of Medical Oncology, Azienda USL 6, Istituto Toscano Tumori,
Livorno, Italy

Silvia Mazzega Sbovata
Department of Chemical Processes of Engineering, University of Padova,
Padova, Italy

Enzo Medico
Division of Molecular Oncology, Institute for Cancer Research and Treatment,
Candiolo, Torino, Italy

Delphine Meynard
Institut Bergonié, Université Victor Segalen, Bordeaux, France

Rino A. Michelin
Department of Chemical Processes of Engineering, University of Padova,
Padova, Italy

Danilo Migoni
Department of Biotechnology and Environmental Science, University of Salento,
Lecce, Italy

Roberta Molteni
Department of Structural and Functional Biology, University of Insubria,
Busto Arsizio, Italy

Elena Monti
Department of Structural and Functional Biology, University of Insubria,
Busto Arsizio, Italy

Michael D. Mueller
Department of Biochemistry, School of Medicine, Morgantown, WV, USA;
Mary Babb Randolph Cancer Center, Robert C. Byrd Health Sciences Center,
West Virginia University, Morgantown, WV, USA

Franco M. Muggia
Division of Medical Oncology, New York University School of Medicine,
New York, NY, USA;
NYU Cancer Institute, New York, NY, USA

Daniela Musio
Department of Radiation Oncology, University "Sapienza," Rome, Italy

Stefania V.L. Nicoletti
Department of Oncology and Oncohematology, Infermi Hospital, Rimini, Italy

David Nowotnik
Access Pharmaceuticals Inc., Dallas, TX, USA

Domenico Osella
Department of Environmental and Life Sciences, University of Piemonte
Orientale "A. Avogadro," Alessandria, Italy

Ilaria Panzini
Department of Oncology and Oncohematology, Infermi Hospital, Rimini, Italy

Maximilian Papi
Department of Oncology and Oncohematology, Infermi Hospital, Rimini, Italy

Giuseppe Parisi
Department of Radiation Oncology, University "Sapienza," Rome, Italy

Enzo Pasquini
Department of Oncology, Cervesi Hospital, Cattolica, Italy

Nick Pavlakis
Bill Walsh Cancer Research Laboratories, Department of Medical Oncology, Royal North Shore Hospital, Sydney, Australia;
The University of Sydney, Lidcombe, NSW, Australia

Anna F.A. Peacock
Department of Chemistry, University of Warwick, Coventry, UK

Paola Perego
Department of Experimental Oncology, Fondazione IRCCS Istituto Nazionale Tumori, Milan, Italy;
Department of Experimental Oncology and Laboratories, Preclinical Chemotherapy and Pharmacology Unit, Istituto Nazionale per lo Studio e la Cura dei Tumori, Milan, Italy

Aurélie Pétain
EA3035, Institut Claudius-Regaud, Toulouse, France

Cinzia Possenti
Department of Oncology and Oncohematology, Infermi Hospital, Rimini, Italy

Denis Querleu
Department of Surgical Oncology, Institut Claudius Regaud, Toulouse, France
Paul Sabatier University, University of Toulouse; Toulouse, France

Nicola Raffetto
Department of Radiation Oncology, University "Sapienza," Rome, Italy

Srinivas Ramachandran
Department of Biochemistry and Biophysics, School of Medicine, Lineberger Comprehensive Cancer Center, University of North Carolina, Chapel Hill, NC, USA

Alberto Ravaioli
Department of Oncology and Oncohematology, Infermi Hospital, Rimini, Italy

Raffaella Ravizza
Department of Structural and Functional Biology, University of Insubria, Busto Arsizio, Italy

Eric Raymond
RayLab and Department of Medical Oncology, Beaujon University Hospital, Clichy, France

Eddie Reed
Division of Cancer Prevention and Control, National Center for Chronic Disease Prevention and Health Promotion, Centers for Disease Control and Prevention, Atlanta, GA, USA

Keyvan Rezaï
Rene Huguenin Cancer Center, Saint-Cloud, France

Riccardo Riccardi
Division of Pediatric Oncology, Department of Pediatric Sciences, Catholic
University of Rome, Rome, Italy

Jacques Robert
Institut Bergonié, Université Victor Segalen, Bordeaux, France

Alessandro Romano
Department of Biotechnology and Environmental Science, University of Salento,
Lecce, Italy

Britt Rudnas
Department of Oncology and Oncohematology, Infermi Hospital, Rimini, Italy

Antonio Ruggiero
Division of Pediatric Oncology, Department of Pediatric Sciences, Catholic
University of Rome, Rome, Italy

Peter J. Sadler
Department of Chemistry, University of Warwick, Coventry, UK

Roohangiz Safaei
Department of Medicine and the Moores Cancer Center, University of California,
San Diego, La Jolla, CA, USA

Lisa Salvatore
Division of Medical Oncology, Azienda USL 6, Istituto Toscano Tumori,
Livorno, Italy

Gianni Sava
Department of Biomedical Sciences, University of Trieste and Callerio Foundation
Onlus, Trieste, Italy

Antonin Schmitt
EA3035, Institut Claudius-Regaud, Toulouse, France

Maria Serova
RayLab and Department of Medical Oncology, Beaujon University Hospital,
Clichy, France

Shantanu Sharma
Department of Biochemistry and Biophysics, School of Medicine, University
of North Carolina, Chapel Hill, NC, USA

Ding-Wu Shen
Laboratory of Cell Biology, National Cancer Institute, National Institutes
of Health, Bethesda, MD, USA

Emily A. Short
Department of Medicine, Indiana University School of Medicine,
Indianapolis, IN, USA

Sarah C. Shuck
Department of Biochemistry and Molecular Biology, Indiana University
School of Medicine, Indianapolis, IN, USA

Katia Sparnacci
Department of Environmental and Life Sciences, University of Piemonte
Orientale "A. Avogadro," Alessandria, Italy

Gian Paolo Spinelli
Department of Experimental Medicine and Pathology, University "Sapienza,"
Rome, Italy

Irene Stasi
Division of Medical Oncology, Azienda USL 6, Istituto Toscano Tumori,
Livorno, Italy

Britta Stordal
Bill Walsh Cancer Research Laboratories, Department of Medical Oncology,
Royal North Shore Hospital, Sydney, Australia
The University of Sydney, Lidcombe, NSW, Australia

Emiliano Tamburini
Department of Oncology and Oncohematology, Infermi Hospital, Rimini, Italy

Saverio Tardito
Unit of General and Clinical Pathology, Department of Experimental Medicine,
University of Parma, Parma, Italy

Kevin Tay
Medical Oncology Branch, National Cancer Institute, National Institutes
of Health, Bethesda, MD, USA

Brenda Temple
Department of Biochemistry and Biophysics, School of Medicine, University
of North Carolina, Chapel Hill, NC, USA

Fabienne Thomas
EA3035, Institut Claudius Regaud, Toulouse, France
Paul Sabatier University, University of Toulouse, Toulouse, France

Ryan C. Todd
Department of Chemistry, Massachusetts Institute of Technology, Cambridge,
MA, USA

John J. Turchi
Department of Medicine and Department of Biochemistry and Molecular Biology,
Indiana University School of Medicine, Indianapolis, IN, USA

Sabine H. van Rijt
Department of Chemistry, University of Warwick, Coventry, UK

Enrico Vasile
Division of Medical Oncology, Azienda USL 6, Istituto Toscano Tumori,
Livorno, Italy;
Department of Oncology, Transplantations and New Technologies in Medicine,
University of Pisa, Italy

Vita M. Vecchio
Department of Biotechnology and Environmental Science, University of Salento,
Lecce, Italy

Tiziano Verri
Department of Biotechnology and Environmental Science, University of Salento,
Lecce, Italy

Yibing Wu
Department of Biochemistry and Biophysics, School of Medicine,
University of North Carolina, Chapel Hill, NC, USA

Qing-Wu Yan
Department of Biochemistry, School of Medicine, Morgantown, WV, USA
Mary Babb Randolph Cancer Center, Robert C. Byrd Health Sciences Center,
West Virginia University, Morgantown, WV, USA

Jing Jie Yu
Department of Biochemistry, School of Medicine, Morgantown, WV, USA
Mary Babb Randolph Cancer Center, Robert C. Byrd Health Sciences Center,
West Virginia University, Morgantown, WV, USA

Jun Qing Yu
Discipline of Biomedical Sciences, Cumberland Campus, The University
of Sydney, Lidcombe, NSW, Australia

Wainer Zoli
The Scientific Institute of Romagna for the Study and Treatment of Cancer,
Meldola, Forlì-Cesena, Italy

Franco Zunino
Department of Experimental Oncology, Fondazione IRCCS Istituto Nazionale
Tumori, Milan, Italy;
Department of Experimental Oncology and Laboratories, Preclinical
Chemotherapy and Pharmacology Unit, Istituto Nazionale per lo Studio e
la Cura dei Tumori, Milan, Italy

Platinum Compounds: The Culmination of the Era of Cancer Chemotherapy

Franco M. Muggia

Abstract The history of cancer chemotherapy is considered part of a chapter of empiricism that is coming to a close. However, the effect of cisplatin on germ cell tumors and, to a lesser extent, on epithelial ovarian cancer has captivated scientists and oncologists, and continues to expand its therapeutic horizons as more is learned. This is the Tenth Symposium on Platinum and Other Metal Coordination Compounds in Cancer Chemotherapy, and its highlights provide further confirmation of the value of scientific investment in this area of therapeutic research.

Keywords Chemotherapy; Cisplatin; Carboplatin; Germ cell and testicular tumors; Ovarian cancer

Various reviews have recounted the history of cancer chemotherapy, and its dawn at the beginning of the twentieth century with the introduction of "the magic bullet" concept against infectious pathogens and tumors by the brilliant German pathologist, Paul Ehrlich. The introduction of sulfonamides against bacteria and the effects of hormones against certain tumors constituted early validation of this concept. Modern chemotherapy, however, is usually traced to the sensational 2 December 1943 incident (1, 2) that occurred at the harbor of Bari, Italy. An air raid destroyed 17 allied ships, including one containing mustard "bombs" (being stored as possible retaliation to the threat of chemical warfare); exposed personnel experienced the marrow hypoplasia and involution of lymphoid tissue previously reported with sulfur mustard gas during World War I (3–5). In fact, the medicinal studies of the related nitrogen mustard by the U.S. governmental agencies, in concert with biomedical researchers at academic institutions such as Yale, had already started in 1942 (6). Fleming's unique discovery of penicillin in 1928 – a powerful stimulus for drug development – was followed by the search for drugs effective against

F.M. Muggia
Division of Medical Oncology, New York University School of Medicine and NYU Cancer Institute, NY, USA
e-mail: Franco.Muggia@nyumc.org

A. Bonetti et al. (eds.), *Platinum and Other Heavy Metal Compounds in Cancer Chemotherapy*, DOI: 10.1007/978-1-60327-459-3_1,
© Humana Press, a part of Springer Science + Business Media, LLC 2009

1

tuberculosis. This constellation of events led to the creation of the U.S. National Institutes of Health and the National Cancer Institute (NCI), which were to play a pivotal role in launching the era of anticancer chemotherapy. These government entities had the ability to sponsor scientific exchanges with other national and international institutions functioning largely unencumbered by profit motives. They succeeded as a clearing house of ideas to combat cancer, despite the rather primitive understanding of neoplastic cell and molecular biology.

The Initial Phases of Systematic Anticancer Drug Discovery

With the support of Congress and as a part of the U.S. government's Public Health Service, the NCI organized itself to utilize evolving knowledge of tumor biology for the bold idea of identifying drugs for cancer treatment. Activity against carcinogen-induced L1210 and P388 leukemias in mice became a criterion for selectivity of a drug against these rapidly dividing tumor cells, without irreparably harming the host (7). A number of drugs related to nitrogen mustard and biochemically designed antimetabolites were established to have clinical activity and, in spite of the shortcomings of random screening, successes could be claimed against some human malignancies (8). Collaboration with other governmental agencies (e.g., the Department of Agriculture) and the pharmaceutical industry also led to the selection of useful natural products such as the vincas, camptothecins, and taxanes – the vincas mostly developed by industry, and camptothecins, and taxanes through the perseverance of NCI-sponsored investigations. Another landmark achievement was the identification, by Heidelberger and colleagues, of 5-fluorouracil and its eventual potential in the treatment of breast and gastrointestinal cancers (9).

Clinical Investigators

It was important to link such therapeutic drug discovery efforts with physicians skilled in diagnosis, and eventually with experience in dealing with supportive care and management of complications of malignancies and drug treatments. It is not a coincidence that early pioneers in cancer treatment focused either on hematologic diseases (following their training in internal medicine), or on certain solid tumors (following their training in surgery and its specialties). In either case, these physicians considered clinical investigation the final common pathway for anticancer drug development and, in the course of patient care, began to apply them systematically in situations that, until that time, had been considered hopeless. Documentation of their success in clinical trials became a major important step in these efforts (reviewed by DeVita and Chu) (10).

Often unrecognized is one such pioneer: Ezra Greenspan (1919–2004), best known for developing the foundations of combination chemotherapy against advanced breast and ovarian cancers (11, 12). His optimistic outlook – as stated in the autobiographical notes he left to his colleagues – derived from having survived pneumonia while attending college at Cornell, because his physician opted to treat him with the recently obtained Prontosyl (a classmate who had preceded him in the hospital died without such intervention). Subsequently, upon finishing his medical studies at NYU, he was exposed to his first clinical trial under the mentorship of Isidore Snapper: the use of urethane (ethyl carbamate) in multiple myeloma (5) that included attempts to correlate clinical benefit with serial bone marrow examinations. When recruited into the Army in 1947, he became a physician at the Tumor Service at Walter Reed, where he describes adding the first available drugs (nitrogen mustard, triethylene melamine, and methotrexate) to radiation therapy for the treatment of testicular cancers and Hodgkin's disease. As the NCI opened its first clinical unit, Greenspan became the first clinical investigator in this fledgling program, and teamed up with the preclinical scientist, Abraham Goldin, who was to develop many of the principles of chemotherapy based on optimizing dose-scheduling of a drug in mouse leukemia models (13, 14). This experience with new therapeutic agents provided Greenspan with the unwavering optimism he demonstrated in facing the challenges of his long career as a clinical oncologist at Mount Sinai Hospital in New York.

Greenspan was the first to exploit the antitumor effects of methotrexate for the treatment of solid tumors, and document positive results in combination with alkylating agents (11, 12). In the 1950s and 1960s, a number of other physicians in academic centers began to develop clinical units devoted to the treatment of cancer, but met with resistance and disdain, particularly from Departments of Medicine that were skeptical of investing human resources in coupling the semi-empirical identification of anticancer drugs with the science of clinical trials (10). Despite this, clinical oncology began to flourish in the 1950s under the leadership of Alfred Gellhorn at Columbia and David Karnofsky at Memorial Sloan-Kettering, to be followed in the 1960s by a number of prominent specialists in hematology, general internal medicine, and surgery that were to become the key developers of Medical Oncology, followed by other oncologic specialties (10).

In the meantime, the NCI with its Chemotherapy Program led by C. Gordon Zubrod (himself a product of pharmacology research first devoted to antituberculous drugs), and its Medicine Branch staffed with clinical investigators such as Emil Frei and Emil (Jay) Freireich, concentrated its efforts on finding therapeutic regimens useful against leukemias (15). These efforts were later expanded to the treatment of Hodgkin's and other lymphomas, and subsequently to breast and ovarian cancers, with investigators such as Vincent DeVita, Paul Carbone, George Canellos, Robert Young, Philip Schein, and Bruce Chabner (10, 16–19). The success of the NCI intramural programs, coupled with a dramatic extramural expansion via cooperative groups (initially under the leadership of James Holland, Bernard Fisher, and John Durant, among others) and its phase I/II working groups, led to widening of the clinical testing of anticancer drugs, thereby accelerating changes in cancer treatment worldwide. The investment of the pharmaceutical industries in this area, long considered a risky proposition, grew rapidly in the 1970s, with substantial programs being developed in the U.S. by Bristol Myers, in Europe by Burroughs Welcome, Farmitalia, Rhone Poulenc, Roche, and Sandoz, and in Japan.

Curable Tumors as the "Stalking Horse" of Drug Discovery

Joseph Burchenal, who headed Developmental Therapeutics at Memorial Sloan-Kettering for approximately 40 years, starting from the 1950s (pairing up with David Karnofsky, who ran the Chemotherapy service), used the imagery of a "stalking horse" to describe Burkitt's lymphoma as an identifier of strategies applicable to leukemia in his 1966 presidential address to the American Association for Cancer Research. Early experience in testicular cancer has similarly served to validate treatment strategies: "prophylactic" radiation to the retroperitoneal space (20), and Greenspan's addition of alkylating agents to men he treated in 1947–1949 at Walter Reed's tumor service. Twenty-five years after the Walter Reed experience, complete responses to cisplatin in advanced testicular cancer were documented by Higby et al. (21) in Holland's group at Roswell Park, convincing initially skeptical investigators that it was worthy of further development. Shortly thereafter, trials performed at Memorial Sloan-Kettering (22) and at Indiana University with collaborators from the Southeastern Cancer Study Group (23) defined cisplatin-based treatments as curative. In the setting of recurrence, Einhorn and his group established the usefulness of certain anticancer drugs (e.g., etoposide and ifosfamide) (24), and also tested whether cisplatin dose-intensification would be a reasonable strategy. If such intensification did not prove useful in testicular cancer, it certainly would not be useful against cancers that are much less sensitive to platinums (25).

The impressive activity of cisplatin against germ-cell tumors, leading to cures in advanced disease conditions (exemplified by Lance Armstrong's extraordinary saga), should continue to influence our notions on how to succeed in drug development. Although it has been fashionable to speak about "personalized therapy," such a concept belies the fact that unparalleled successes can take place without individualized knowledge on the deranged pathways involved in tumorigenesis. Platinum contributions are not confined to this most impressive example; the extraordinary sensitivity of ovarian cancer to cisplatin and carboplatin is nothing short of remarkable, if one considers the very advanced presentations that are commonplace in this disease. In addition, the strides achieved during the past decade in the treatment of colorectal cancer owe as much to the introduction of oxaliplatin-based combinations as to the monoclonal antibodies against VEGF and EGFR (26). Emphasizing such contributions is not designed to shift the focus back to cytotoxic drug development, but to reiterate that research into mechanisms of platinum resistance and their manipulation may lead to therapeutic developments of the magnitude now preferentially expected from "targeted therapies." In fact, in an animal model of ovarian cancer from Dinulescu's laboratory (27), cisplatin is able to achieve cures that are beyond the reach of targeted agents directed against the targets that were implicated in the model. Similar observations have been made in the engineered mouse model of triple negative breast cancer (28).

Platinums in the Era of "Targeted Agents"

One might ask: What is it that continues to bring together chemists, basic scientists, and oncologists to hold meetings on platinums? For those of us who have attended a number of these events, the answer appears to be that platinums represent the culmination of anticancer drug development to date, and their achievements have continued to expand over the years (see Table 1). As an example, the 2007 meeting showcased a new generation of "targeted" drugs, such as poly (ADP-ribose) polymerase-1 (PARP-1) inhibitors and the proteasome inhibitor bortezomib, which are reversing important mechanisms that mediate resistance to platinums, such as DNA-repair and intracellular transport, respectively. The involvement of chemists and experimental biologists gleaned from these publications stimulates clinical investigations, and vice versa.

For an oncologist, the overview of these meetings epitomizes the satisfaction of being part of scientific advances that have the potential of bringing about major improvements in outcomes where inexorable progression of a cancerous tumor was once the rule. The pioneers that led the field of cancer chemotherapy in the early days were undoubtedly similarly inspired. Learning more about platinum drugs continues to provide us with an expanding number of patients that can attain the most successful outcome: a cure.

Table 1 Highlights of the ten international symposia on platinum coordination compounds in cancer chemotherapy (ISPCC), from 1971 to 2007

Year	Site	Chair(s)	Highlights and/or (ref)
1971	Prague	Barnett Rosenberg	Cisplatin: discovery and preclinical activity (29)
1973	Oxford	Tom Connors and John Roberts	(30)
1976	Dallas	Joseph Hill	Phase II studies by NCI and the Wadley Institute (31, 32)
1983	Burlington	Irwin Krakoff	Carboplatin introduced (33)
1987	Padova	Mario Nicolini	(34)
1991	San Diego	Stephen Howell	(35)
1995	Amsterdam	Herbert Pinedo and Jan Schornagel	(36)
1999	Oxford	Lloyd Kelland and IR Judson	Oxaliplatin highlighted (37)
2003	New York	Nicholas Farrell and Franco Muggia	Copper transporters; clinical results in gynecologic and colorectal cancers
2007	Verona	Andrea Bonetti and Roberto Leone	Current publication

References

1. Diel V. Hodgkin's disease – from pathology specimen to cure. N Eng J Med 2007;357: 1968–71.
2. Papac RJ. Chemotherapy plus involved-field radiation in early-stage Hodgkin's disease. N Eng J Med 2008;358:742–3 (letter).
3. Hirsh J. An anniversary for cancer chemotherapy. JAMA 2006;296:1518–20.
4. Krumbaar EB. Role of the blood and the bone marrow in certain forms of gas poisoning. 1. Peripheral blood changes and their significance. JAMA 1919;72:3941.
5. Goodman LS, Gilman A. Drugs used in the chemotherapy of neoplastic disease. In: Goodman LS, Gilman A, eds. The Pharmacological Basis of Therapeutics (2nd edn). New York, US: The Macmillan Company, 1958:1414–50.
6. Goodman LS, Wintrobe MM, Dameshek W, Goodman MJ, Gilman A, McLennan MT. Nitrogen mustard therapy. JAMA 1946;132:126–32.
7. Skipper HE. Cancer chemotherapy is many things: G.H.A. Clowes Memorial Lecture. Cancer Res 1971;31:1173–9.
8. Zubrod CG. Agents of choice in neoplastic disease. In: Sartorelli AC, Johns DG, eds. Antineoplastic and Immunosuppressive Agents I. New York, US: Springer, 1974:1–11.
9. Heidelberger C, Chaudhuari NK, Danenberg P, et al. Fluorinated pyrimidines: a new class of tumor inhibitory compounds. Nature 1957;179:663–6.
10. DeVita VT, Chu E. History of cancer chemotherapy. Cancer Res 2008;68:(in press).
11. Greenspan EM, Fieber M. Combination chemotherapy of advanced ovarian carcinoma with the antimetabolite methotrexate and the alkylating agent thio-TEPA. J Mt Sinai Hosp 1962;29:48–62.
12. Greenspan EM, Fieber M, Lesnick G, Edelman S. Response of advanced breast carcinoma to the combination of the antimetaboite, methotrexate and the alkylating agent, thio-TEPA. J Mt Sinai Hosp 1963;30:246–67.
13. Goldin A, Mantel N, Greenhouse SW, Venditti JM, Humphreys SR. Estimation of the anti-leukemic potency of the antimetabolite aminopterin, administered alone, and in combination with citrovorum factor or folic acid. Cancer Res 1953;13:843–50.
14. Goldin A, Mantel N, Greenhouse SW, Venditti JM, Humphreys SR. Factors influencing the specificity of action of an acute leukemia agent (aminopterin). Time of treatment and dosage schedule. Cancer Res 1954;14:311–4.
15. Frei E III, Freireich EJ, Gehan E, et al. Studies of sequential and combination antimetabolite therapy in acute leukemia: 6-mercaptopurine and methotrexate: from acute leukemia group A. Blood 1961;18:431–4.
16. DeVita VT, Serpick AA, Carbone PP. Combination chemotherapy in the treatment of advanced Hodgkin's disease. Ann Intern Med 1970;73:881–95.
17. DeVita VT, Canellos GP, Chabner B, Schein P, Young RC, Hubbard SM. Advanced diffuse histiocytic lymphoma: a potentially curable disease. Results with combination chemotherapy. Lancet 1975;1:248–54.
18. Fisher B, Carbone P, Economou SG, et al. L-phenylalaninine mustard (L-PAM) in the management of primary breast cancer. N Eng J Med 1975;292:122.
19. Young RC, Hubbard SP, DeVita VT. The chemotherapy of ovarian cancer. Cancer Treat Rev 1974;1:99–110.
20. Boden GL, Gibb R. Radiotherapy and testicular neoplasms. Lancet 1951;2:1195–7.
21. Higby DJ, Wallace HJ, Albert D, Holland JF. Diamminedichloroplatinum: a phase I study showing responses in testicular and other tumors. Cancer 1974;33:1219–25.
22. Cheng E, Cvitkovic E, Wittes RE, et al. Germ cell tumor: VABII in metastatic testicular cancer. Cancer 1978;42:2162–8.
23. Einhorn LH, Donahue JP. Cis-diamminedichloroplatinum, vinblastine, and bleomycin combination chemotherapy in disseminated testicular cancer. Ann Intern Med 1977;87:293–8.

24. Loehrer PJ, Einhorn LH, Williams SD. Salvage therapy for refractory germ cell tumors with VP-16, ifosfamide, and cisplatin. J Clin Oncol 1986;4:528–36.
25. Nichols CR, Williams SD, Loehrer PJ, Einhorn LH. Cisplatin dose-intensity in testicular cancer treatment: analysis of randomized clinical trials. In: Howell SB, ed. Platinum and Other Metal Coordination Compounds in Cancer Chemotherapy. New York, US: Plenum Press, 1991: 409–20.
26. Mathe G, Kidani Y, Triana K, et al. A phase I trial of trans-1-diaminocyclohexane oxalate-platinum (l-OHP). Biomed Pharmacother 1986;40:372–6.
27. Dinulescu DM, Ince TA, Quade BJ, Shafer SA, Crowley D, Jacks T. Role of K-ras and Pten in the development of mouse models of endometriosis and endometrioid ovarian cancer. Nat Med 2005;11:63–70.
28. Rottenberg S, Nygren AO, Pajic M, et al. Selective induction of chemotherapy resistance of mammary tumors in a conditional mouse model for hereditary breast cancer. Proc Natl Acad Sci USA 2007;104:12117–22.
29. Rosenberg B. Cisplatin: its history and possible mechanisms of action. In: Prestayko AW, Crooke ST, Carter SK, eds. Cisplatin: Current Status and New Developments. New York, US: Academic Press, 1980:9–20.
30. Connors TA, Roberts JJ. Platinum Coordination Complexes in Cancer Chemotherapy. Heidelberg, Germany: Springer, 1974.
31. Rozencweig M, Von Hoff DD, Slavik M, Muggia FM. Cis-diamminedichloroplatinum II (DDP): a new anticancer drug. Ann Intern Med 1977;86:803–12.
32. Rosenberg B. Cisplatin. J Clin Hematol Oncol (Wadley Bull) 1977;7:817–27.
33. Hacker MP, Double EB, Krakoff IH. Platinum Coordination Complexes in Cancer Chemotherapy. Boston, US: Martinus Nihjoff, 1984.
34. Nicolini M. Platinum and Other Metal Coordination Compounds in Cancer Chemotherapy. Boston, US: Martinus Nihjoff, 1988.
35. Howell SB. Platinum and other metal coordination compounds in cancer chemotherapy. New York, US: Plenum, 1991.
36. Pinedo HM, Schornagel JH. Platinum and other metal coordination compounds in cancer chemotherapy. New York, US: Plenum, 1996.
37. Kelland LR, Farrell NP. Platinum-based drugs in cancer therapy. Totowa, NJ, US: Humana, 2000.

Section A
Novel Platinum Analogues, Original Formulations and Other Heavy Metals

Studies on New Platinum Compounds

Fazlul Huq, Jun Qing Yu, and Philip Beale

Abstract This chapter provides a review of the activities of a number of recently synthesized planaramineplatinum(II) complexes and platinum compounds with multiple metal centers against human ovarian cancer cell lines. Planaramineplatinum complexes code named YH12 and CH1 are found to be significantly more active than cisplatin in the resistant ovarian cancer cell lines A2780^{cisR} and A2780^{ZD0473R}. The compound code-named CH3 contains three 3-hydroxypyridine ligands bound to platinum(II) and therefore can only form a monofunctional Pt(G) adduct and is found to be significantly active, thus indicating that the formation of bifunctional adducts with DNA may not be an essential requirement for activity. Among compounds containing multiple metal centers, DH6Cl and TH1 are much more active than cisplatin.

Keywords Planaramineplatinum complexes; Ovarian cancer cell lines

Introduction

Widespread use in clinics and increasing volume of sales indicate that even in the postgenomic age there is a need for the type of shotgun chemotherapy provided by platinum drugs. Although thousands of cisplatin analogues have been prepared by changing the nature of the leaving groups and carrier ligands, resulting in much reduced toxicity, only a limited change in the spectrum of activity has been achieved. Therefore attention is currently being given to rule-breaker platinum compounds, with the aim of widening the spectrum of activity and reducing the side effects associated with platinum-based chemotherapy (1–4). Two such classes

F. Huq (✉), J.Q. Yu, and P. Beale
Discipline of Biomedical Sciences, Cumberland Campus,
The University of Sydney, Lidcombe
e-mail: F.Huq@usyd.edu.au

A. Bonetti et al. (eds.), *Platinum and Other Heavy Metal Compounds
in Cancer Chemotherapy*, DOI: 10.1007/978-1-60327-459-3_2,
© Humana Press, a part of Springer Science + Business Media, LLC 2009

of compounds are *trans*-planaramineplatinum(II) complexes and compounds containing two or more platinum centers. One of the main reasons for the limited spectrum of activity of platinum drugs is the drug resistance that may be intrinsic and/or acquired. This paper provides a review of the work on new mononuclear and multinuclear platinum complexes carried out in our laboratory. Some of the complexes were found to be significantly more active than cisplatin against ovarian cancer cell lines (5–18).

Planaramineplatinum(II) Complexes

Figure 1 gives the structures of a number of planaramineplatinum(II) complexes of the forms: Pt(L)(NH$_3$)Cl$_2$, PtL$_2$X$_2$ and PtL$_3$X (where L = a planaramine ligand and X = Cl$^-$ except in the case of AH8 where X = I$^-$) that have been synthesized, characterized, and investigated for activity against human ovarian cancer cell lines A2780, A2780^{cisR} and A2780^{ZD0473R}. The cell uptake and level of binding with nuclear DNA have also been determined. Table 1 gives the IC$_{50}$ values of YH9, YH10, YH11, YH12, CH1, CH2, CH3 and CH4 against the human ovarian cancer cell lines A2780, A2780^{cisR} and A2780^{ZD0473R}.

Although *cis*-planaramineplatinum(II) complexes (with the exception of the totally inactive compound AH8 that has two iodide leaving groups) are found to be more active than the corresponding *trans*-planaramineplatinum(II) complexes, their resistance factors are generally larger. For example, AH5 is more active than YH12 against the A2780 cell line but less so against the A2780^{cisR} cell line. The results indicate that *cis*-planaramineplatinum(II) complexes have greater cross-resistance with cisplatin than the corresponding *trans* compounds. The results may also be seen to provide support to the idea that the increased DNA repair is a dominant mechanism of resistance operating in the ovarian cancer cell lines. As *cis*-planaramineplatinum(II) complexes, like cisplatin, are expected to form mainly bifunctional intrastrand Pt(GG) adducts and *trans*-planaramineplatinum(II) complexes are more likely to form interstrand Pt(GG) adducts, it follows that the DNA repair in *cis*-planaramineplatinum(II) complexes may involve the removal of intrastrand Pt(GG) adducts. Absence of any activity in TH8 (even though the compound is found to have a high level of binding with nuclear DNA) indicates that the compound may not form any significant amount of the critical bifunctional intrastrand Pt(GG) adduct, possibly because of the greater covalent character of Pt–I bond. It should, however, be noted that the formation of a bifunctional adduct is not an essential requirement for activity since CH3 (that has three 3-hydroxypyridine ligands bound to platinum and therefore can only form monofunctional adduct with DNA) is also found to be significantly active. One of the *trans*-planaramineplatinum(II) complexes, namely YH12, was found to be more active against the resistant cell line A2780^{cisR}, indicating its lack of cross-resistance with cisplatin. When the activities of compounds with different planaramine ligands are compared, it was found that 3-hydroxypyridine and imidazo(1,2-α)

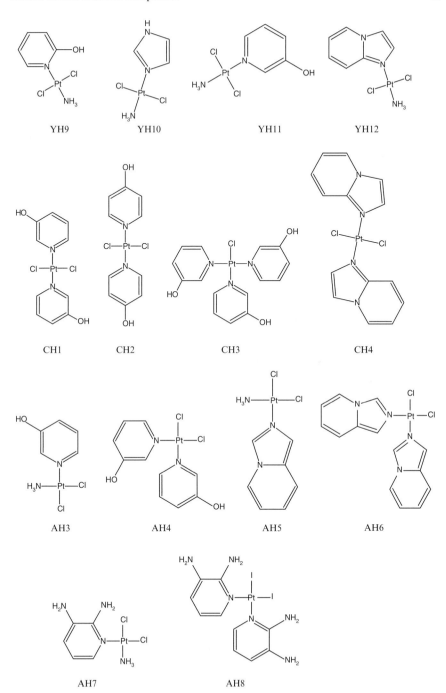

Fig. 1 Structure of synthesized *cis*- and *trans*-planaramineplatinum(II) complexes

Table 1 IC$_{50}$ values of YH9, YH10, YH11, YH12, AH3, AH5, AH6, AH7 and AH8 against the human ovarian cancer cell lines A2780, A2780^{cisR} and A2780^{ZD0473R}

Compound	IC$_{50}$ values (µM)			RF (A2780 vs. A2780^{cisR})	RF (A2780 vs. A2780^{ZD0473R})
	A2780	A2780^{cisR}	A2780^{ZD0473R}		
Cisplatin	0.45 ± 0.1	4.4 ± 0.6	1.2 ± 0.2	9.8	4.8
YH9	15.0 ± 9	18.5 ± 13.5	11.0 ± 1	1.2	0.8
YH10	13.2 ± 1.5	16.5 ± 3.4	17.9 ± 3.5	1.4	1.4
YH11	11.7 ± 1.9	15.0 ± 1.9	16.2 ± 1.6	1.4	1.4
YH12	4.4 ± 1.6	2.3 ± 0.5	4.9 ± 0.3	0.5	1.1
CH1	1.5 ± 0.8	2.7 ± 0.6	1.2 ± 0.8	1.8	0.8
CH2	3.4 ± 1.2	10.2 ± 1.0	5.7 ± 0.6	3.0	1.7
CH3	3.3 ± 1.2	6.1 ± 0.7	3.4 ± 0.7	1.8	1.0
CH4	0.9 ± 0.6	7.2 ± 0.7	4.3 ± 1.0	8.0	4.8
AH3	0.8 ± 1.0	7.1 ± 1.0	2.7 ± 1.0	8.9	3.4
AH4	1.8 ± 0.6	20.6 ± 0.7	8.0 ± 0.6	11.4	2.8
AH5	0.9 ± 0.1	6.5 ± 0.7	3.3 ± 0.6	7.2	2.8
AH6	2.0 ± 0.1	8.0 ± 0.5	3.6 ± 0.6	4.0	3.0
AH7	3.1 ± 0.3	9.9 ± 1.3	4.5 ± 1.0	3.2	3.8
AH8	N/A	N/A	N/A	N/A	N/A

pyridine act as activating ligands whereas 4-hydroxypyridine acts as a deactivating ligand. DH4 that has two 2-methylimidazole ligands in a *trans*-geometry is found to be significantly more active than cisplatin against all the three ovarian cancer cell lines.

Platinum Complexes with Multiple Metal Centers

Figure 2 gives the structures of a number of trinuclear Pt–Pd–Pt and Pt–Pt–Pt complexes that have been synthesized and investigated for activity against human ovarian cancer cell lines A2780, A2780^{cisR} and A2780^{ZD0473R}. Table 2 gives the IC$_{50}$ values of DH4Cl, DH5Cl, DH6Cl, DH7Cl, TH1 and TH8 against the human ovarian cancer cell lines A2780, A2780^{cisR} and A2780^{ZD0473R}. DH6Cl and TH1 are found to be significantly more active than cisplatin against the ovarian cancer cell lines A2780, A2780^{cisR} and A2780^{ZD0473R}. Although DH6Cl is more active than TH1, the former has larger resistance factors than the latter; these may be the result of noncovalent interactions involving 3-hydroxypyridine ligands. Among DH4Cl, DH5Cl, DH6Cl and DH7Cl, it was found that DH7Cl has the highest cellular level but DH6Cl has the highest level of nuclear binding in line with its highest activity in all the three ovarian cancer cell lines.

Finally, it should be noted that YH12, CH3, DH4, DH6Cl and TH1 have the potential for development as novel platinum-based anticancer drugs with a spectrum of activity different from that of cisplatin.

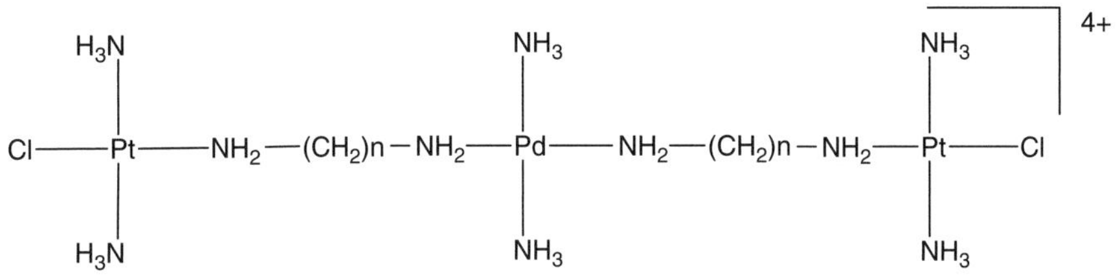

n=4, 5, 6, 7 for DH4Cl, DH5Cl, DH6Cl and DH7Cl respectively

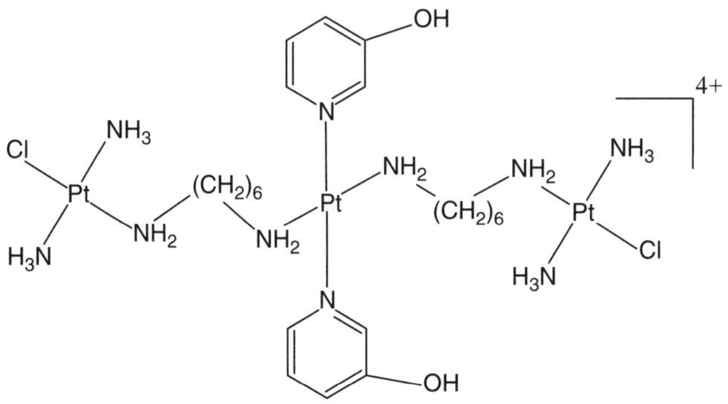

TH1

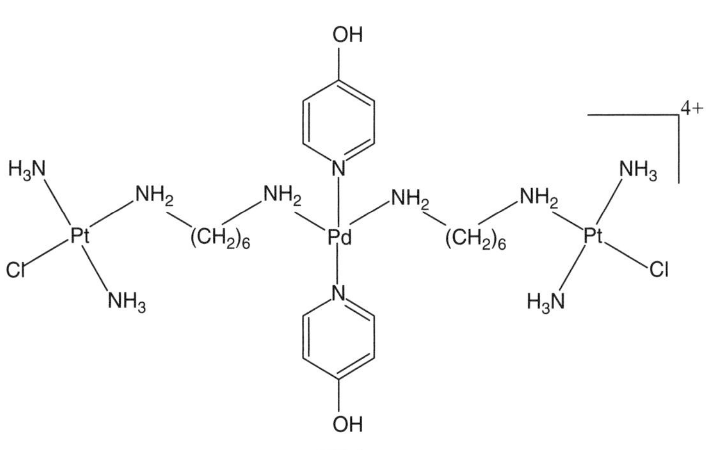

TH8

Fig. 2 Structure of synthesized platinum complexes with multiple metal centres

Table 2 IC$_{50}$ values of DH4Cl, DH5Cl, DH6Cl, DH7Cl, TH1 and TH8 against the human ovarian cancer cell lines A2780, A2780^{cisR} and A2780^{ZD0473R}

Compound	IC$_{50}$ values (µM)			RF (A2780 vs. A2780^{cisR})	RF (A2780 vs. A2780^{ZD0473R})
	A2780	A2780^{cisR}	A2780^{ZD0473R}		
Cisplatin	0.45 ± 0.1	4.4 ± 0.6	1.2 ± 0.2	9.8	4.8
DH4Cl	3.24 ± 0.2	3.66 ± 0.3	5.31 ± 0.4	1.1	0.7
DH5Cl	3.42 ± 0.4	3.99 ± 0.3	4.49 ± 0.7	1.2	1.3
DH6Cl	0.05 ± 0.01	0.25 ± 0.01	0.23 ± 0.01	5.2	1.4
DH7Cl	1.03 ± 0.10	2.91 ± 0.5	4.91 ± 0.2	2.8	1.1
TH1	0.26 ± 0.20	0.50 ± 0.20	0.27 ± 0.10	1.9	0.4
TH8	2.3 ± 0.40	3.2 ± 0.20	9.1 ± 1.1	1.39	2.1

References

1. Farrell N. Platinum anti-cancer drugs. In: Sessler JA, Doctorow SE, McMurry TJ, and Lippard SJ, eds. From Laboratory to Clinic. ACS Symposium Series 903. Medicinal Inorganic Chemistry, 2005:62–79.
2. Farrell N, Kelland LR, Roberts JD, Van Beusichem M. Activation of the trans geometry in platinum antitumor complexes: a survey of the cytotoxicity of trans complexes containing planar ligands in murine L1210 and human tumor panels and studies on their mechanism of action. Cancer Res 1992;52:5065–72.
3. Farrell N. Polynuclear platinum drugs. Met Ions Biol Syst 2004;41:252–96.
4. Farrell N. Polynuclear charged platinum as a new class of anticancer agents: toward a new paradigm. In: Kelland LR, Farrell NP, eds. Platinum-Based Drugs in Cancer Therapy. Totowa, New Jersey: Humana Press, 2000:321–38.
5. Huq F, Daghriri H, Yu JQ, Beale P, Fisher K. Studies on the synthesis and characterization of four *trans*-planaramineplatinum(II) complexes of the form *trans*-PtL(NH$_3$)Cl$_2$ where L = 2-hydroxypyridine, 3-hydroxypyridine, imidazole, and imidazo(1,2-α)pyridine. Eur J Med Chem 2004;39:691–7.
6. Huq F, Yu JQ, Daghriri H, Beale P. Studies on activities, cell uptake and DNA binding of four trans-planaramineplatinum(II) complexes of the form: *trans*-PtL(NH$_3$)Cl$_2$ where L = 2-hydroxypyridine, imidazole, 3-hydroxypyridine and imidazo(1,2-α)pyridine. J Inorg Biochem 2004;98:1261–70.
7. Chowdhury MA, Huq F, Abdullah A, Beale P, Fisher K. Synthesis, characterization and binding with DNA of four planaramineplatinum(II) complexes of the form: *trans*-PtL$_2$Cl$_2$ and PtL$_3$Cl where L = 3-hydroxypyridine, 4-hydroxypyridine and imidazo(1,2-α)pyridine. J Inorg Biochem 2005;99:1098–112.
8. Huq F, Abdullah A. Studies on the synthesis and characterization, and binding with DNA of two *cis*-planaramineplatinum(II) complexes of the forms: cis-PtL$_2$Cl$_2$ and *cis*-PtL(NH$_3$)Cl$_2$ where L = 3-hydroxypyridine and imidazo(1,2-α)pyridine respectively. Int J Pure Appl Chem 2006;1:91–100.
9. Huq F, Abdullah A. Studies on the synthesis and characterization, binding with DNA and activity of *cis*-bis{imidazo(1,2-α)pyridine}dichloroplatinum(II). Asian J Chem 2006;18:1637–48.
10. Abdullah A, Huq F, Chowdhury A, Tayyem H, Beale P, Fisher K. Studies on the Synthesis, Characterization, Binding with DNA and Activities of two *cis*-planaramineplatinum(II) complexes of the form: *cis*-PtL(NH$_3$)Cl$_2$ where L = 3-hydroxypyridine and 2,3-diaminopyridine. BMC Chem Biol 2006;6:3. doi:10.1186/1472-6769-6-3; http://www.biomedcentral.com/1472-6769/6/3.

11. Huq F, Abdullah A. Antitumour activity of *cis*-bis{imidazo(1,2-α)pyridineplatinum(II). Int J Cancer Res 2006;2:367–75.
12. Huq F, Daghriri H, et al. Syntheses and characterisation of four trinuclear complexes of the form: [{*trans*-PtCl(NH$_3$)$_2$}$_2$ *u-{trans*-Pd(NH$_3$)$_2$(H$_2$N(CH$_2$)$_n$NH$_2$)$_2$]Cl$_4$ where n = 4 to 7. Int J Pure Appl Chem 2006;1:493–507.
13. Tayyem H, Huq F, Yu JQ, Beale P, Fisher K. Synthesis and activity of a novel trinuclear platinum complex: [{*trans*-PtCl(NH$_3$)$_2$}$_2$µ-{*trans*-Pt(3-hydroxypyridine)$_2$(H$_2$N(CH$_2$)$_6$NH$_2$)$_2$}]Cl$_4$ in ovarian cancer cell lines. Chem Med Chem 2008;3:145–51.
14. Huq F, Daghriri H, Yu JQ, Tayyem H, Beale P, Zhang M. Synthesis, characterization, activities, cell up take and DNA binding of [{trans-PtCl(NH$_3$)$_2$}{µ-(H$_2$N(CH$_2$)$_6$NH$_2$)}{trans-PdCl(NH$_3$)$_2$](NO$_3$)Cl. Euro J Med Chem 2004;39:947–58.
15. Daghriri H, Huq F, Beale P. Studies on activities, cell up take and DNA binding of four multi-nuclear complexes of the form: [{*trans*-PtCl(NH$_3$)$_2$}$_2${µ-*trans*-Pd(NH$_3$)$_2$-(H$_2$N(CH$_2$)$_n$NH$_2$)$_2$]Cl$_4$ where n = 4 to 7. J Inorg Biochem 2004;98(11):1722–33.
16. Cheng H, Huq F, Beale P, Fisher K. Synthesis, characterization, activities, cell uptake and DNA binding of the trinuclear complex: [{*trans*-PtCl(NH$_3$)}$_2$µ-{*trans*-Pt(NH$_3$)(2-hydroxypyridine)-(H$_2$N(CH$_2$)$_6$NH$_2$)$_2$]Cl$_4$. Euro J Med Chem 2005;40:772–81.
17. Huq F, Daghriri H, et al. Syntheses and characterization of four trinuclear complexes of the form: [{*trans*-PtCl(NH$_3$)$_2$}$_2$µ-{*trans*-Pd(NH$_3$)$_2$(H$_2$N(CH$_2$)$_n$NH$_2$)$_2$]Cl$_4$ where n = 4 to 7. Intern J Pure Appl Chem 2006;1:493–507.
18. Huq F, Tayyem H. Synthesis and characterization and binding of amine-palladium(II) complexes and their interaction with DNA. Asian J Chem 2006;18:65–78.

Assessment of the In Vivo Antiproliferative Activity of a Novel Platinum Particulate Pharmacophore

Elena Monti, Marzia B. Gariboldi, Raffaella Ravizza, Roberta Molteni, Elisabetta Gabano, Katia Sparnacci, Michele Laus, and Domenico Osella

Abstract The development of synthetic polymer drug-delivery systems is a promising strategy to improve the therapeutic index of effective but highly toxic anti-cancer agents, such as cisplatin, by taking advantage of the peculiar characteristics of tumor blood and lymphatic circulation, often referred to as the enhanced permeability and retention (EPR) effect. In the present study, water-soluble, biocompatible core–shell nanospheres (ZN2) obtained from polymethylmethacrylate (PMMA), with a shell featuring positively charged quaternary ammonium groups, were used as noncovalently linked pharmacophores for the anionic platinum-containing moiety, $[PtCl_3NH_3]^-$ (PtA). The resulting adduct (PtA-ZN2), at the estimated maximum tolerated dose (MTD) of 25 mg Pt/kg/day for 5 consecutive days was significantly more effective than cisplatin, also at the MTD of 3.25 mg Pt/kg/day×5, in inhibiting the growth of B16 murine melanoma in mice, in the absence of signs of general toxicity. In contrast, treatment with free PtA did not significantly affect tumor growth as compared to control mice. *In vivo* efficacy of the three Pt-containing species was found to correlate with Pt intratumor accumulation, as evaluated by ICP-MS following tumor tissue mineralization. PtA-ZN2 was also found to be superior to PtA in the *in vitro* cytotoxicity assays on cultured B16 cells (IC_{50} values at 5 days: 1.78 ± 0.79 μg Pt/ml for PtA-ZN2 and 10.47 μg Pt/ml for PtA), where the EPR effect is not an issue. This suggests that polymer conjugation can also enhance Pt efficacy at the single-cell level, possibly by facilitating Pt uptake; determinations of intracellular Pt levels following in vitro incubation of B16 cells with PtA and PtAZN2 and of internalization of fluorescent ZN2 nanospheres seem to support this hypothesis.

Keywords Platinum complexes; Drug targeting and delivery; B16 melanoma

E. Monti (✉)[1], M.B. Gariboldi[1], R. Ravizza[1], R. Molteni[1], E. Gabano[2], K. Sparnacci[2], M. Laus[2], and D. Osella[2]
[1]Department of Structural and Functional Biology, University of Insubria, Busto Arsizio, Italy
[2]Department of Environmental and Life Sciences, University of Piemonte Orientale "A. Avogadro", Alessandria, Italy
e-mail: elena.monti@uninsubria.it

A. Bonetti et al. (eds.), *Platinum and Other Heavy Metal Compounds in Cancer Chemotherapy*, DOI: 10.1007/978-1-60327-459-3_3,
© Humana Press, a part of Springer Science + Business Media, LLC 2009

Introduction

Synthetic polymer-drug systems hold promise as passive tumor-targeting and delivery vehicles for improving the therapeutic index of effective but highly toxic anticancer agents such as cisplatin (1). Attachment of drugs to polymeric carriers significantly modifies cellular uptake with respect to the free drug, prolongs its plasma half-life and enhances the drug tumor/healthy tissue ratio by taking advantage of the peculiar characteristics of tumor blood flow and lymphatic circulation that allow the leakage and subsequent accumulation of relatively high molecular weight species into the tumor interstitium (Enhanced Permeability and Retention, or EPR, effect) (2). So far, only polymers covalently linked to cytotoxic Pt-containing drugs have been tested in the clinic. Some of the resulting polymer-drug conjugates, including AP5346, a N-(2-hydroxypropyl)methacrylamide (HPMA)-conjugate of a diaminocyclohexane-platinum derivative, have shown enhanced tumor/healthy tissue ratios and favorable toxicity profiles as compared to the parent drugs (3).

In the present study, we explored the potential viability of a novel concept in conjugate design, namely, the attachment of a negatively charged cisplatin derivative ($[PtCl_3NH_3]^-$, henceforth abbreviated as PtA) to positively charged polymethylmethacrylate core-shell nanoparticles (ZN2) by means of ionic interactions. The activity of the resulting drug conjugate, named PtA-ZN2, was tested in B16 murine melanoma cells, grown as monolayer cultures and as subcutaneous tumors in mice, and compared with the activity of cisplatin (CDDP) and that of free (unconjugated) PtA.

Results and Discussion

Polymethylmethacrylate core–shell nanospheres (ZN2) were synthesized as detailed elsewhere (4) which exhibited the following characteristics: average SEM diameter, 145 ± 40 nm; hydrodynamic radius, evaluated by dynamic light scattering (DLS), 188 ± 1 nm; ζ-potential, $+69.0 \pm 2$ mV; charge density 347 ± 33 μmol/g. The negatively charged species PtA was synthesized according to the procedure described by Giandomenico $et~al.$ (5). The presence of positively charged ammonium groups in ZN2 allows multiple electrostatic interactions with the negatively charged PtA units, thus yielding the drug-loaded polymer PtA-ZN2 (Fig. 1). The estimated Pt content was 344 ± 18 μmol Pt/g PtA-ZN2, indicating an almost complete loading of the polymer.

The antitumor activity of PtA-ZN2 was assessed in C57BL mice inoculated subcutaneously with B16 murine melanoma cells (10^6 cells/mouse). Drug treatment was initiated as soon as the tumors became palpable and was repeated once daily for 5 consecutive days; the animals were then monitored daily for tumor growth, body weight gain and general toxicity for one additional week at the end of which they were euthanized. Preliminary experiments allowed definition of the

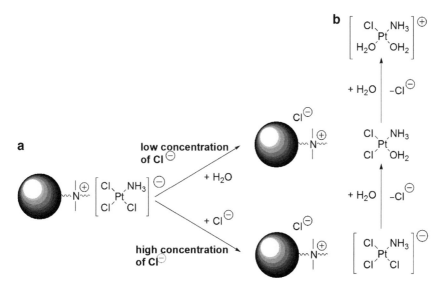

Fig. 1 Mechanism of platinum release from PtA-ZN2

maximum-tolerated i.p. dose (MTD) which was 25 mg Pt/kg/day for PtA-ZN2 and 3.25 mg Pt/kg/day for CDDP. Accordingly, two of the four experimental groups received PtA-ZN2 and CDDP at their respective MTDs, whereas one of the two remaining groups received unconjugated PtA (at the same dose as CDDP, i.e., 3.25 mg Pt/kg/day for 5 days) and the other served as control and was treated with vehicle (saline) only on the same schedule.

The results of this in vivo experiment are shown in Fig. 2 Tumor growth was significantly impaired in mice receiving CDDP or PtA-ZN2 as compared to control mice, whereas unconjugated PtA was inactive (Fig. 2a). This last observation was not unexpected, based on the SAR rules defined by Cleare-Hoeschele (6), predicting that, in principle, neutral CDDP is the most active among Pt(II) chloroamine derivatives. Interestingly, at the end of the observation period, the tumor mass was slightly but significantly smaller in PtA-ZN2-treated mice than in those treated with CDDP. Determination of Pt, performed by inductively coupled plasma mass spectrometry (ICP-MS) on mineralized tumor tissues at the end of the, indicated that some degree of correlation exists between Pt intratumor accumulation and antitumor activity (Fig. 2c). Body weight gain was transiently impaired in PtA-ZN2-treated animals during the 5 days of drug administration, but promptly resumed after the last dose (Fig. 2b); none of the four experimental groups displayed signs of general toxicity at necropsy at the end of the experiment. Thus, the results of this preliminary experiment suggest that, in principle, tumor growth inhibition can be achieved in the absence of significant side-toxicity using a Pt-polymer conjugate involving electrostatic rather than covalent interactions between the cytotoxic moiety and the polymeric matrix, and that this effect is likely due to increased Pt accumulation in tumor tissue.

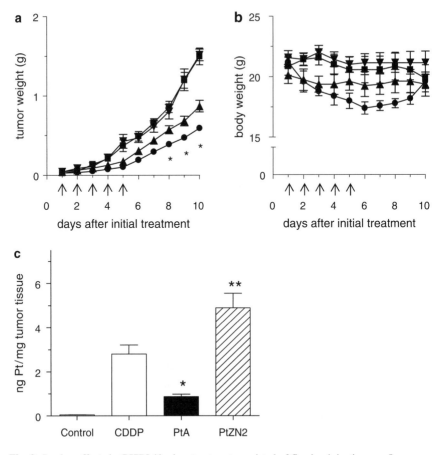

Fig. 2 In vivo effects in C57BL/6 mice; treatment consisted of five i.p. injections on 5 consecutive days (arrows). (**a**) Time course of tumor growth; (**b**) time course of body weight. *filled square* control (saline) *filled triangle* CDDP (3.25 mg Pt/kg/day, Pt equivalent); *filled inverted triangle* PtA (3.25 mg Pt/kg/day); *filled circle* Pt-ZN2 (25 mg Pt/kg/day). (**c**) Intratumor Pt content at the end of the experiment, assessed by ICP-MS; each value is the mean ± SEM of 4 replications. * p < 0.05 vs. CDDP; ** p < 0.05 vs. CDDP and PtA (statistical analysis performed by two-way analysis of variance for repeated measures and Bonferroni's *t* test)

To investigate the stability of PtA-ZN2, the rate of release of PtA from the nanospheres was evaluated in solutions containing 100 and 5 mM NaCl, mimicking chloride concentrations in plasma and in the cytosol, respectively. The residual Pt content in the nanospheres recovered at different time points up to 2 h was assessed by thermogravimetric analysis (TGA) and ICP-MS, whereas the hydrolysis of PtA was monitored by means of UV-vis spectroscopy and RP-HPLC. In 100 mM NaCl, about 50% of PtA is released from PtA-ZN2 in 2 h, likely because of replacement of PtA by chlorides as counter-ions for the ammonium groups on the nanospheres (Fig. 1). In contrast, only 10% of PtA is released in 5 mM NaCl within 2 h; at this low chloride concentration, aquation reactions are likely to prevail, leading first to the loss of the negative charge of PtA and then to its dissociation from the polymer, and subsequently to the formation of DNA-interacting species (Fig. 1).

Two possible scenarios may follow the systemic administration of PtA-ZN2: (a) the conjugate is distributed quickly and preferentially to the tumor site (because of EPR effect), where most of the PtA is released and enters the cell in an unconjugated form. If this were the case, cytotoxicity assays should yield similar results, whether PtA is used as free or as conjugated species; (b) the rate of nanosphere uptake by tumor cells is of the same order of magnitude as the rate of PtA release, and thus part of the compound enters the cells still attached to the nanospheres. In this latter case, the *in vitro* cytotoxicities of PtA and PtA-ZN2 would not necessarily be similar; namely, if the cellular uptake of the Pt-containing moiety were somehow facilitated by its conjugation to the polymer, a more potent cytotoxic effect would be expected of PtA-ZN2.

To determine which of the two hypotheses is more likely to apply to our delivery system, we proceeded to assess the comparative cytotoxicities of PtA and PtA-ZN2 *in vitro*, using CDDP as a reference compound. Dose/response curves were obtained from the results of MTT assays performed on B16 cells grown as monolayers after a 5-day exposure to the different Pt-containing species and the following IC_{50} values (based on Pt content) were estimated: $0.41 \pm 0.14 \mu$g Pt/ml for CDDP, 10.47μg Pt/ml for PtA and $1.78 \pm 0.79 \mu$g Pt/ml for PtA-ZN2. One-way analysis of variance of these data indicates that PtA is significantly less potent than both CDDP and PtA-ZN2 ($p < 0.01$); this strongly suggests that, in spite of the fast rate of PtA dissociation at high chloride concentrations, such as those present in the culture medium, PtA released extracellularly from PtA-ZN2 cannot be the only causative agent of cytotoxicity.

To test hypothesis (b), we evaluated the rate of uptake of ZN2 nanospheres labeled with a FITC-derived fluorophore by B16 cells, by assessing intracellular fluorescence both qualitatively by confocal microscopy and quantitatively by flow cytometry (see Fig. 3), following incubation for different time, from 30 min to 24 h. With both techniques, a significant increase in intracellular fluorescence was observed at 2 h; this was enhanced at 6 h but no further significant increase occurred up to 24 h. These observations suggest that ZN2 uptake achieves a steady state within 6 h. The fact that at 2 h, when only 50% of PtA had been released from the polymer (see above) a non-negligible amount of nanoparticles was detected intracellularly suggests that PtA may be partially internalized together with the polymer.

To conclude our preliminary study on PtA-ZN2, we assessed the intracellular Pt content of B16 cells, following *in vitro* exposure for 5 days to equitoxic concentrations of CDDP, PtA and PtA-ZN2 (corresponding to their respective IC_{50} values). The results of these measures, shown in Fig. 4a, indicate that to achieve half-maximal inhibition of cell growth, similar amounts of intracellular Pt have to be present in cells exposed to PtA and PtA-ZN2, which suggests that for both compounds the same species, i.e., PtA, is probably involved in the observed antiproliferative effect. However, a significantly higher concentration of extracellular

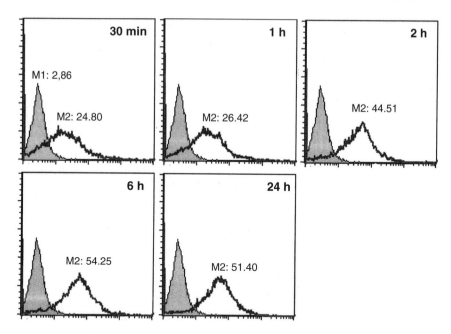

Fig. 3 Uptake of fluorescent ZN2 nanospheres in B16 cells. Cells were exposed to ZN2 nano-spheres (30 µg/ml) labeled with a FITC-derived fluorophore; at the indicated times, they were collected, washed with ice-cold PBS and analyzed with a FACScalibur flow cytometer (Becton Dickinson) equipped with a 15-mW, 488-nm, air-cooled argon ion laser. Fluorescent emissions from 10^4 events/sample were collected through a 530-nm band-pass filter for fluorescein; M1 indicates the median fluorescence for grey peaks (control cells), while M2 indicates the corresponding value for white peaks (cells exposed to fluorescent ZN2)

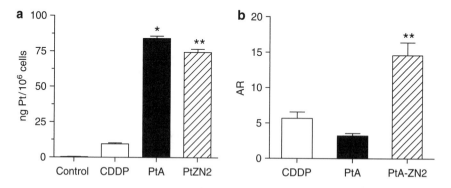

Fig. 4 (**a**) Intracellular Pt levels following in vitro incubation for 5 days with equitoxic concentrations (corresponding to the IC_{50}) of CDDP, PtA and PtA-ZN2. Each value is the mean ± SEM of 6–7 replications. (**b**) Accumulation ratio (AR), i.e., the ratio between intra- and extracellular Pt concentration (7). * $p < 0.01$ vs. CDDP; ** $p < 0.05$ vs. CDDP and PtA (statistical analysis performed by one-way analysis of variance for repeated measures and Bonferroni's t test)

Pt must be present in the case of PtA than in the case of PtA-ZN2 to obtain similar intracellular Pt levels (and similar cytotoxic effects). This observation is reflected by their respective AR values, reported in Fig. 4b [AR: accumulation ratio, i.e., the ratio between intra- and extracellular Pt concentration (7)], which seems to support the hypothesis that when cells are exposed to PtA-ZN2, Pt uptake may occur at least in part by endocytotosis of the conjugated form, and that this process is quantitatively more efficient than the uptake of the negatively charged PtA. In contrast, CDDP has a lower AR value than PtA-ZN2, but is slightly more potent in inhibiting cell growth. This suggests that the electrophilic species generated from CDDP hydrolysis interact more efficiently with their intracellular targets (mainly DNA) than the corresponding species generated from PtA (Fig. 1b). Further investigations are required, especially to determine the DNA platination; however, the behavior of PtA-ZN2 *in vitro* is in good agreement with its observed effects *in vitro* and supports the potential antitumor efficacy of Pt-conjugates based on electrostatic interactions.

References

1. Duncan R. Polymer conjugates as anticancer nanomedicines. Nat Rev Cancer 2006;6: 688–701.
2. Iyer AK, Khaled G, Fang J, Maeda H. Exploiting the enhanced permeability and retention effect for tumor targeting. Drug Discov Today 2006;11:812–8.
3. Rice JR, Gerberich JL, Nowotnik DP, Howell SB. Preclinical efficacy and pharmacokinetics of AP5346, a novel diaminocyclohexane-platinum tumor-targeting drug delivery system. Clin Cancer Res 2006;12:2248–54.
4. Laus M, Sparnacci K, Lelli M, Vannini R, Tondelli L. Core-shell functional nanospheres for oligonucleotide delivery. II. J Polym Sci Part A Polym Chem 2000;38:1110–7.
5. Giandomenico CM, Abrams MJ, Murrer BA, et al Carboxylation of kinetically inert platinum(IV) hydroxy complexes. An entrée into orally active platinum(IV) antitumor agents. Inorg Chem 1995;34:1015–21.
6. Cleare MJ, Hoeschele JD. Anti-tumour platinum compounds. relationship between structure and activity. Platinum Metals Rev 1973;17:2–13.
7. Gabano E, Ravera M, Colangelo D, Osella D. Bioinorganic chemistry: the study of the fate of platinum-based antitumor drugs. Current Chem. Biol. 2007;1:278–89.

Nanocapsules of Platinum-Based Anticancer Drugs

Irene H.L. Hamelers and Anton I.P.M. de Kroon

Abstract One of the strategies to reduce the side effects of platinum anticancer drugs is encapsulation of the drug in a lipid formulation. Nanocapsules represent a novel lipid-based drug delivery system, with high encapsulation efficiencies of cisplatin and carboplatin. The encapsulation in nanocapsules, dramatically improves the in vitro cytotoxicity of the platinum drugs towards carcinoma cell lines. The nanocapsule technology may generally be applicable to platinum drugs with limited water solubility and low lipophilicity, and improve the therapeutic index and profile of these drugs.

Keywords Cisplatin; Carboplatin; Nanocapsule; Liposome; Drug delivery; Phospholipids

Lipid-Based Delivery Vehicles for Platinum Anticancer Drugs

One of the strategies to reduce the systemic toxicity of platinum anticancer drugs is to encapsulate the drug in a carrier that selectively targets the tumor. Currently, research focuses on the bioactive platinum complexes linked to biocompatible water-soluble macromolecular carriers (described elsewhere in this volume), and on the lipid formulations of platinum drugs. The potential of the latter is demonstrated by Doxil (ALZA Corp.), the clinically applied liposomal formulation of doxorubicin. The carrier should protect the platinum drug from inactivation in the plasma, and should have a circulation half-life that permits it to accumulate in the tumor by the enhanced permeability and retention (EPR) effect. The leaky vasculature of neoplastic tissues allows for extravasation of the carrier, while the limited lymphatic drainage in most

I.H.L. Hamelers and A.I.P.M. de Kroon (✉)
Biochemistry of Membranes, Bijvoet Institute and Institute of Biomembranes,
Utrecht University, Utrecht, The Netherlands
e-mail: a.i.p.m.dekroon@uu.nl

A. Bonetti et al. (eds.), *Platinum and Other Heavy Metal Compounds in Cancer Chemotherapy*, DOI: 10.1007/978-1-60327-459-3_4,
© Humana Press, a part of Springer Science + Business Media, LLC 2009

tumors ensures its retention (1). In the tumor, the carrier should release its content either in the interstitial space or intracellular space after endocytosis. As an additional advantage, the drug delivery vehicle could overcome the mechanisms of intrinsic and acquired platinum resistance by delivering a high dose of the drug in the tumor.

Liposomes have been extensively investigated as a potential delivery vehicle for platinum drugs. Liposomes are micro-particulate or colloidal carriers, typically 0.05–0.5 μm in diameter, which form spontaneously when certain lipids are hydrated. They are made of nontoxic, biodegradable material, and consist of an aqueous volume entrapped by one or more bilayers of natural and/or synthetic lipids. In the liposomal formulation SPI-077, cisplatin is enclosed as a solute in the aqueous core of sterically stabilized polyethylene glycol-coated (PEGylated or "stealth") liposomes, with an average particle size of 110 nm (2). PEG is a physiologically stable water-soluble polymer that prevents the access of plasma proteins to the membrane-surface by steric hindrance, thus prolonging the liposomes' circulation time. Preclinical studies show that SPI-077 exhibits an extended circulation time, increased antitumor efficacy, and reduced toxicity compared to the free drug (2). However, in phase I and II studies, SPI-077 exhibited essentially no antitumor activity (3), which was attributed to the limited bioavailability of cisplatin in the tumor. Due to cisplatin's poor solubility in water, the encapsulation efficiency of cisplatin in SPI-077 is low. Moreover, drug release in the tumor is very slow (4).

Lipoplatin, another liposomal formulation of cisplatin, did exhibit antitumor efficacy in phase I and II studies, with reduced side effects compared to the free drug (5), and is currently being tested in phase III studies. Liposomal encapsulation of oxaliplatin by similar technology yielded Lipoxal, which was found to greatly reduce the side effects of oxaliplatin in a phase I trial, without losing efficacy (6).

Aroplatin represents a promising liposomal formulation of the oxaliplatin analogue *cis*-bis-neodecanoato-*trans-R,R*-1,2-diaminocyclohexane platinum (II) (NDDP) (7), that was recently tested in a phase II clinical trial (8). Due to its lipophilic character, NDDP partitions in the membrane resulted in improved efficiency of encapsulation as compared to that of the parent drug.

Cisplatin Nanocapsules

While preparing liposomes enclosing cisplatin for the purpose of studying the dependence of cisplatin membrane permeation on lipid composition, Koert Burger and Rutger Staffhorst serendipitously discovered a new method for encapsulating cisplatin in a lipid bilayer coat with superior efficiency (9). During the freeze–thaw cycles that are part of the procedure, they observed the appearance of rapidly precipitating yellow particles, when it was applied to an equimolar mixture of zwitterionic phosphatidylcholine (PC) and anionic phosphatidylserine (PS) hydrated in 5 mM cisplatin in water. Analysis of the phospholipid and platinum content of the yellow particles yielded an unprecedented cisplatin-to-lipid molar ratio of around ten. An examination by the electron microscopy revealed bean-shaped, electron-dense particles, containing nanoprecipitates of cisplatin

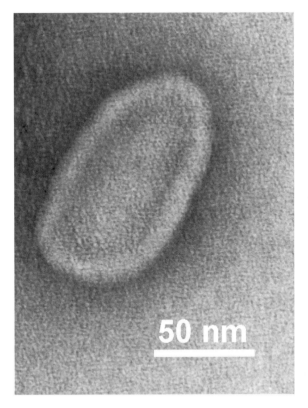

Fig. 1 Negative stain electron micrograph of a typical cisplatin nanocapsule

coated with a lipid bilayer (Fig. 1), which were named cisplatin nanocapsules (9). Nanocapsule formation requires the presence of negatively charged phospholipids, and is incompatible with high chloride concentration and alkaline pH, indicating that electrostatic interaction between the positively charged species of cisplatin and the negatively charged lipids is crucial.

The molecular architecture of the cisplatin nanocapsules was solved by NMR techniques using ^{15}N-labeled cisplatin (10). ^{15}N- and ^{2}H-NMR demonstrated the solid nature of the cisplatin core that is essentially devoid of free water. The magic angle spinning NMR and mass spectrometry revealed the chemical composition of the nanocapsules' solid core: 90% consists of the dichlorido species of cisplatin with the remainder contributed by a newly identified positively charged chloride-bridged dinuclear species (10). The physical properties of the surrounding lipid bilayer of nanocapsules are distinctly different from those of liposomes with a corresponding lipid composition. ^{31}P-NMR showed that the phospholipid head groups in the bilayer coat of cisplatin nanocapsules are motionally restricted compared to liposomal lipids, with part of the lipids fully immobilized (10). This is most likely due to the strong electrostatic interaction between the negatively charged PS head group and the positively charged solid core.

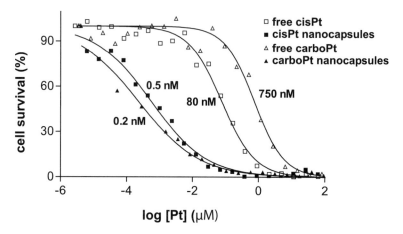

Fig. 2 In vitro cytotoxicity towards IGROV-1 human ovarian carcinoma cells of cisplatin and carboplatin nanocapsules compared to that of the free drugs. The IC50 values are indicated

Based on the data summarized above a model for the formation of nanocapsules was proposed (9–11). During freezing, cisplatin is concentrated in the residual fluid, giving rise to nanoprecipitates of dichloro-cisplatin that are covered by positively charged chloride-bridged dinuclear species of cisplatin. The latter most likely originates from a reaction between dichlorido and aquated species, facilitated by the increasing concentrations during freezing (10). The negatively charged PC/PS vesicles interact with the positively charged nanoprecipitates and reorganize to wrap them. Nanoprecipitates of cisplatin that are completely wrapped in a phospholipid bilayer do not redissolve upon thawing.

The cytotoxicity of the cisplatin nanocapsules towards human ovarian carcinoma cells was tested and compared to that of free cisplatin (9). As shown in Fig. 2, the IC50 value of cisplatin administered as nanocapsules, is two orders of magnitude smaller than that of the free drug. The bilayer coat protecting cisplatin from inactivation by components of the extracellular environment, contributes to the enhanced cytotoxicity of the nanocapsules. The increased intracellular accumulation of cisplatin resulting from endocytic uptake of the nanocapsules (Hamelers et al., 2008, Clin. Cancer Res., in press) is probably the main cause.

Carboplatin Nanocapsules

The applicability of the nanocapsule technology to other platinum anticancer drugs was first tested on carboplatin. Compared to cisplatin, carboplatin has different chemical properties: the molecule is more hydrophobic due to the substitution of the chloride leaving groups by cyclobutanedicarboxylate, the solubility of carboplatin in water is fivefold higher (12), and the rate of hydrolysis of carboplatin is much slower (13). Application of this protocol, developed for cisplatin, to carboplatin, with minor modifications, yielded a lipid formulation enriched in carboplatin (14). Similar to cisplatin nanocapsules, the formation of carboplatin nanocapsules depends strictly on the freeze–thaw steps and the presence of negatively charged lipids, suggesting a common mechanism of formation. However, interestingly, the drug-to-lipid molar ratio of the carboplatin nanocapsules is lower (0.7:1; (14)) than that of the cisplatin nanocapsules (11:1; (9)), which is reflected by a different particle structure (our unpublished results).

The encapsulation in nanocapsules strongly improves the cytotoxicity of carboplatin towards ovarian (Fig. 2), renal, and nonsmall cell lung carcinoma cells in vitro (14). The increased cytotoxicity of the carboplatin nanocapsules, compared to that of free carboplatin, results from enhanced cellular uptake by endocytosis (14).

Concluding Remarks

With their unsurpassed encapsulation efficiency and favorable antitumor cell efficacy in vitro, nanocapsules present a promising formulation platform for platinum drugs. The ability of the nanocapsules to dump a high concentration of the platinum drug intracellularly may circumvent mechanism(s) of intrinsic and acquired drug resistance (15).

For future clinical application, the stability, particle size, and surface charge of the nanocapsule formulations require optimization. PEGylation as used in liposomes was shown to prolong the life-time of cisplatin nanocapsules in serum, without affecting encapsulation efficiency and in vitro cytotoxicity (16). Compared to cisplatin nanocapsules, the carboplatin nanocapsules are more stable (our unpublished results). Moreover, the content of negatively charged lipids in the formulation of carboplatin could be lowered to 20% without a loss of yield or cytotoxicity (14), which should reduce the rate of clearance from circulation by the reticulo-endothelial system. Testing the pharmacological behavior of the nanocapsule formulations in vivo in appropriate animal models will be the next step.

Acknowledgments The authors thank Drs. Koert Burger, Ben de Kruijff, Vladimir Chupin, Maria Velinova and Mr. Rutger Staffhorst for their contributions to the research on nanocapsules, and acknowledge the financial support by the Dutch Cancer Society (KWF Kankerbestrijding) and by NanoNed, a national nanotechnology program coordinated by the Dutch Ministry of Economic Affairs.

References

1. Gabizon AA, Shmeeda H, Zalipsky S. Pros and cons of the liposome platform in cancer drug targeting. J Liposome Res 2006;16:175–83.
2. Newman MS, Colbern GT, Working PK, Engbers C, Amantea MA. Comparative pharma-cokinetics, tissue distribution, and therapeutic effectiveness of cisplatin encapsulated in

long-circulating, pegylated liposomes (SPI-077) in tumor-bearing mice. Cancer Chemother Pharmacol 1999;43:1–7.

3. Meerum Terwogt JM, Groenewegen G, Pluim D, et al. Phase I and pharmacokinetic study of SPI-77, a liposomal encapsulated dosage form of cisplatin. Cancer Chemother Pharmacol 2002;49:201–10.

4. Zamboni WC, Gervais AC, Egorin MJ, et al. Systemic and tumor disposition of platinum after administration of cisplatin or STEALTH liposomal-cisplatin formulations (SPI-077 and SPI-077 B103) in a preclinical tumor model of melanoma. Cancer Chemother Pharmacol 2004;53:329–36.

5. Stathopoulos GP, Boulikas T, Vougiouka M, et al. Pharmacokinetics and adverse reactions of a new liposomal cisplatin (lipoplatin): phase I study. Oncol Rep 2005;13:589–95.

6. Stathopoulos GP, Boulikas T, Kourvetaris A, Stathopoulos J. Liposomal oxaliplatin in the treatment of advanced cancer: a phase I study. Anticancer Res 2006;26:1489–93.

7. Abra RM, Bankert RB, Chen F, et al. The next generation of liposome delivery systems: recent experience with tumor-targeted, sterically-stabilized immunoliposomes and active-loading gradients. J Liposome Res 2002;12:1–3.

8. Dragovich T, Mendelson D, Kurtin S, Richardson K, Von Hoff D, Hoos A. A phase 2 trial of the liposomal DACH platinum L-NDDP in patients with therapy-refractory advanced colorectal cancer. Cancer Chemother Pharmacol 2006;58:759–64.

9. Burger KN, Staffhorst RW, de Vijlder HC, et al. Nanocapsules: lipid-coated aggregates of cisplatin with high cytotoxicity. Nat Med 2002;8:81–4.

10. Chupin V, de Kroon AI, de Kruijff B. Molecular architecture of nanocapsules, bilayer-enclosed solid particles of cisplatin. J Am Chem Soc 2004;126:13816–21.

11. Hamelers IH, de Kroon AI. Nanocapsules: a novel formulation technology for platinum-based anticancer drugs. Future Lipidol 2007;2:445–53.

12. Riley CM, Sternson LA Cisplatin. In: Florey K, ed. Analytical Profiles of Drug Substances, vol. 14. New York: Academic Press, 1985:78–105.

13. Knox RJ, Friedlos F, Lydall DA, Roberts JJ. Mechanism of cytotoxicity of anticancer platinum drugs: evidence that *cis*-diamminedichloroplatinum(II) and *cis*-diammine-(1,1-cyclobutanedicarboxylato)platinum(II) differ only in the kinetics of their interaction with DNA. Cancer Res 1986;46:1972–9.

14. Hamelers IH, van Loenen E, Staffhorst RW, de Kruijff B, de Kroon AI. Carboplatin nanocapsules: a highly cytotoxic, phospholipid-based formulation of carboplatin. Mol Cancer Ther 2006;5:2007–12.

15. Helleman J, Burger H, Hamelers IH, et al. Impaired cisplatin influx in an A2780 mutant cell line: evidence for a putative, *cis*-configuration-specific, platinum influx transporter. Cancer Biol Ther 2006;5:943–9.

16. Velinova MJ, Staffhorst RW, Mulder WJ, et al. Preparation and stability of lipid-coated nanocapsules of cisplatin: anionic phospholipid specificity. Biochim Biophys Acta 2004; 1663:135–42.

The Design and Development of the Tumor-Targeting Nanopolymer Dach Platinum Conjugate AP5346 (Prolindac™)

Stephen B. Howell

Abstract AP5346 (Prolindac™) is a macromolecule consisting of a biocompatible and water soluble polymer to which a DACH-Pt is bound via a pH-sensitive chelating group. It was rationally designed to increase delivery of the DACH Pt moiety to tumors by taking advantage of the increased permeability of tumor capillaries. Studies in murine and human tumor xenograft models demonstrated that the design goals were achieved. AP5436 was shown to have activity superior to oxaliplatin in most models and be capable of increasing Pt delivery to the tumor by 16-fold and to the tumor DNA by 14-fold in the B16 murine melanoma model. A phase 1 trial of AP5346 demonstrated activity in patients with far advanced cancers and documented a favorable toxicity and pharmacokinetic profile. AP5346 is now being tested in patients with Pt-sensitive ovarian cancers in a phase 2 trial.

Keywords AP5346 (Prolindac™); DACH platinum; Oxaliplatin

Introduction

The diaminocyclohexane (DACH) platinum drugs are of interest because they have antitumor activity in some diseases that are resistant to cisplatin and carboplatin. Oxaliplatin, the only DACH platinum drug with marketing approval in the USA and EU countries, has emerged as a key component of modern treatment programs for colorectal carcinoma. It has activity against some cell lines with intrinsic or acquired cisplatin or carboplatin resistance (1), and against cell lines with mismatch repair deficiency, which confers resistance to cisplatin and carboplatin (2, 3). Oxaliplatin also has a different pattern of toxicity; the major toxicity associated with multiple

S.B. Howell
Department of Medicine and the Moores Cancer Center,
University of California,
San Diego, USA
e-mail: showell@ucsd.edu

A. Bonetti et al. (eds.), *Platinum and Other Heavy Metal Compounds in Cancer Chemotherapy*, DOI: 10.1007/978-1-60327-459-3_5,

cycles of treatment with oxaliplatin is the development of acral paraesthesias and dysesthesias that are exacerbated by cold.

In order to further improve the therapeutic index of a DACH platinum, a project was initiated to develop a drug delivery system capable of increasing the amount of the drug reaching the tumor while at the same time reducing systemic exposure and toxicity. The aim of this project was to increase DACH platinum delivery to the DNA of the tumor by at least tenfold, employing a platform that could be used to deliver other drugs if the DACH platinum was successful. Success in this endeavor would result in a drug that would be expected to have better activity in diseases for which oxaliplatin is currently used, and possibly in diseases with intrinsic or acquired resistance to the platinum drugs.

AP5346 was designed as a nanopolymer to take advantage of the "enhanced permeability and retention" (EPR) effect (4). Tumors have abnormal capillaries that are hyper-permeable to a variety of macromolecules. This, in combination with the very poor development of lymphatics in the central part of tumors, results in a situation where a macromolecule is trapped and concentrated in the tumor once it escapes from vascular circulation into the tumor extracellular fluid (5). Drugs conjugated to such polymers can reach concentrations that are 10–100 times higher in a tumor tissue than those attained following administration of a free drug (6). In addition, the polymer can be chemically engineered so that it both protects the attached drug while in the systemic circulation and renders it inactive until it arrives in the tumor, resulting in reduced toxicity to normal tissues in the body (6).

There were four design objectives for AP5346. The first was to keep the drug largely confined to the systemic circulation, until it encountered a highly abnormal and permeable capillary such as those found in tumors (4, 5). The second was to achieve a very prolonged plasma half-life, so that the drug would continue to be delivered to the extracellular fluid of the tumor for a long period of time. The third was to keep the drug in an inactive state while in systemic circulation and allow it to become activated when it entered the tumor. Finally, the fourth objective was to allow the polymer-based drug to eventually be excreted from the body.

AP5346 Structure and Characteristics

AP5346 was rationally designed as a nanopolymer to which a DACH-platinum is bound via a pH-sensitive chelating group (Fig. 1). The water-soluble biocompatible polymer backbone is a 90:10 random copolymer of: N-(2-hydroxypropyl) methacrylamide (HPMA) and a methacrylamide monomer, substituted with a triglycine aminomalonate group that provides the primary binding site for the DACH-platinum moiety (7). The conjugate contains ~10% platinum by weight and has an average molecular weight of 25 kDa. This molecular weight was selected to be small enough to allow renal excretion while being large enough to benefit from EPR.

The release of the DACH-platinum moiety in neutral solutions is very slow but is increased at the lower pH found in the extracellular space of hypoxic tumors and

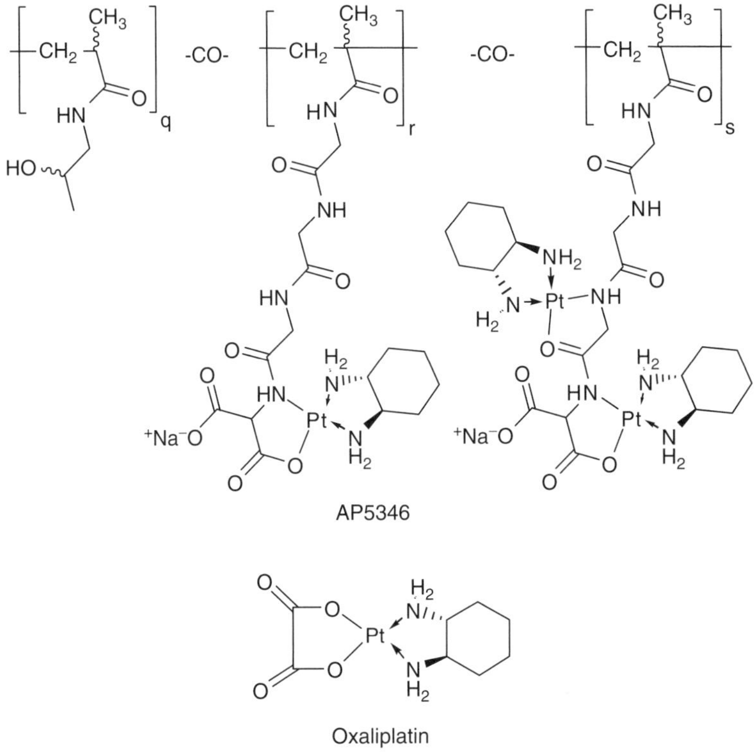

AP5346

Oxaliplatin

Fig. 1 Chemical structure of AP5346 and oxaliplatin

the intracellular lysosomal compartment (8). When AP5346 was dissolved with 5% dextrose in water, there was very little release of free Pt-containing species even after 24 h (9). Chloride displaces both oxygen and nitrogen from the Pt complex and the rate at which the leaving group is displaced from the Pt complex is a direct function of the chloride concentration. Thus, as expected, when AP5346 was dissolved in phosphate buffered saline containing a physiologic concentration of chloride at pH 7.4, there was a slow release of the DACH Pt species that reached 3.5 ± 0.1 (SD, $N = 3$)% by 24 h. However, when AP5346 was dissolved in phosphate/citrate buffered saline at pH 5.4 23.6 ± 0.1 (SD, $N = 3$)% was released within 24 h. Thus, the aminomalonate-Pt chelate was found to function as a pH-sensitive linker with the result that AP5346 is expected to be mostly inert in the systemic circulation and in the extracellular fluid of normal tissues because of the stability of the DACH Pt linkage at pH 7.4, and to release the DACH Pt at a more rapid rate in malignant tissues where extracellular fluid pH is often very much lower. In the tumor some fraction of the DACH platinum may be released in the extracellular fluid, following which the free DACH enters the cell on one or more transporters. In addition, AP5346 may be endocytosed and the bulk of the DACH platinum released as the resulting endosomes are acidified as part of normal cellular metabolism (10). No data is currently available as to the relative contributions of the two mechanisms.

Nonclinical Studies of AP5346

The antitumor activity of AP5346 was evaluated in both syngeneic murine and human tumor xenograft models (9). In C57BL/6 mice bearing subcutaneously implanted B16F10 tumors, the maximum tolerated dose (~10% weight loss at the nadir) of oxaliplatin, given as a single IP injection, was 5 mg Pt/kg and the maximum tolerated dose of AP5346 was 100 mg Pt/kg, indicating that AP5346 was ~20-fold less toxic to normal mouse tissues. AP5346 was tested in a total of 11 tumor models. It produced markedly greater tumor growth inhibition and prolonged growth delay compared to equitoxic doses of oxaliplatin and/or carboplatin in B16 melanoma, 2008 human ovarian, and the cisplatin-resistant form of the M5076 tumors. It was also superior in three human colon xenograft models including Colo-26, HT-29, and HCT116 human colon, as well as in the L1210 murine leukemia and 0157 hybridoma models. AP5346 had similar activity in the cisplatin-sensitive M5076, Lewis lung, and P815 mastocytoma models. Thus, it was not less effective than oxaliplatin in any model.

Detailed pharmacokinetic studies of the ability of AP5346 to enhance delivery of platinum to the tumor and tumor DNA were carried out in the B16 melanoma model using IP injection of equitoxic doses of AP5346 (100 mg Pt/kg) and oxaliplatin (5 mg Pt/kg) (9). AP5346 produced higher and more sustained plasma levels of total Pt than oxaliplatin. The C_{max} was 25-fold higher for AP5346. The terminal half-life was 23.2 h for AP5346 and 15 h for oxaliplatin. In the case of AP5346, this long terminal excretion phase appears to reflect the kinetics of the intact drug whereas in the case of oxaliplatin it probably reflects the kinetics of inactive drug bound to plasma proteins (11). The $AUC_{(0-\infty)}$ was 93 times higher for AP5346 than for oxaliplatin. The volume of distribution of AP5346 was only 33%, and the clearance only 21%, of that for oxaliplatin consistent with the much greater molecular weight of AP5346. No Pt was detected in the plasma ultrafiltrates generated using a 3-kDa MW cut-off filter, suggesting that the DACH Pt moiety remained on the polymer while in the blood.

The delivery of Pt to the tumor and to tumor DNA was determined by measuring the time course of the appearance and disappearance of Pt from SC implanted B16F10 melanomas (9). Following IP injection of oxaliplatin, Pt appeared in the tumor rapidly and peaked at 2 h at 8.8 ± 8.2 (SEM) ng Pt/mg tumor wet weight. The Pt level then declined rapidly in parallel with the initial rapid decline in the total plasma Pt concentration. The estimated half-life was 73 h. Following injection of AP5346 the Pt content of the tumor also increased rapidly and peaked at 2 h at 28.2 ± 12.1 (SEM) ng Pt/mg, a level 3.2 times higher than that produced by oxaliplatin. In contrast to the rapid decline in the tumor, the Pt level observed following injection of oxaliplatin, and the Pt content of the tumor following injection of AP5346 remained elevated for a much longer period of time, and both the initial and terminal rates of loss of Pt from the tumor were lower. The estimated terminal half-life was 220 h. The ratio of the $AUC_{(0-168)}$ for the tumor Pt content following AP5346 to that for oxaliplatin was 16.3. Thus, when both drugs were injected at their respective maximum tolerated doses, AP5346 markedly increased delivery of the DACH Pt to the tumor.

The time course of the appearance of Pt in DNA isolated from the same tumors for which the total tumor Pt was measured was also determined (9). Following the injection of oxaliplatin, tumor DNA Pt content initially peaked at 8 h at 3.1 ± 2.6 (SEM) pg Pt/mg DNA but declined by 90.1% within 24 h. In contrast, following injection of AP5346 the Pt content of tumor DNA continued to increase for at least 6 days, peaking at 71.1 ± 16.4 (SEM) pg Pt/mg DNA and remaining near this value even until day 7. The ratio of the tumor DNA content $AUC_{(1-168h)}$ for AP5346 to that of oxaliplatin was 14.3. Thus, the ability of AP5346 to maintain a high plasma concentration for a prolonged period of time and the slow loss of AP5346 from the tumor resulted in a very large increase in the amount of Pt delivered to the DNA of the tumor.

In the *in vivo* preclinical models, elevated doses of AP5346 exhibited a toxicity profile typical of platinum compounds, with the dose-limiting toxicity being impairment of renal function and myelosuppression (9). No adverse events outside those already identified for platinum cytotoxic agents were observed.

Phase 1 Trial

Based on the success of AP5346 in increasing the delivery of Pt to the tumor and tumor DNA in the B16 melanoma model, and its favorable activity in other tumor models, AP5346 was advanced into clinical development. For the first phase 1 trial, AP5346 was given as a 1h infusion administered weekly for 3 out of every 4 weeks. This schedule was selected, based on the observation that efficacy and drug delivery to the tumor and tumor DNA improved with the more prolonged exposure attainable with weekly dosing of this long-half drug, and prior clinical experience with AP5280, a polymer carrying cisplatin rather than a DACH platinum (12). The primary objective was to determine the pattern of adverse events and the maximum tolerated dose (MTD) in patients with advanced solid tumors. The secondary objectives were to determine the recommended dose for subsequent Phase II studies, characterize the pharmacokinetic profile and undertake a preliminary assessment of the antitumor activity.

This trial was open to patients with advanced solid tumors that had failed all therapy of established merit, who were age ≥18 years with a performance status ≤ 2 a life expectancy ≥ 3 months who were not receiving any other anticancer treatments, and who had adequate bone marrow, hepatic and renal function (13). Seven dose levels were explored: 40-mg platinum (Pt)/m^2 (1 patient); 80 (1 patient); 160 (3 patients); 320 (3 patients); 640 (6 patients); 850 (6 patients); and, 1,280 (6 patients) mg Pt/m^2. A total of 26 patients received 41 cycles (median 1/patient, range 1–4). No dose-limiting toxicities occurred at doses up to 320 mg Pt/m^2. There was one dose-limiting toxicity in the 6 patients treated at 640 mg Pt/m^2 (renal insufficiency) and two such toxicities in the 6 patients treated at 850 mg Pt/m^2 (vomiting; fatigue). There were a total of five, dose-limiting toxicities in the 6 patients treated at the 1,280 mg Pt/m^2

dose level (neutropenic infection with diarrhea; neutropenia with vomiting; vomiting with fatigue; renal insufficiency; fatigue). Two deaths occurred due to renal insufficiency at the 640 mg Pt/m^2 dose level; in both cases patients had disease in or surrounding genitourinary tract whose contribution to the renal insufficiency could not be accurately discerned. Grade 1–2 creatinine abnormalities occurred in 7 patients. Nausea/emesis was frequent (92%), reaching grade 3–4 (23%), but adequately controlled by antiemetics. The 850 mg/m^2 dose level was considered the maximum tolerated dose. The myelosuppressive effect of AP5346 was moderate with no neutropenia observed below 850 mg Pt/m^2, and thrombocytopenia grade 1–2 occurring in only 4 patients (20%) below that dose level. Allergic reactions occurred during infusion in 4 patients (15%) in dose levels 160–640 mg Pt/m^2, reaching grade 3–4 in 2 cases, with one episode of anaphylactic shock and respiratory arrest in a patient with a history of allergy to carboplatin. No ototoxicity was reported, and there was no significant development of persistent peripheral neuropathy although the total number of cycles received by any patient was too limited to adequately assess the potential of AP5346 to produce the neurotoxicity typical of oxaliplatin.

Sixteen of the patients in this trial were evaluated for response to this treatment. Evidence of antitumor activity was observed at doses of 320 mg Pt/m^2 and above. Two patients obtained a partial response as defined by the RECIST guidelines, one with far advanced ovarian cancer and one with metastatic melanoma. In addition, a patient with adenocarcinoma of unknown primary, suspected to be of ovarian origin, had normalization of CA-125 3 weeks after her last AP5346 infusion, with an attained 5-month clinical and biological response to the follow-up treatment with a single-agent oxaliplatin.

Pharmacokinetics was assessed in 26 patients following the first infusion. The total plasma Pt exhibited biphasic elimination, while ultrafiltrate Pt concentrations displayed a secondary peak at 24 h post-infusion. C_{max} and $AUC_{0-1 wk}$ for total plasma platinum increased linearly with dose over the entire range of doses studied for total plasma platinum; the correlation coefficients for C_{max} and AUC_{0-162} were 0.903 and 0.870, respectively, indicating excellent correlation of the parameters for total platinum with dose. For the ultrafiltrate Pt the correlation coefficients were 0.346 and 0.511 for C_{max} and AUC_{0-162}, respectively, indicating moderate correlation of the pharmacokinetic parameters with dose. Only a very small fraction of the total platinum was present free in the plasma; the ultrafiltrate Pt $AUC_{0-1 wk}$ averaged only 0.6% of the total platinum AUC. Mean terminal half-life was 72.3 ± 16.9 h for total platinum and 56.7 ± 14.7 h for ultrafiltrate platinum at doses ≥320 mg/m^2 and the terminal half-life did not vary with dose.

Discussion

AP5346 was rationally designed to increase the delivery of a DACH Pt moiety to tumors. The drug was designed to take advantage of the ability of the flexible water soluble HPMA polymer to become trapped and accumulate in the extracellular compartment of tumors, and to include a chelator for the DACH Pt that released the drug only very slowly at the pH of plasma but more rapidly at the lower pH values typically found in tumors and lysosomes. The aim of markedly increasing Pt delivery to the tumor and tumor DNA was achieved by this strategy as evidenced by the results of studies in the B16 murine melanoma model, and that the drug has shown activity in a phase 1 trial in patients with far advanced disease. AP5436 has now entered a phase 2 trial in patients with Pt-sensitive ovarian cancer; the design of this trial allows exploration of changes in both schedule and dose, to further define both the safety and efficacy of this new entity.

Whether AP5346 can increase Pt delivery to tumors in patients to the extent that it did in the B16 model, and whether such an increase will translate into an improved response rate, is yet to be established. It is reasonable to expect that there will be large differences between tumors in the extent of AP5346 accumulation, based on current information, on the variability of tumor capillary permeability and the fluid dynamics of the extracellular space in human tumors. Nevertheless, AP5346 represents an innovative approach to the challenge of targeting drug to tumors, and one of a very small number of drugs in development that utilize the polymer strategy to take advantage of the EPR effect.

References

1. Rixe O, Ortuzar W, Alvarez M, et al. Oxaliplatin, tetraplatin, cisplatin, and carboplatin: spectrum of activity in drug-resistant cell lines and in the cell lines of the National Cancer Institute's Anticancer Drug Screen panel. Biochem Pharmacol 1996;52:1855–65.
2. Vaisman A, Varchenko M, Umar A, et al. The role of hMLH1, hMSH3, and hMSH6 defects in cisplatin and oxaliplatin resistance: correlation with replicative bypass of platinum-DNA adducts. Cancer Res 1998;58:3579–85.
3. Aebi S, Kurdi-Haidar B, Gordon R, et al. Loss of DNA mismatch repair in acquired resistance to cisplatin. Cancer Res 1996;56:3087–90.
4. Matsumura Y, Maeda H. A new concept for macromolecular therapeutics in cancer chemotherapy: mechanism of tumoritropic accumulation of proteins and the antitumor agent smancs. Cancer Res 1986;46:6387–92.
5. Seymour LW. Passive tumor targeting of soluble macromolecules and drug conjugates. Crit Rev Ther Drug Carrier Sys 1992;6:135–87.
6. Duncan R. Polymer therapeutics for tumour specific delivery. Chem Ind 1997;7:262–4.
7. Rice JR, Howell SB. AP5346: polymer-delivered platinum complex. Drugs Future 2004;29:561–6.
8. Mukherjee S, Ghosh RN, Maxfield FR. Endocytosis. Physiol Rev 1997;77:759–803.
9. Rice JR, Gerberich JL, Nowotnik DP, Howell SB. Preclinical efficacy and pharmacokinetics of AP5346, a novel diaminocyclohexane-platinum tumor-targeting drug delivery system. Clin Cancer Res 2006;12:2248–54.
10. Izumi H, Torigoe T, Ishiguchi H, et al. Cellular pH regulators: potentially promising molecular targets for cancer chemotherapy. Cancer Treat Rev 2003;29:541–9.
11. Ehrsson H, Wallin I, Yachnin J. Pharmacokinetics of oxaliplatin in humans. Med Oncol 2002;19:261–5.
12. Rademaker-Lakhai JM, Terret C, Howell SB, et al. A Phase I and pharmacological study of the platinum polymer AP5280 given as an intravenous infusion once every 3 weeks in patients with solid tumors. Clin Cancer Res 2004;10:3386–95.
13. Campone M, Rademaker-Lakhai JM, Bennouna J, et al. Phase I and pharmacokinetic trial of AP5346, a DACH-platinum-polymer conjugate, administered weekly for three out of every four weeks to advanced solid tumor patients. Cancer Chemother Pharmacol 2007; 60:523–33.

In vitro Anti-proliferative Effects of ProLindac™, a Novel Dach-Platinum-Linked Polymer Compound, as a Single Agent and in Combination with Other Anti-cancer Drugs

Maria Serova, Aïda Ghoul, Keyvan Rezaï, François Lokiec, Esteban Cvitkovic, David Nowotnik, Sandrine Faivre, and Eric Raymond

Abstract ProLindac (AP5346) is a novel hydrophilic biocompatible co-polymer acting as a macromolecular carrier of bioactive DACH-platinum (Pt) complexes and has recently entered clinical trials. The pH-dependent polymer delivery system is intended to improve the safety profile of the DACH-Pt by exploiting the "leaky" nature of tumour angiogenesis, allowing for the possibility of high drug concentrations at the acidic hypoxic sites of the tumour. In our study, ProLindac displayed concentration- and time-dependent cytotoxic effects against a broad range of human cancer cell lines. The cytotoxicity profile, along with a number of preclinical experiments, showed cellular and molecular effects of ProLindac closely related to oxaliplatin, but different from cisplatin. We observed that expression of several genes of the DNA repair mechanism and the drug metabolism (MLH1, MDR1, GSTP1) seem to correlate with ProLindac cytotoxicity in a panel of human cancer cell lines. Exposure to 120 μM ProLindac (300 ng/mL Pt) led to incorporation of ~0.1 μg Pt per mg of DNA. Similar to that of oxaliplatin, ProLindac induced p21 expression and 48-h exposure to IC_{50} concentrations of ProLindac led to the accumulation of cells in the G2/M phase of cell cycle and apoptosis induction in p53-mutated HT29, as well as in wild-type p53 HCT116. In summary, ProLindac displayed molecular and cellular effects similar to that of oxaliplatin in most cancer cell lines.

Keywords DACH-platinum; ProLindac; Cytotoxicity

Introduction

Four platinum compounds (cisplatin, carboplatin, tetraplatin and oxaliplatin) have been extensively studied against in vitro and in vivo models, with a special emphasis on the 60-cell-line panel of the National Cancer Institute (NCI) (1). Rixe et al.

M. Serova (✉), A. Ghoul, K. Rezaï, F. Lokiec, E. Cvitkovic,
D. Nowotnik, S. Faivre, and E. Raymond
RayLab and Department of Medical Oncology, Beaujon University Hospital, Clichy
e-mail: mlserova@yahoo.fr

A. Bonetti et al. (eds.), *Platinum and Other Heavy Metal Compounds in Cancer Chemotherapy*, DOI: 10.1007/978-1-60327-459-3_6,
© Humana Press, a part of Springer Science + Business Media, LLC 2009

have established the comparative *in vitro* cytotoxicity profiles of these agents, and have shown strong similarities between cisplatin and carboplatin (first and second generation platinums), and between oxaliplatin and tetraplatin, and, both the latter with the diaminocyelohexane (DACH) non-leaving chemical moiety.

This clear-cut distinction between the two groups of platinum compounds can be interpreted as a consequence of the existence of different mechanisms of action of those compounds, or at least a difference in their respective mechanisms of resistance. This prompted us to explore the molecular determinants of the activity of these compounds by establishing relationships between gene expression profiles and sensitivity to platinum compounds of tumour models (2). Several markers identified as significantly correlated to the cytotoxicity of platinum compounds were previously known as determinants of drug activity (2). This is the case for the functionality of the p53 pathway or for the expression of ERB-B2 or BCL-XL proteins. For instance, highly significant correlation between tetraplatin sensitivity and topoisomerase II expression has been observed. Furthermore, DNA mismatch repair (MMR) proteins MLH1 and MSH2, which have been found to be deficient in cisplatin-resistant cell lines, positively correlated with cytotoxicity of tetraplatin and oxaliplatin (2).

Oxaliplatin became the lead compound for a third generation platinum anti-tumour analogue in which 1,2-diaminocyclohexane (DACH) ligand substitutes for the amine groups of cisplatin (3). Oxaliplatin has demonstrated a broad spectrum of activity in a wide range of human tumours in vitro and in vivo. The toxicity profile of oxaliplatin differs from that of cisplatin and carboplatin, and in various clinical situations was preferred to cisplatin by virtue of a superior therapeutic index coupled with activity against cisplatin-resistant tumours (4). Oxaliplatin shares several properties with that of cisplatin. Both drugs react with the same GC-rich sites in naked DNA and similarly prefer GC-enriched regions of cellular DNA. Like cisplatin, oxaliplatin not only induces intrastrand crosslinks but also forms interstrand crosslinks (ISC) and DNA-protein crosslinks (DPC) in cellular DNA (5). All these oxaliplatin-induced DNA lesions are likely to play a role in cell growth inhibition. Several studies repeatedly showed that oxaliplatin was markedly less reactive with naked DNA and forms fewer adducts with cellular DNA than equimolar cisplatin (6). It was shown that DNA fragmentation produced by DACH-platinum compounds determines their cytotoxicity (6).

ProLindac (AP5346)

ProLindac appears as a further improvement of DACH-platinum drugs, comprising a novel hydrophilic biocompatible co-polymer to which a DACH-platinum compound is attached by an amidomalonato chelating group and triglycine spacer. The pH-dependent polymer prodrug has been designed to improve the specificity of platinum delivery to acidic tumour sites. The low pH of hypoxic regions of tumours enables sustained release of the active DACH-platinum compound, thus increasing its concentration preferentially within the tumour (7). This higher concentration of platinum may improve the therapeutic index of ProLindac as compared to that of oxaliplatin and cisplatin. ProLindac is currently undergoing phase I/II clinical evaluation (8). The aim of our study was to determine the ProLindac anti-proliferative effects in our panel of cancer cell lines, to study its molecular mechanisms of action. To improve the clinical use of ProLindac we tried to identify the predictive factors of sensitivity as well as the effects of ProLindac on gene expression as a molecular signature of drug action.

Cytotoxicity of ProLindac in a Panel of Cancer Cell Lines

The cytotoxicity of ProLindac was compared to that of cisplatin and oxaliplatin in a panel of cancer cell lines including colon, breast, lung, ovarian, prostate and leukaemic cell lines (Fig. 1). ProLindac displayed time- and concentration-dependent cytotoxicity with IC_{50s} ranging 3–85 μM for 48 h exposure. The cytotoxicity profile of ProLindac was similar to that of oxaliplatin. In addition ProLindac was active against several cisplatin resistant cell lines. After 48 h exposure to IC_{50} concentrations, ProLindac induced apoptosis and gave rise to an increased number of cells in the G2/M phase in colon and ovarian cancer cells. While less pronounced, these effects were similar to those for cisplatin or oxaliplatin, which also normally block the cells in G2/M phase.

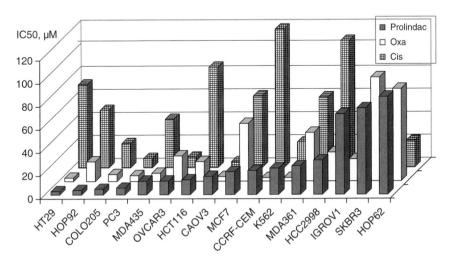

Fig. 1 The cytotoxicity of ProLindac, oxaliplatin and cisplatin given for 48 h to a panel of cancer cell lines

Molecular Mechanisms of Action of ProLindac

To study the role of pH on platinum release from ProLindac, the drug was incubated for 1, 4 and 24 h in cell-free media adjusted to different pH levels. The amount of platinum released was quantified by atomic absorption spectroscopy (Fig. 2). An acidic pH 5.4 caused an increase of platinum release by 24 h compared to neutral pH conditions. At pH 3.0, about 70% of the total platinum in ProLindac was released over 4 h. We have demonstrated that this increase of platinum release at acidic pH was associated with an increase of the Pt-DNA content. ProLindac was pre-incubated for 4h at pH 7, 5.4, and 3 and then exposed to the cells. Concentration levels of platinum in DNA was slightly higher when pre-incubated in pH 5.4, than at pH 7.0. When ProLindac was pre-incubated at pH 3.0; the platinum DNA level was about 20-fold greater. This result indicates that pre-incubation of ProLindac in acidic conditions favours platinum release and associated Pt incorporation in DNA that determines the cytotoxic effects.

We then studied the intracellular distribution of platinum after a 4h ProLindac treatment, compared to oxaliplatin and cisplatin at equiplatinum concentrations (Table 1). Despite the fact that the high molecular weight of ProLindac might be

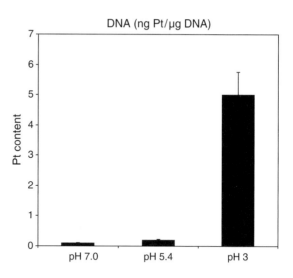

Fig. 2 DNA platinum content after pre-incubation of ProLindac at different pHs

Table 1 Intracellular platinum distribution after 4-h exposure to equiplatinum ProLindac, oxaliplatin and cisplatin

Drug	Pt content after 4h incubation with 300 µg/mL Pt	
	Total cell lysate (µg/mL)	DNA (ng/µg)
ProLindac	1	0.1
Oxaliplatin	4.1	0.8
Cisplatin	4.6	2.6

expected to inhibit DACH-platinum entering the cell, the percentage of platinum adducts formed with ProLindac is similar to that induced by oxaliplatin that is already known to be inferior to that of cisplatin (5). On the other hand the 4h-exposure may be a too short period of time to obtain maximum platinum release, platinum-D incorporation for longer exposures being currently investigated.

Predictive Factors and Biomarkers of ProLindac Activity

We have further assessed the expression level of potential factors implicated in drug transport, metabolism and repair in a panel of ten cancer cell lines and cor-related the expression level with ProLindac cytotoxicity (IC_{50s}). We have shown a clear correlation between ProLindac sensitivity and low expression level of MLH1, MDR1 and MRP genes. We have also demonstrated a slight correlation between low GSTP1, XPA and high KI67 gene expression levels and ProLindac sensitivity. Expression levels of ERCC1, hMSH2, and Rb1 genes were not correlated with sensitivity to ProLindac.

It was recently shown (9) that exposure to oxaliplatin in colon cancer cells induced significant changes in expression of many genes implicated in drug transport, DNA repair and cell cycle regulation. We compared the genetic effects induced by ProLindac with those induced by oxaliplatin and cisplatin in HCT116 cell line. We have shown that 48-h exposure to ProLindac induces p21 and XPA expression and decreases expression of Ki67 and TOP2A significantly (Fig. 3).

To determine more precisely the role of MMR genes on these effects, we compared the isogenic cell line HCT116-CH3 (which carries an additional chromosome 3) with several MMR genes (10). The effects of ProLindac were retained in the HCT116-CH3 cell line. When we used another isogenic cell line HCT116-p53 with 53 inactivation, the effects of ProLindac on gene expression were

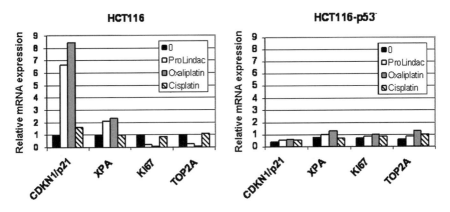

Fig. 3 The effects of ProLindac, oxaliplatin and cisplatin on gene expression

completely abolished in p53 defective cells. This allows us to consider a role for p53 in ProLindac's anti-tumour activity.

ProLindac in Combination with Gemcitabine, 5-FU, Docetaxel and SN38

As platinum agents are generally used in combination with other anti-cancer compounds, we explored the anti-proliferative potential of ProLindac in combination with gemcitabine, 5-FU, docetaxel and SN38 in colon and ovarian cancer cell lines. Effects of sequential and simultaneous schedules of exposure were determined by median effect plot analysis (Chou & Talalay test) (Table 2). When combined with other cytotoxics such as 5-FU, gemcitabine, and SN-38, ProLindac showed synergistic effects for several administration schedules. When ProLindac was given after gemcitabine and 5-FU, the resulting cytotoxic effects were higher than those of other dosing sequences. The effects of several schedules of administration were in general similar to those of oxaliplatin combinations in colon and ovarian cancer cell lines (11).

Table 2 Summary table of ProLindac (PLD)-based combination effects

Combination	Optimal schedules	HCT116	HT29
PLD – 5FU	5-FU prior PLD	Synergy	Synergy
PLD – Gemcitabine	Gem prior PLD	Additive/synergy	Synergy
PLD – Docetaxel	Doc prior PLD Simultaneous	Additive/synergy Additive/synergy	Additive Additive/synergy
PLD – SN38	PLD prior SN38, SN38 prior PLD	Synergy Additive/ Synergy	Additive/synergy Synergy

Conclusions

The novel DACH-platinum compound ProLindac demonstrated superior cytotoxicity to that of cisplatin, and similar cytotoxicity to that of oxaliplatin in a panel of human cancer cell lines associated with apoptosis and an increase of G2/M phase. Anti-proliferative effects of ProLindac were associated with induction of p21 expression and with a decrease of Ki67 and TOP2A mRNA. The rate of Pt release from the ProLindac polymer is a function of the pH, with increasing amounts of Pt per mg of DNA being observed with decreasing pH. Some proteins implicated in DNA-repair and metabolism may be considered as predictive factors of ProLindac cytotoxicity. ProLindac may display synergistic effects with other cytotoxic drugs, including 5-FU, gemcitabine and SN38. These results provide an early indication that ProLindac can effectively substitute for oxaliplatin in combination therapies.

References

1. Rixe O, Ortuzar W, Alvarez M, et al. Oxaliplatin, tetraplatin, cisplatin and carboplatin: spectrum of activity in drug-resistant cell lines and in the cell lines of the National Cancer Institute anticancer drug screen panel. Biochem Pharmacol 1996;52:1855–65.
2. Vekris A, Meynard D, Haaz MC, Bayssas M, Bonnet J, Robert J. Molecular determinants of the cytotoxicity of platinum compounds: the contribution of in silico research. Cancer Res 2004;64:356–62.
3. Raymond E, Faivre S, Woynarowski J, Chaney S. Oxaliplatin: mechanism of action and antineoplastic activity. Semin Oncol 1998;25:4–12.
4. Misset JL, Bleiberg H, Sutherland W, Bekradda M, Cvitkovic E. Oxaliplatin clinical activity: a review. Crit Rev Oncol Hematol 2000;35:75–93.
5. Woynarowski JM, Faivre S, Herzig MC, et al. Oxaliplatin-induced damage of cellular DNA. Mol Pharmacol 2000;58:920–7.
6. Faivre S, Chan D, Salinas R, Woynarowska B, Woynarowski JM. DNA strand breaks and apoptosis induced by oxaliplatin in cancer cells. Biochem Pharmacol 2003;66:225–37.
7. Rice JR, Gerberich JL, Nowotnik DP, Howell SB. Preclinical efficacy and pharmacokinetics of AP5346, a novel diaminocyclohexane-platinum tumour-targeting drug delivery system. Clin Cancer Res 2006;12:2248–54.
8. Campone M, Rademaker-Lakhai JM, Bennouna J, et al. Phase I and pharmacokinetic trial of AP5346, a DACH-platinum-polymer conjugate, administered weekly for three out of every 4 weeks to advanced solid tumour patients. Cancer Chemother Pharmacol 2007;60:523–33.
9. Voland C, Bord A, Péleraux A, et al. Repression of cell cycle-related proteins by oxaliplatin but not cisplatin in human colon cancer cells. Mol Cancer Ther 2006;5:2149–57.
10. Colella G, Marchini S, D'Incalci M, Brown R, Broggini M. Mismatch repair deficiency is associated with resistance to DNA minor groove alkylating agents. Br J Cancer 1999;80:338–43.
11. Raymond E, Faivre S, Chaney S, Woynarowski J, Cvitkovic E. Cellular and molecular pharmacology of oxaliplatin. Mol Cancer Ther 2002;1:227–35.

Synthesis of Cisplatin Analogues: Cytotoxic Efficacy and Anti-tumour Activity of Bis-Amidine and Bis-Iminoether Pt(II) Complexes

Roberta Bertani, Silvia Mazzega Sbovata, Valentina Gandin, Rino A. Michelin, and Cristina Marzano

Abstract A series of new platinum(II) bis-amidine derivatives were prepared by addition of primary and secondary aliphatic amines to coordinated nitrile ligands in *cis*- and *trans*-[PtCl$_2$(NCR)$_2$] (R = Me, Ph, CH$_2$Ph). The bis-amidine complexes were tested for their *in vitro* cytotoxicity on a panel of various human cancer cell lines. The results indicated that the *trans* isomers are more effective than the *cis* species, and in particular the benzamidine complex *trans*-[PtCl$_2${*E*-N(H)=C(NMe$_2$) Ph}$_2$] was the most active derivative and was able to circumvent acquired cisplatin resistance, thus suggesting a different mechanism of action compared to that exhibited by cisplatin. New benzyliminoether derivatives *cis*- and *trans*-[PtCl$_2${*E*-N(H)=C(OMe)CH$_2$Ph}$_2$] were also prepared by addition of MeOH to *cis*- and *trans*-[PtCl$_2$(NCCH$_2$Ph)$_2$] and the cytotoxic properties were evaluated in terms of cell growth inhibition against a panel of different types of human cancer cell lines. The complex *cis*-[PtCl$_2${*E*-N(H)=C(OMe)CH$_2$Ph}$_2$] was significantly more potent than cisplatin against all tumour cell lines, including cisplatin-resistant ones. Moreover, the in vivo studies, performed on two transplantable tumour models, showed that *cis*-[PtCl$_2${*E*-N(H)=C(OMe)CH$_2$Ph}$_2$] exhibited a marked activity against murine L1210 leukaemia and Lewis lung carcinoma in terms of survival prolongation and tumour growth inhibition, respectively.

Keywords Amidine platinum(II) complexes; Iminoether platinum(II) complexes; Anti-tumour activity; Drug resistance

The investigation of the relationship between the chemical properties and the pharmacological activity of cisplatin analogues has guided the development of several hundreds of compounds designed to optimize their anti-tumour potential. Within

R. Bertani (✉), S.M. Sbovata, V. Gandin, R.A. Michelin, and C. Marzano
Department of Chemical Processes of Engineering,
University of Padova, Padova, Italy
e-mail: roberta.bertani@unipd.it

A. Bonetti et al. (eds.), *Platinum and Other Heavy Metal Compounds in Cancer Chemotherapy*, DOI: 10.1007/978-1-60327-459-3_7,
© Humana Press, a part of Springer Science + Business Media, LLC 2009

this research area, a relevant class of biologically active Pt(II)-based drugs has been prepared from the synthetically useful organonitrile Pt(II) complexes *cis*- and *trans*-[PtCl$_2$(NCR)$_2$] (R = Me, Ph, CH$_2$Ph) by taking advantage of their ability to undergo nucleophilic addition (1, 2) of alcohols (3, 4) and amines (5–8) at the C≡N triple bond to achieve iminoether (iminoether = (H)N=C(OMe)CH$_2$Ph) and amidine (amidine = (H)N=C(NHR′)R and (H)N=C(NR′$_2$)R, where R = Me, Ph, CH$_2$Ph; R′ = Me, Et, Pr^i) derivatives, respectively. The interest in these classes of compounds arises from their ready synthetic availability and from the possibility to modify the following parameters: (a) the *cis* or *trans* stereogeometry of the metal complexes; (b) the *E* or *Z* conformation of the ligands; (c) the chemical nature of R and R′ groups able to modify the lipophylicity of the metal drug.

The addition of primary aliphatic amines R′NH$_2$ (R′ = Me, Et, Pr^i) to *cis*- and *trans*-[PtCl$_2$(NCR)$_2$] (R = Me, Ph, CH$_2$Ph) leads to the formation of the amidine complexes *cis*- and *trans*-[PtCl$_2${N(H)=C(NHR′)R}$_2$], where both amidine ligands are preferentially in the *Z* configuration and are characterized by the presence of strong intramolecular hydrogen bonds between each chlorine atom and the imino proton of the NHR′ moiety forming a six-member ring as confirmed by the X-ray diffraction analysis of *trans*-[PtCl$_2${Z-N(H)=C(NHMe)Me}$_2$] (Fig. 1a) (5). The reactions of *cis*- and *trans*-[PtCl$_2$(NCR)$_2$] (R = Me, Ph, CH$_2$Ph) with secondary aliphatic amines R$_2$NH (R = Me, Et) afford the corresponding bis-amidine

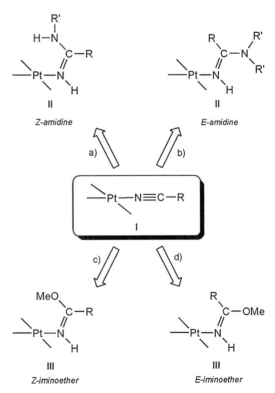

Fig. 1 Schematic representation of the addition reactions of amines and alcohols to coordinated nitrile ligands in *cis*- or *trans*-[PtCl$_2$(NCR)$_2$] complexes (I) to give amidine (II) and iminoether (III) derivatives, respectively. The metal fragment represents a *cis*- or *trans*-[PtCl$_2$(ligand)] unit, where ligand = RCN (I), amidine (II), iminoether (III). (**a**) +R′NH$_2$(5-fold exc) (R′ = Me, Et, Pr^i), CH$_2$Ph, CH$_2$Cl$_2$, −10°C, 5 h, R = Me, Ph, CH$_2$Ph; (**b**) +R′$_2$NH$_{(5-fold exc)}$ (R′ = Me, Et), CH$_2$Cl$_2$, −10°C, 5 h, R = Me, Ph, CH$_2$Ph; (**c**) +MeOH, KOH$_{(cat)}$, CH$_2$Cl$_2$, RT, 1 h, R = CH$_2$–C$_6$H$_4$-*p*-X, X = H, Me, OMe, F; (**d**) +MeOH, KOH$_{(cat)}$, CH$_2$Cl$_2$, RT, 1 day, R = CH$_2$–C$_6$H$_4$-*p*-X, X = H, Me, OMe, F

derivatives *cis*- and *trans*-[PtCl$_2${N(H)=C(NR$'_2$)R}$_2$], in which both amidine ligands have preferentially the *E* configuration as confirmed by the X-ray diffraction analysis of *trans*-[PtCl$_2${*E*-N(H)=C(NMe$_2$)Me}$_2$] (Fig. 1b) (6).

The benzyl di-nitrile complexes *cis*- and *trans*-[PtCl$_2$(NCCH$_2$-*p*-C$_6$H$_4$-X)$_2$] (where X = H, CH$_3$, OCH$_3$, F) dissolved in a mixture of dichloromethane/methanol and in the presence of a catalytic amount of KOH undergo the formation at room temperature of the bis-iminoether derivatives *cis*- and *trans*-[PtCl$_2${N(H)=C(OMe)CH$_2$-*p*-C$_6$H$_4$-X}$_2$] (9, 10) with a similar procedure previously reported by Natile et al. (3). Detailed nuclear magnetic resonance (NMR) studies demonstrated that the iminoether ligands are initially formed in the kinetically favoured *Z* configuration (Fig. 1c), which can be converted, in the presence of OH$^-$ ions, into the more thermodynamically stable *E* form, which is also obtained under prolonged reaction times (Fig. 1d) (4).

The biological activity of the bis-amidine and bis-iminoether complexes has been evaluated against a panel of human tumour cell lines. IC$_{50}$ values, calculated from the dose–survival curves obtained after a 24- or 48-h drug treatment by 3-(4,5-dimethyl-thiazol-2-yl)-2,5-diphenyltetrazolium bromide (MTT) (11, 12), are reported in Table 1. It is observed that the benzamidine derivatives of the type [PtCl$_2${N(H)=C(NR$'$R$''$) Ph}$_2$] (R$'$ = H, Me; R$''$ = Me) show a growth inhibitory potency markedly higher

Table 1 Evaluation of in vitro cytotoxic activity of the platinum(II) amidine and iminoether complexes towards some established human tumour cell lines by the 3-(4,5-dimethylthiazol-2-yl)-2,5-diphenyltetrazolium bromide (MTT) test

Compound	IC$_{50}$[a](μM) ± SD[b]		
	HL60	A549	A375
cis-[PtCl$_2${Z-N(H)=C(NHMe)Ph}$_2$][c]	>100	>100	>100
trans-[PtCl$_2${Z-N(H)=C(NHMe)Ph}$_2$][c]	6.10 ± 0.99	32.9 ± 1.66	62.88 ± 2.04
cis-[PtCl$_2${*E*-N(H)=C(NMe$_2$)Ph}$_2$][c]	>100	>100	>100
trans-[PtCl$_2${*E*-N(H)=C(NMe$_2$)Ph}$_2$][c]	4.75 ± 0.44	13.07 ± 1.16	24.05 ± 1.42
cis-[PtCl$_2${*E*-N(H)=C(OMe)CH$_2$Ph}$_2$][d]	8.59 ± 2.7	2.33 ± 1.7	9.15 ± 1.2
trans-[PtCl$_2${*E*-N(H)=C(OMe)CH$_2$Ph}$_2$][d]	89.98 ± 1.2	87.90 ± 2.6	77.55 ± 1.8
cis-[PtCl$_2${*E*-N(H)=C(OMe)CH$_2$-*p*-C$_6$H$_4$-CH$_3$}$_2$][d]	8.0 ± 1.2	6.2 ± 1.1	10.3 ± 0.9
trans-[PtCl$_2${*E*-N(H) = C(OMe)CH$_2$-*p*-C$_6$H$_4$-CH$_3$}$_2$][d]	58.4 ± 2.1	61.1 ± 0.8	65.5 ± 2.5
cis-[PtCl$_2${*E*-N(H)=C(OMe)CH$_2$-*p*-C$_6$H$_4$-OCH$_3$}$_2$][d]	21.1 ± 0.6	35.0 ± 1.2	28.4 ± 1.9
trans-[PtCl$_2${*E*-N(H)=C(OMe)CH$_2$-*p*-C$_6$H$_4$-OCH$_3$}$_2$][d]	66.0 ± 2.0	79.5 ± 2.5	71.3 ± 1.4
cis-[PtCl$_2${*E*-N(H)=C(OMe)CH$_2$-*p*-C$_6$H$_4$-F}$_2$][d]	6.7 ± 1.8	12.7 ± 1.1	13.5 ± 0.9
trans-[PtCl$_2${*E*-N(H)=(OMe)CH$_2$-*p*-C$_6$H$_4$-F}$_2$][d]	27.3 ± 1.2	39.5 ± 1.6	57.2 ± 0.5
Cisplatin[c]	19.55 ± 0.26	38.37 ± 1.79	50.05 ± 2.03
Cisplatin[d]	15.91 ± 1.55	29.21 ± 1.92	20.28 ± 1.3

[a]IC$_{50}$ values were calculated by probit analysis ($p < 0.05$, χ^2 test)
[b]*SD* standard deviation
[c]Cells ((3–8) × 10^4 ml^{-1}) were treated for 24h with increasing concentrations of the tested compound
[d]Cells ((3–8) × 10^4 ml^{-1}) were treated for 48h with increasing concentrations of the tested compound

than the corresponding acetamidine derivatives of the type [PtCl$_2${N(H)=C(NR'R'')Me}$_2$] (R' = H, Me; R'' = Me), possibly owing to the more lipophylic properties of the phenyl ring. Moreover, the benzamidine complexes derived from the addition reactions of secondary amines are more effective than those obtained from primary amines. In these latter, the presence of strong intramolecular hydrogen bonds between the chlorine atom and the imino proton of the NHR' moiety likely prevents further hydrogen interactions involving the Pt-NH moiety. Among the benzamidine derivatives, those endowed with higher cytotoxicity are those with *trans* geometry, and within them the complex *trans*-[PtCl$_2${E-N(H)=C(NMe$_2$)Ph}$_2$] appeared the most effective derivative. It shows a growth inhibitory potency markedly higher than that of cisplatin and exhibits a different cross-resistance profile from that of cisplatin, being able to circumvent acquired resistance as suggested by resistance factors (RFs) calculated on three different cell line pairs that have been selected for their resistance to cisplatin (RF = 0.53 towards 2008/C13* cell lines; 0.96 towards A431/A431-Pt cell lines; 1.25 towards U2OS/U2OS-Pt cell lines) (11). The results obtained by cellular uptake indicate that *trans*-[PtCl$_2${E-N(H)=C(NMe$_2$)Ph}$_2$] enters the cells more easily than cisplatin, possibly owing to the marked lipophylicity of the benzamidine ligands. Moreover, *trans*-[PtCl$_2${E-N(H)=C(NMe$_2$)Ph}$_2$] shows a marked inhibitory effect on DNA and RNA synthesis, whereas it is unable to directly affect protein synthesis. Studies performed *in vitro* on pBR322 DNA treated with *trans*-[PtCl$_2${E-N(H)=C(NMe$_2$)Ph}$_2$] and digested by different restriction endonucleases indicate that it shows a marked preference for GG-rich DNA sequences, which are the preferred DNA binding sequences of cisplatin. In contrast, DNA alkaline elution experiments demonstrate that *trans*-[PtCl$_2${E-N(H)=C(NMe$_2$)Ph}$_2$] does not form detectable interstrand DNA cross-link (ISC) amounts on cellular DNA but induces a frequency of DNA–protein cross-link (DPC) significantly higher than that of cisplatin, suggesting a different anti-proliferative action with respect to cisplatin, but similar to that previously reported for *trans*-iminoether complexes for which the formation of DPC is involved in the termination of DNA polymerization (13). It is also important to observe that this new amidine *trans*-Pt(II) complex could represent the lead compound of a new class of platinum anti-tumour drugs in which activation of the *trans* geometry is associated with an increased efficiency to form DPC, thereby acting by a different mechanism from cisplatin. NMR and electrospray ionization (ESI) mass spectrometric studies demonstrated the formation of a new cationic species in which the substitution by dimethyl sulfoxide (DMSO) of one chlorine atom in the platinum coordination sphere takes place. Reasonably, this species is involved in the ligand exchange processes occurring in the biological medium (11).

In the case of the benzyliminoether derivatives of the type [PtCl$_2${E-N(H)=C(OMe)CH$_2$-p-C$_6$H$_4$-X}$_2$] (X = H, CH$_3$, OCH$_3$, F), the data reported in Table 1 show that the *cis* isomers are significantly more cytotoxic than the corresponding *trans* derivatives (9, 13). In particular, the complex *cis*-[PtCl$_2${E-N(H)=C(OMe)CH$_2$Ph}$_2$] appears to be much more cytotoxic than cisplatin on both cisplatin-sensitive and -resistant sublines, exhibiting RF values significantly lower than those calculated for cisplatin (RF = 2.1 toward 2008/C13* cell lines; 0.9 toward A431/A431-Pt cell lines; 1.9 toward U2OS/U2OS-Pt cell lines; 1.4 toward L1210/L1210-Pt cell lines). The overcoming of cross-resistance in all cisplatin phenotypes supports the hypothesis of a different pathway of action of this benzyliminoether platinum complex with respect to cisplatin, through the occurrence of different types of DNA lesions or less efficiently repaired by DNA mismatch repair systems (14). Moreover, regarding the inhibition of the macromolecular synthesis, cis-[PtCl$_2${E-N(H)=C(OMe)CH$_2$Ph}$_2$] exhibits a strong dose-dependent decrease of ^{3}H-thymine incorporation, reducing DNA synthesis by about 60% even at the lowest concentration, while RNA and protein syntheses are less inhibited, showing a trend very similar to that exhibited by cisplatin. Finally, the investigation of cell death mechanism on 2008 cells treated with cis-[PtCl$_2${E-N(H)=C(OMe)CH$_2$Ph}$_2$] showed that it induces apoptosis in a dose-dependent manner accompanied by the activation of caspase-3 (15). On the basis of the *in vitro* studies, cis-[PtCl$_2${E-N(H)=C(OMe)CH$_2$Ph}$_2$] was selected for *in vivo* studies. The toxicity was assessed from the lethality in BALB/c mice within 30 days; the median lethal dose (55 mg kg^{-1}) attests a noticeably lower systemic toxicity than that of cisplatin (11.4 mg kg^{-1}). The anti-tumour activity of cis-[PtCl$_2${E-N(H)=C(OMe)CH$_2$Ph}$_2$] was evaluated at four dose levels (i.e., 2.5, 5, 7.5, and 10 mg kg^{-1}) in two murine tumour models, L1210 leukaemia and Lewis lung carcinoma, and compared with that of cisplatin (9). Against murine leukaemia L1210, it was found that cis-[PtCl$_2${E-N(H)=C(OMe)CH$_2$Ph}$_2$], at the highest dose, significantly prolonged the life span of the treated animals, demonstrating an anti-tumour effect about 1.5-fold higher (%T/C = 245.6) than that of cisplatin (%T/C = 159.9) with a body weight loss significantly lower (Fig. 2). In L1210/R,

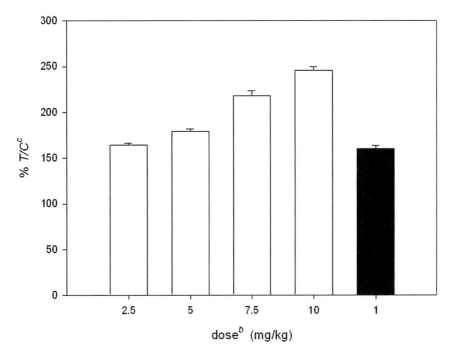

Fig. 2 *In vivo* anti-tumour activity of the complex cis-[PtCl$_2${E-N(H)=C(OMe)CH$_2$Ph}$_2$] *square* and cisplatin *filled square* in murine L1210 leukaemia[a]

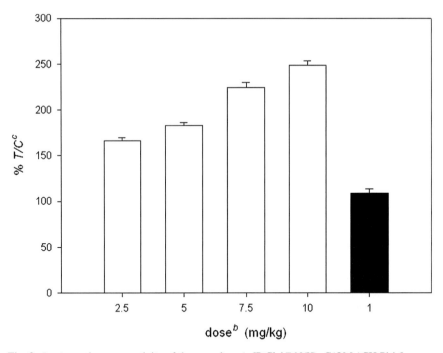

Fig. 3 *In vivo* anti-tumour activity of the complex *cis*-[PtCl$_2${*E*-N(H)=C(OMe)CH$_2$Ph}$_2$] *square* and cisplatin *filled square* in murine L1210/R leukaemia[a]

the %*T/C* values (248.7) obtained in mice treated with *cis*-[PtCl$_2${*E*-N(H)=C(OMe)CH$_2$Ph}$_2$] were similar to those obtained in mice implanted with L1210, confirming the cisplatin resistance overcoming effect (Fig. 3). Chemotherapy performed on Lewis lung carcinoma demonstrated that complex *cis*-[PtCl$_2${*E*-N(H)=C(OMe)CH$_2$Ph}$_2$] has, at 5 mg kg^{-1} dose, a significant tumour growth inhibition (64.88%) in comparison to untreated controls, and this anti-tumour effect appears similar to that showed by cisplatin. At the highest dose, the anti-tumour activity (87.9% of tumour growth inhibition) is about 1.3 times higher than that of the reference drug (65.65%) (Fig. 4). This data reveals for the first time that an iminoether of *cis* geometry shows higher biological activity than the corresponding *trans* species. In terms of high cytotoxic activity, overcoming of acquired and intrinsic cisplatin resistance, delineation of an apoptotic cell-death mechanism and noticeable *in vivo* anti-tumour activity against transplantable tumour models, *cis*-[PtCl$_2${*E*-N(H)=C(OMe)CH$_2$Ph}$_2$] represent a very interesting candidate for the development of a new class of Pt-based anti-tumour drugs.

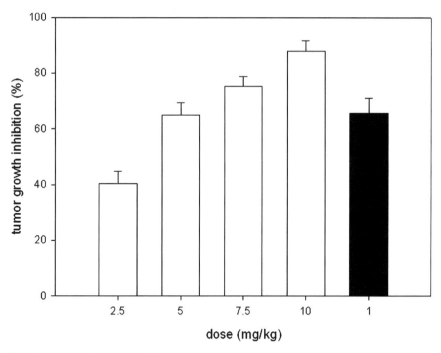

Fig. 4 *In vivo* anti-tumour activity of the complex *cis*-[PtCl$_2$\{*E*-N(H)=C(OMe)CH$_2$Ph\}$_2$] *open square* and cisplatin *filled square* in the murine Lewis Lung Carcinoma

References

1. Michelin RA, Mozzon M, Bertani R. Reactions of transition metal-coordinated nitriles. Chem. Rev 1996;147:299–338.
2. Kukushkin VY, Pombeiro AJL. Additions to metal-activated organonitriles. Chem. Rev 2002;102:1771–802.
3. Fannizzi FP, Intini FP, Natile G. Nucleophilic attack of methanol on bis(benzonitrile)dichloroplatinum: Formation of mono- and bis-imido ester derivatives. J. Chem. Soc. Dalton Trans. 1989;5:947–51.
4. Cini R, Caputo P A, Intini FP, Natile G. Mechanistic and stereochemical investigation of imino ethers formed by alcoholysis of coordinated nitriles: X-ray crystal structures of *cis*- and *trans*-bis(1-imino-1-methoxyethane)dichloroplatinum(II). Inorg. Chem. 1995;34:1130–7.
5. Bertani R, Catanese D, Michelin RA, Mozzon M, Bandoli G, Dolmella A. Reactions of platinum(II)-nitrile complexes with amines. Synthesis, characterization and X-ray structure of the platinum(II)-amidine complex *trans*-[PtCl$_2$\{Z-N(H)=C(NHMe)Me\}$_2$]. Inorg. Chem. Commun. 2000;3:16–18.
6. Michelin RA, Bertani R, Mozzon M, et al. Cis addition of dimethylamine to the coordinated nitriles of *cis*- and *trans*-[PtCl$_2$(NCMe)$_2$]. X-ray structure of the amidine complex *cis*-[PtCl$_2$\{*E*-N(H)=C(NMe$_2$)Me\}$_2$]·CH$_2$Cl$_2$. Inorg. Chem. Commun. 2001;4:275–80.
7. Belluco U, Benetollo F, Bertani R, et al. Stereochemical investigation of the addition of primary and secondary aliphatic amines to the nitrile complexes *cis*- and *trans*-[PtCl$_2$(NCMe)$_2$]. X-ray structure of the amidine complexes *trans*-[Pt(NH$_2$Pr^i)$_2$\{Z-N(H)=C(NHPr^i)Me\}$_2$]Cl$_2$·4H$_2$O and *trans*-[PtCl$_2$(NCMe)\{*E*-N(H)=C(NMeBut)Me\}]. Inorg. Chim. Acta 2002;330:229–39.

8. Belluco U, Benetollo F, Bertani R, et al. Addition reactions of primary and secondary aliphatic amines to the benzonitrile ligands in *cis*- and *trans*-[PtCl$_2$(NCPh)$_2$] complexes. X-ray structure of the amidine complex *trans*-[PtCl$_2${*Z*-N(H)=C(NHBut)Ph}$_2$]. Inorg. Chim. Acta 2002;334:437–47.
9. Mazzega Sbovata S, Bettio F, Mozzon M, et al. Cisplatin and transplatin complexes with benzyliminoether ligands: Synthesis, characterization, structure-activity relationship, and in vitro and in vivo antitumor efficacy. J. Med. Chem. 2007;50:4775–84
10. Mazzega Sbovata S, Bettio F, Marzano C, et al. Synthesis, characterization and cytotoxic activity of substituted benzyl iminoether Pt(II) complexes of the type *cis*- and *trans*-[PtCl$_2${*E*-N(H)= C(OMe)CH$_2$-*p*-C$_6$H$_4$-R}$_2$] (X = Me, OMe, F). X ray structure of *trans*-[PtCl$_2${*E*-N(H)=C(OMe) CH$_2$-*p*-C$_6$H$_4$-F}$_2$]. J. Inorg. Biochem. 2008;102:882–91.
11. Marzano C, Mazzega Sbovata S, Bettio F, et al. Solution behaviour and biological activity of bisamidine complexes of platinum(II). J. Biol. Inorg. Chem. 2007;12:477–93.
12. Mazzega Sbovata S, Bettio F, Marzano C, et al. Benzylamidine complexes of platinum(II) derived by nucleophilic addition of primary and secondary amines. X ray crystal structure of *trans*-[PtCl{*Z*-N(H)=C(NHMe)CH$_2$Ph}$_2$]. Inorg. Chim. Acta 2008;361:3109–16.
13. Coluccia M, Natile G. Trans-platinum complexes in cancer therapy. Anti-cancer Agents Med. Chem. 2007;7:111–3.
14. Perego P, Camerini C, Gatti L, et al. A novel trinuclear platinum complex overcomes cisplatin resistance in an osteosarcoma cell system. Mol. Pharmacol. 1999;55:528–34.
15. Khazanow E, Barenholz Y, Gibson D, Najajreh Y. Novel apoptosis-inducing trans-platinum piperidine derivatives: Synthesis and biological characterization. J. Med. Chem. 2002;45:5196–204.

Ruthenium Drugs for Cancer Chemotherapy: An Ongoing Challenge to Treat Solid Tumours

Gianni Sava and Alberta Bergamo

Abstract Ruthenium-based pharmaceuticals have brought some important insights in the chemotherapy of cancer. The knowledge acquired about the chemistry and biological interactions of these inorganic chemicals has allowed us to understand the limits of targeting DNA to achieve selective and innovative drugs. After a number of attempts to copy platinum drugs with a system claimed to be selective because of transferrin transportation and activation to cytotoxic species in tumour cells by a reduction mechanism, new innovative ideas are emerging such as those of using Ruthenium to structure organic ligands to enzyme or receptor targets responsible for tumour cell pathways associated to cell survival. Besides the staurosporine mimetics capable of inhibiting GSKbeta and inducing p53-mediated apoptosis, one example of this new wave is NAMI-A, a compound capable of controlling solid tumour metastases through the modulation of integrins and cell cytoskeleton. These data open up the interesting perspective of achieving potent agents to control tumour malignancy by selectively targeting tumour cells.

Keywords Ruthenium; Chemotherapy; Metastasis

From Metal-Coordinated to Organometallic Drugs

The most important studies on ruthenium anticancer compounds are those performed at the University of Vienna and at Trieste (University and Callerio Foundation), leading to the identification of indazolium bis-indazoletetrachloro ruthenate (KP1019, FFC14A) and imidazolium *trans*-imidazoledimethylsulfox idetetrachlororuthenate (NAMI-A), respectively (1, 2). In spite of the structural and chemical similarities, these two ruthenium(III) complexes show a consistently different anti-tumour behaviour. KP1019 is cytotoxic in vitro, causing apoptosis in

G. Sava (✉) and A. Bergamo
Callerio Foundation Onlus, Trieste, Italy
e-mail: g.sava@callerio.org

A. Bonetti et al. (eds.), *Platinum and Other Heavy Metal Compounds in Cancer Chemotherapy*, DOI: 10.1007/978-1-60327-459-3_8,
© Humana Press, a part of Springer Science + Business Media, LLC 2009

the treated cells, particularly on colorectal tumours (3, 4). NAMI-A is completely free of direct cell cytotoxicity (in conventional in vitro experiments where cells are typically exposed to the test drug) but it selectively kills metastasis in almost all the solid tumours metastasising to the lungs, including human xenografts, on which it had been tested so far (5, 6).

Today, NAMI-A benefits from an extensive literature, particularly on drug protein interactions and on the chemical reactivity in biological fluids, extended also to analogues with other metals, and also from studies on theoretical physics, giving the reader quite a clear picture of its fate upon intravenous administration to living beings, including humans (7–13). Binding to serum albumin and serum transferrin appears to be an important step of the pharmacological behaviour in vivo of NAMI-A (11, 14) and also of KP1019 (15, 16). Binding to albumin explains the persistence of the drug in the body, renal elimination being the most important way to reduce blood concentrations (11, 16). Binding to transferrin permits discussions on a large part of the selectivity claimed for ruthenium compounds, i.e., the capacity of these compounds to be transported with this carrier to cells greedy for iron such as fast growing tumour cells. Conversely, the chemical reactivity of the ruthenium centre at +3 oxidation state allows for the discussion of the other part of the selectivity claimed for ruthenium-based drugs, i.e., the capacity to undergo activation by a reduction mechanism. It is commonly accepted that ruthenium(III) compounds are rather inert while their ruthenium(II) counterparts are much more reactive towards biological targets, a theory developed and exhaustively explained by Michael Clarke with some ruthenium-chloro tetra- or penta-ammine derivatives (17, 18). Given that solid tumours are accredited of an hypoxic environment, activation of ruthenium(III) (relatively inert) compounds to ruthenium(II) reactive species is supposed to occur in the tumour masses much better than in normally oxidising healthy tissues. Reduction of Ruthenium(III) to Ruthenium(II) also governs the solution chemistry of these compounds as shown by experimental and theoretical studies (9, 10, 19, 20).

Besides KP1019 and NAMI-A, a plethora of compounds were prepared and tested for anti-tumour activity in cultured tumour cells in vitro worldwide, some with the metal at +3, as expected for the reasons given above, and some others, with different reasons, at +2 oxidation state. Examples are those with the bidentate beta-diketonato ligands, such as acetylacetonate and trifluoroacetylacetonate which showed good cytotoxicity on cisplatin sensitive and resistant osteosarcoma (U2-OS and U2-OS/Pt) and A2780 cells with a significant apoptosis induction on these latter, leading to cell accumulation in S phase and decrease of the percent of G_1 and G_2 cells (21). Gonzalez-Vilchez et al. showed the DNA binding of cis-dichloro-1,2-propylenediamine-N,N,N',N'-tetraacetato ruthenium (III) was persisting after removal of the compound from the culture medium, suggesting a strong cytotoxicity for the target cells (22). Also, bis(1,10-phenanthroline-2,2'-bipyridine) ruthenium(II) complexes containing ligands such as 1-thiocarbamoyl-3,5-diphenyl-2-pyrazoline, 2-(3,5-diphenyl-4,5-dihydropyrazol-1-yl)-4-phenylthiazole, 2-hydroxyphenyl benzimidazole or benzoin thiosemicarbazone, coordinate throughout nitrogen, sulphur and oxygen atoms to DNA and showed significant activity in mice with Ehrlich ascites carcinoma, prolonging the life expectancy of the tumour bearing hosts and reducing tumour burden while sparing RBC and WBC in the same animals (23). The use of 2,2'-bipyridine and aryl-beta-diketonato ligands has also brought a series of complexes of Ru(II)-2,2'-bipyridyl with substituted diazopentane-2,4-diones, showing the compound with naphtyldiazopentane-2,4-dione as a co-ligand endowed with an interesting cytotoxicity on a discrete panel of tumour cells in vitro (24). Djinovic' et al. have conversely pursued the goal to treat astrocytomas with a new ruthenium(III) complex, $K_2[Ru(N,N\text{-dimethylglycine})Cl_4]\cdot2H_2O$, a compound equally effective in confluent and non confluent C6 cells but not on rat astrocytes or macrophages, suggesting selectivity for tumour cells in vivo (25). In 2002, Anna Hotze, in the group of Reedijk, at the Leiden Institute of Chemistry, explored the chemical and biological activity of water-soluble bis(2-phenylazopyridine) ruthenium(II) complexes, a group of isomers endowed with an interesting cytotoxicity on ovarian tumour cells in vitro (A2780 and A2780cisR). With the exception of the beta isomers, all the other compounds showed a similar activity on sensitive and platinum-resistant cells, comparable to that showed by cisplatin and superior to that of carboplatin in the sensitive cells (26).

In 2001, the group of Peter Sadler developed a new group of organometallic arene ruthenium(II) diamine compounds which showed a strong cytotoxicity on cancer cells in vitro associated to a parallel DNA interaction, as determined in cell free media (27–30). A detailed study aimed at evaluating the effects of one of these complexes, namely RM175 $[(\eta^6\text{-}C_6H_5C_6H_5)RuCl\ (H_2NCH_2CH_2NH_2\text{-}N,N')]^+PF_6^-$, on the apoptosis controlling machinery in HCT116 colorectal cancer cells, showed that the generation of a p53-dependent early growth arrest and apoptotic response via p21/WAF1 and Bax induces a long-term loss of clonogenicity; nevertheless this latter effect was observed also in HCT116 p53 null cells, underlining the difficulty of understanding the primary cytotoxic lesion (31). In this respect it is interesting to study the work by Gaiddon et al., who used some new organometallic ruthenium(II) compounds to show the p53-dependent and p53-independent mechanism of cyto-toxicity to glioblastoma and neuroblastoma cell lines with G_1 arrest and apoptosis induction. Accumulation of p53 and p73 proteins correlated with an increase in p21 and Bax expression (32).

Conversely, Paul Dyson at EPFL developed in 2004 a new series of organo-metallics characterized by the presence of the phosphoadamantane moiety (PTA), called RAPTA compounds (33–35). These compounds, unlike the previous series, are only weakly cytotoxic on tumour cells in vitro and often completely free of cytotoxicity on healthy cells up to millimolar concentrations and 72 h exposure. Interestingly, when challenged with a solid tumour in vivo, they showed some capacity to reduce metastasis formation without affecting the growth of the primary tumour. This activity, in some way similar to that of NAMI-A, gives this family of organometallics some interest and a detailed study of the effects of this group in vitro shows an important inhibition of the steps of invasion and metastasis (Bergamo et al., manuscript in preparation).

The approach of Eric Meggers who synthesised a class of organometallic ruthenium(II) complexes with the characteristics of mimicking staurosporine analogues but showing a stronger selectivity for enzyme inhibition than staurosporine appears to be much more interesting. One of these compounds, nicknamed DW1/2, is selective for glycogen synthase kinase 3β, and shows the capacity to reactivate p53 in otherwise highly chemoresistant human melanoma cells, leading to the induction of apoptosis with a mechanism involving the down-regulation of Mdm2 and Mdm4 (36). This is the first demonstration of the possibility to use metal-based drugs to target tumour cell pathways and to get innovative drugs directed to tumour cell targets different than DNA. The fact that neither DW1/2 nor other compounds of this group had ever been reported to be active in vivo probably highlights the need for a more complete chemical work to allow the molecule to have a pharmacokinetics suitable for drug administration.

Also the selective metastasis inhibition of NAMI-A appears to be due to an interaction with a cellular target different than DNA. Although no univocal proof has been given yet, the results of several experiments support the hypothesis that metastasis reduction is due to the modulation of cell cytoskeleton, leading to inhibition of the invasion processes. This effect is also associated in vitro and in vivo to the activation of a checkpoint responsible for the control of cell cycle, thus leading to the widely described arrest at the G_2-M pre-mitotic phase, a step of cell division at which cells are particularly prone to undergo apoptotic death (Bergamo et al., unpublished data).

Phase-I Studies Completed

There are two studies of ruthenium complexes in humans and these studies concern the two most important drugs that have been developed in preclinical studies, NAMI-A and KP1019.

NAMI-A underwent a phase I clinical trial with an i.v. infusion over 3 h, daily for 5 days every 3 weeks in 24 patients with solid tumours. The drug was in general well tolerated. The disabling effects of nausea and vomiting, particularly severe at the highest dosages tested, were fully controlled with granisentron, and dexamethasone controlled the hypersensitivity reactions observed. Of particular attention is that renal toxicity was completely reversed 3 weeks after the end of drug administration and did not result in drug administration delay. The maximum tolerated dose was established at $300 \, mg/m^2/day$ on this schedule, and the main dose-limiting toxicity was blister formation, lasting for some weeks, on the hands and feet. Ruthenium concentration in these blisters was below the limit of detection. Pharmacokinetic analysis revealed a weak linear relationship between dose and AUC, with accumulation of the drug as protein bound in plasma. Ruthenium revealed linear elimination based on the linear relationship between NAMI-A dose, AUC and C_{max} of total and unbound drug, and the half-life time of elimination was shorter after the first dose than after the fifth dose. Disease stabilization was observed in heavily pre-treated patients with advanced NSCLC, a finding that may have a relevant clinical meaning in choosing this tumour for a Phase II study (37).

Also KP1019 underwent a clinical trial and the most relevant findings are that the pharmacokinetic profile looks very close to that of NAMI-A, although this compound could not reach a true maximum tolerated dose because of problems of solubility and the dose-escalation had to be stopped at 600 mg/patient (starting dose was 25 mg/patient), given intravenously twice a week over 3 weeks (1). Interestingly, some patients with colorectal cancer had stabilization of the disease, confirming the observations of the preclinical work (3, 4).

Perspectives for Ruthenium Drugs in Cancer Chemotherapy

Apparently, ruthenium complexes are important as a basis for drugs active in cancer chemotherapy mainly because they represent an attractive alternative to platinum drugs, not because of a better specified lower toxicity but showing the same ligand-exchange kinetics to those of platinum(II) anti-tumour drugs. The two 'plus' attributed to ruthenium complexes are the facility to mimic the binding of iron to biologically relevant molecules, allowing their transportation across the body, and the capacity to interact with the biological changes occurring on solid tumours leading to a more hypoxic environment that may activate 'inert' prodrugs to highly reactive and cytotoxic species. Due to their ligand geometries, ruthenium complexes bind to DNA affecting its conformation differently than cisplatin and its analogues. Thus ruthenium complexes may offer the potential of a non-cross resistance with platinum drugs and a different spectrum of activity, an activity that is anyhow correlated, in many instances, to their ability to bind DNA (38). This aspect is viewed as a fundamental ground to stress the potential role of ruthenium complexes to replace platinum drugs in clinical practice (39).

The role of the redox potential in the anti-tumour activity of ruthenium complexes has been shown, among others, by the group of Keppler who, in a series of complexes of the general formula [Ru(III)Cl(6–n)(ind)n](3–n)- (n = 0–4; ind = indazole; counterions = Hind+ or Cl-) proved that with colorectal cancer (SW480) and ovarian cancer (CH1) there is a strict correlation of the cell cytotoxicity with the reduction potential of these compounds (40). In this respect, an elegant work was done by Reisner et al., to demonstrate the possibility to tune the redox potential of ruthenium drugs to get compounds more suitable to the selective activation in the hypoxic environment of solid tumours (41). A pioneering suggestion in that direction comes from the work of Frühauf and Zeller who suggested that in hypoxic tumour tissue the Ru(III)-ion of *trans*-indazolium-tetrachlorobisindazole-ruthenate(III) (IndCR, KP1019, FFC14A) might be reduced to Ru(II), which is shown to be more reactive to DNA (42).

Besides the scientific interest raised by the aspects of transferrin transportation and activation by reduction, none of the ruthenium compounds being used up today to treat tumours in laboratory or in the clinics may be accredited of an activity clearly involving these mechanisms. Also, these ruthenium drugs suffer from at least two important biases. From the one side, they are being developed with the rules written with the experience accumulated with some thousands of platinum drugs, and from the other side, they are conceived with the principle to give strong bonding with the target. The similarities with platinum analogues led researchers to restrict their scientific fantasy to compounds that have to bind DNA and possibly to cause some kind of distortions, preferably different than those of cisplatin to circumvent platinum resistance (43). Conversely, the search for drugs capable of strong bonding with their targets does not fulfil the key requirements for agents that need to cross a number of biologically relevant structures prior to interacting specifically with the selected target.

Yet, the occupation of the relevant biological space with metals offers opportunities that none of the classical organic compounds can ever reach. If Barbara Kirchner et al. try to focus attention on the astonishing array of intricate electronic structures of metal radical systems that may lead to molecular level insights into reaction mechanisms that were hardly conceivable only few years ago (44), Ott and Gust on one side, and Zhang and Lippard on the other, limit their attention to an aseptic analysis of the existent compounds and of what have been shown by those who have described their activity (45, 46). Conversely, interesting aspects are raised by Bertini and Rosato who highlighted the 'extremely exciting and challenging' possibility to develop areas of medical, environmental and nanotechnology sciences, concluding that metal-binding to proteins might help to unravel the metabolic pathways and the mechanisms of life (47). These aspects appear to be of great importance, giving the challenges of the so called 'second golden era' of cancer chemotherapy focused on cancer genomics and particularly to targeting molecules selectively expressed or overexpressed by the disregulation of cell genome during cancer differentiation and growth, to achieve a kind of personalized therapy (48), provided that every cancer might represent a unique biological situation (49). In fact, targeting the disorganized tissue architecture at the primary site, and the restoration of the cell death program in cancer cells appears to create new opportunities in drug design. Also the cytoskeleton, which represents a dynamic set due to its plasticity and multiplicity, seems to be a promising target in anticancer therapy. Moreover, the evolving knowledge of the role of metastasis suppressor genes in regulating cancer cell growth at the secondary site suggests that they could serve as new targets for therapeutic interventions (50). Metal-organic compounds have the ability to form structures with unique and defined shapes for the design of small molecule drugs where the metal can organize and orient the organic ligands in a three-dimensional space leading to the discovery of drugs with superior biological activities (51). These aspects are stressed also by Finney and O'Halloran who suggested that the different coordination numbers, types of coordinating residues and solvent accessibilities of proteins essential to cell functioning are providing insights into inorganic chemistry (52). The examples of the ruthenium organometallics mimicking staurosporine and revealing a unique inhibitory activity of kinases leading to switches of cellular pathways (53–55), and that of NAMI-A targeting integrins in their active site and leading to the alteration of the cell cytoskeleton (56, Bergamo et al., unpublished data), are emblematic and represent examples of the feasibility of this approach.

One important aspect concerning the type of bonding metal-based compounds (organometallics included) is to do with their biological targets. Typically, metal-based drugs are conceived to give strong bonding with their target (this is one of the assiomas contained in the relevant literature of inorganic chemistry and of chemotherapy of platinum drugs). Weak bonds with targets are one of the main aspects at which frontier research is looking, for simply copying nature. Nature makes the differences between cells throughout the explosion of the number of 'receptors' involved in cell recognition and the number of bonding with ubiquitary ligands to these receptors. If these bondings were hard, then cells would be inhibited in many of their activities independently on the number of receptors. Then we should reassess the use of ruthenium compounds and the use of ligands to get structures for target interactions aimed at occupying the active site and to induce (or prevent) the activities consequent to this occupancy rather than getting an irreversible metal-target bonding after dissociation of one or more of these ligands. Inorganic chemistry has acquired an enormous bulk of expertise and will certainly accept this challenge and give rise to a fundamental development of new innovative drugs to cure cancer.

Acknowledgements Work done in the frame of COST D39 action. The financial support of MURST, Regione Autonoma Friuli Venezia Giulia and of Fondazione CRTrieste is gratefully appreciated.

References

1. Hartinger CG, Zorbas-Seifried S, Jakupec MA, et al. From bench to bedside – preclinical and early clinical development of the anticancer agent indazolium *trans*-[tetrachlorobis(1*H*-indazole)ruthenate(III)] (KP1019 or FFC14A). J Inorg Biochem 2006;100:891–904.
2. Alessio E, Mestroni G, Bergamo A, et al. Ruthenium antimetastatic agents. Curr Topics Med Chem 2004;4:1525–35.
3. Kapitza S, Pongratz M, Jakupec MA, et al. Heterocyclic complexes of ruthenium(III) induce apoptosis in colorectal carcinoma cells. J Cancer Res Clin Oncol 2005;131:101–10.
4. Kapitza S, Jakupec MA, Uhl M, et al. The heterocyclic ruthenium(III) complex KP1019 (FFC14A) causes DNA damage and oxidative stress in colorectal tumor cells. Cancer Lett 2005;226:115–21.
5. Sava G, Zorzet S, Turrin C, et al. Dual action of NAMI-A in inhibition of solid tumor metastasis: selective targeting of metastatic cells and binding to collagen. Clin Cancer Res 2003;9:1898–905.
6. Bergamo A, Zorzet S, Gava B, et al. Effects of NAMI-A and some related ruthenium complexes on cell viability after short exposure of tumor cells. Anticancer Drugs 2000;11:665–72.
7. Cebrián-Losantos B, Krokhin AA, Stepanenko IN, et al. Osmium NAMI-A analogues: synthesis, structural and spectroscopic characterization, and antiproliferative properties. Inorg Chem 2007;46:5023–33.
8. Barca A, Pani B, Tamaro M, et al. Molecular interactions of ruthenium complexes in isolated mammalian nuclei and cytotoxicity on V79 cells in culture. Mutat Res 1999;423:171–81.
9. Chen J, Chen L, Liao S, et al. A theoretical study on the hydrolysis process of the antimetastatic ruthenium(III) complex NAMI-A. J Phys Chem B 2007;111:7862–9.
10. Vargiu AV, Robertazzi A, Magistrato A, et al. The hydrolysis mechanism of the anticancer ruthenium drugs NAMI-A and ICR investigated by DFT-PCM calculations. J Phys Chem B;112:4401–9.

11. Brouwers EEM, Tibben MM, Rosing H, et al. Determination of ruthenium originating from the investigational anti-cancer drug NAMI-A in human plasma ultrafiltrate, plasma, and urine by inductively coupled plasma mass spectrometry. Rapid Commun Mass Spectrom 2007;21:1521–30.

12. Groessl M, Reisner E, Hartinger CG, et al. Structure-activity relationships for NAMI-A-type complexes (HL)[trans-RuCl₄L(S-dmso)ruthenate(III)] (L = imidazole, indazole, 1,2,4-triazole, 4-amino-1,2,4-triazole, and 1-methyl-1,2,4-triazole): aquation, redox properties, protein binding, and antiproliferative activity. J Med Chem 2007;50:2185–93.

13. Mura P, Camalli M, Messori L, et al. Synthesis, structural characterization, solution chemistry, and preliminary biological studies of the ruthenium(III) complexes [TzH][trans-RuCl₄(Tz)₂] and [TzH][trans-RuCl₄(DMSO)(Tz)]·(DMSO), the thiazole analogues of antitumor ICR and NAMI-A. Inorg Chem 2004;43:3863–70.

14. Bergamo A, Messori L, Piccioli F, et al. Biological role of adduct formation of the ruthenium(III) complex NAMI-A with serum albumin and serum transferrin. Invest New Drugs 2003;21:401–11.

15. Timerbaev AR, Rudnev AV, Semenova O, et al. Comparative binding of antitumor indazolium [trans-tetrachlorobis(1H-indazole)ruthenate(III)] to serum transport proteins assayed by capillary zone electrophoresis. Anal Biochem 2005;341:326–33.

16. Hartinger CG, Hann S, Koellensperger G, et al. Interactions of a novel ruthenium-based anti-cancer drug (KP1019 or FFC14a) with serum proteins – significance for the patient. Int J Clin Pharmacol Ther 2005;43:583–5.

17. Clarke MJ, Bitler S, Rennert D, et al. Reduction and subsequent binding of ruthenium ions catalyzed by subcellular components. J Inorg Biochem 1980;12:79–87.

18. Clarke MJ. Ruthenium metallopharmaceuticals. Coord Chem Rev 2003;236:209–33.

19. Bacac M, Hotze ACG, van der Schilden K, et al. The hydrolysis of the anti-cancer ruthenium complex NAMI-A affects its DNA binding and antimetastatic activity: an NMR evaluation. J Inorg Biochem 2004;98:402–12.

20. Schluga P, Hartinger CG, Egger A, et al. Redox behaviour of tumor-inhibiting ruthenium(III) complexes and effects of physiological reductants on their binding to GMP. Dalton Trans 2006;14:1796–802.

21. Arandjelovic S, Tesic Z, Perego P, et al. Cellular sensitivity to beta-diketonato complexes of ruthenium(III), Chromium(III) and rhodium(III). Med Chem 2006;2:227–37.

22. Vilaplana RA, Delmani F, Manteca C, et al. Synthesis, interaction with double-helical DNA and biological activity of the water soluble complex cis-dichloro-1,2-propylenediamine-N,N,N',N'-tetraacetato ruthenium (III) (RAP). J Inorg Biochem 2006;100:1834–41.

23. Rathinasamy S, Karki SS, Bhattacharya S, et al. Synthesis and anticancer activity of certain mononuclear Ru (II) complexes. J Enzyme Inhib Med Chem 2006;21:501–7.

24. Mishra L, Yadaw AK, Bhattacharya S, et al. Mixed-ligand Ru(II) complexes with 2,2'-bipyridine and aryldiazo-β-diketonato auxillary ligands: synthesis, physico-chemical study and antitumour properties. J Inorg Biochem 2005;99:1113–8.

25. Djinovic V, Momcilovic M, Grguric-Sipka S, et al. Novel ruthenium complex K₂[Ru(dmgly)Cl₄]·2H₂O is toxic to C6 astrocytoma cell line, but not to primary rat astrocytes. J Inorg Biochem 2004;98:2168–73.

26. Hotze AC, Bacac M, Velders AH, et al. New cytotoxic and water-soluble bis(2-phenylazopyridine) ruthenium(II) complexes. J Med Chem 2003;46:1743–50.

27. Morris RE, Aird RE, Murdoch Pdel S, et al. Inhibition of cancer cell growth by ruthenium(II) arene complexes. J Med Chem 2001;44:3616–21.

28. Novakova O, Chen H, Vrana O, et al. DNA interactions of monofunctional organometallic ruthenium(II) antitumor complexes in cell-free media. Biochemistry 2003;42:11544–54.

29. Chen H, Parkinson JA, Parsons S, et al. Organometallic ruthenium(II) diamine anticancer complexes: arene-nucleobase stacking and stereospecific hydrogen-bonding in guanine adducts. J Am Chem Soc 2002;124:3064–82.

30. Chen H, Parkinson JA, Morris RE, et al. Highly selective binding of organometallic ruthenium ethylendiamine complexes to nucleic acids: novel recognition mechanisms. J Am Chem Soc 2003;125:173–86.

31. Hayward RL, Schornagel QC, Tente R, et al. Investigation of the role of Bax, p21/Waf1 and p53 as determinants of cellular response in HCT116 colorectal cancer cells exposed to the novel cytotoxic ruthenium(II) organometallic agent, RM175. Cancer Chemother Pharmacol 2005;55:577–83.

32. Gaiddon C, Jeannequin P, Bischoff P, et al. Ruthenium (II)-derived organometallic compounds induce cytostatic and cytotoxic effects on mammalian cancer cell lines through p53-dependent and p53-independent mechanisms. J Pharmacol Exp Ther 2005;315:1403–11.

33. Scolaro C, Bergamo A, Brescacin L, et al. In vitro and in vivo evaluation of ruthenium(II)-Arene PTA complexes. J Med Chem 2005;48:4161–71.

34. Scolaro C, Geldbach TJ, Rochat S, et al. Influence of hydrogen-bonding substituents on the cytotoxicity of RAPTA compounds. Organometallics 2006;25:756–65.

35. Scolaro C, Chaplin AB, Hartinger CG, et al. Tuning the hydrophobicity of ruthenium(II)-arene (RAPTA) drugs to modify uptake, biomolecular interactions and efficacy. Dalton Trans 2007;43:5065–72.

36. Smalley KS, Contractor R, Haass NK, et al. An organometallic protein kinase inhibitor pharmacologically activates p53 and induces apoptosis in human melanoma cells. Cancer Res 2007;67:209–17.

37. Rademaker-Lakhai JM, van den Bongard D, Pluim D, et al. A phase I and pharmacological study with imidazolium-*trans*-DMSO-imidazole-tetrachlororuthenate, a novel ruthenium anticancer agent. Clin Cancer Res 2004;10:3717–27.

38. Brabec V, Novakova O. DNA binding mode of ruthenium complexes and relationship to tumor cell toxicity. Drug Resist Update 2006;9:111–22.

39. Brabec V. DNA modifications by antitumor platinum and ruthenium compounds: their recognition and repair. Prog Nucleic Acid Res Mol Biol 2002;71:1–68.

40. Jakupec MA, Reisner E, Eichinger A, et al. Redox-active antineoplastic ruthenium complexes with indazole: correlation of in vitro potency and reduction potential. J Med Chem 2005;48:2831–7.

41. Reisner E, Arion VB, Guedes da Silva MFC, et al. Tuning of redox potentials for the design of ruthenium anticancer drugs – an electrochemical study of [*trans*-RuCl$_4$L(DMSO)]$^-$ and [*trans*-RuCl$_4$L$_2$]$^-$ complexes, where L = imidazole, 1,2,4-triazole, indazole. Inorg Chem 2004;43:7083–93.

42. Frühauf S, Zeller WJ. New platinum, titanium, and ruthenium complexes with different patterns of DNA damage in rat ovarian tumor cells. Cancer Res 1991;51:2943–8.

43. Reedijk J. New clues for platinum antitumor chemistry: kinetically controlled metal binding to DNA. Proc Natl Acad Sci 2003;100:3611–6.

44. Kirchner B, Wennmohs F, Ye S, et al. Theoretical bioinorganic chemistry: the electronic structure makes a difference. Curr Opin Chem Biol 2007;11:134–41.

45. Ott I, Gust R. Non platinum metal complexes as anti-cancer drugs. Arch Pharm Chem Life Sci 2007;340:117–26.

46. Zhang CX, Lippard SJ. New metal complexes as potential therapeutics. Curr Opin Chem Biol 2003;7:481–9.

47. Bertini I, Rosato A. Bioinorganic chemistry in the postgenomic era. Proc Natl Acad Sci 2003;100:3601–4.

48. Mullin R. Personalized medicine. Chem Eng News 2008;86:17–27.

49. Workman P. Genomics and the second golden era of cancer drug development. Mol Biosyst 2005;1:17–26.

50. Dollé L, Depypere HT, Bracke ME. Anti-invasive and anti-metastasis strategies: new roads, new tools and new hopes. Curr Cancer Drug Targets 2006;6:729–51.

51. Meggers E. Exploring biologically relevant chemical space with metal complexes. Curr Opin Chem Biol 2007;11:287–92.

52. Finney LA, O'Halloran TV. Transition metal speciation in the cell: insights from the chemistry of metal ion receptors. Science 2003;300:931–5.

53. Williams DS, Atilla GE, Bregman H, et al. Switching on a signalling pathway with an organoruthenium complex. Angew Chem Int Ed Engl 2005;44:1984–7.

54. Bregman H, Williams DS, Atilla GE, et al. An organometallic inhibitor for glycogen synthase kinase 3. J Am Chem Soc 2004;126:13594–5.
55. Zhang L, Carroll P, Meggers E. Ruthenium complexes as protein kinase inhibitors. Org Lett 2004;6:521–3.
56. Frausin F, Scarcia V, Cocchietto M, et al. Free exchange across cells, and echistatin-sensitive membrane target for the metastasis inhibitor NAMI-A (imidazolium *trans*-imidazole dimethyl sulfoxide tetrachlororuthenate) on KB tumor cells. J Pharmacol Exp Ther 2005;313:227–33.

X-ray Crystal Structure of a Monofunctional Platinum–DNA Adduct, *cis*-{Pt(NH$_3$)$_2$-(Pyridine)}$^{2+}$ Bound to Deoxyguanosine in a Dodecamer Duplex

Ryan C. Todd and Stephen J. Lippard

Abstract Features of the 2.17 Å resolution X-ray crystal structure of *cis*-diammine-(pyridine)chloroplatinum(II) (cDPCP) bound in a monofunctional manner to deoxyguanosine in a DNA duplex are discussed and compared to those of a cisplatin–1,2-d(GpG) intrastrand cross-link in double-stranded DNA. The global geometry of cDPCP-damaged DNA is quite different from that of DNA containing a cisplatin 1,2-d(GpG) cross-link. The latter platinated duplex is bent by ~40° toward the major groove at the site of the adduct; however, the monofunctional Pt–dG lesion causes no significant bending of the double helix. Like the cisplatin intrastrand adduct, however, the cDPCP moiety creates a distorted base pair step to the 5′ side of the platinum site, which may be correlated with its ability to destroy cancer cells. Structural features of monofunctional platinum adducts are analyzed, the results of which suggest that such adducts may provide a new platform for the design and synthesis of Pt anticancer drug candidates.

Keywords cDPCP; X-ray crystallography; Monofunctional platinum compounds

The propensity of *cis*-diamminedichloroplatinum(II), (*cis*-[Pt(NH$_3$)$_2$Cl$_2$] or cisplatin) to form bifunctional intrastrand cross-links on DNA has been linked to its efficacy as an anticancer drug (1). In contrast, the cationic complex *cis*-diammine(pyridine)-chloroplatinum(II) (*cis*-[Pt(NH$_3$)$_2$(pyridine)Cl]$^+$, cDPCP) (see Fig. 1) displays antineoplastic activity in murine tumor models despite violating the classical structure–activity relationships established for platinum antitumor agents (2). cDPCP binds DNA at the N7 position of guanine residues like other Pt compounds; however, cDPCP contains only one chloride-leaving group, so it forms exclusively monofunctional adducts with nucleic acids. Several biochemical experiments have demonstrated that cDPCP adducts are fundamentally different from those of

R.C. Todd and S.J. Lippard (✉)
Department of Chemistry, Massachusetts Institute of Technology, Cambridge, Massachusetts, USA
e-mail: lippard@mit.edu

A. Bonetti et al. (eds.), *Platinum and Other Heavy Metal Compounds in Cancer Chemotherapy*, DOI: 10.1007/978-1-60327-459-3_9,
© Humana Press, a part of Springer Science + Business Media, LLC 2009

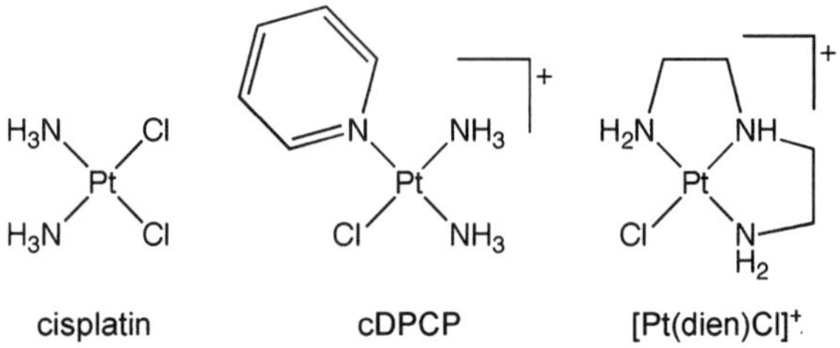

Fig. 1 Chemical structures of
cisplatin, cDPCP, and
[Pt(dien)Cl]⁺

cisplatin   cDPCP   [Pt(dien)Cl]⁺

cisplatin; no bifunctional cross-links arise from loss of the N-donor ligands (3, 4). Thus cDPCP represents one member of a growing class of "rule breakers", platinum complexes with antitumor activity that are incapable of forming the 1,2-intrastrand or any other cross-link.

We were interested to determine the characteristics of cDPCP that confer its cytotoxicity in tumor cells, given that most other monofunctional platinum(II) complexes, including [Pt(dien)Cl]⁺ (dien = diethylenetriamine, Fig. 1) and the trans isomer of cDPCP, are inactive (2). To investigate the structure of cDPCP-modified DNA and compare it with that of DNA damaged by cisplatin, we synthesized a DNA dodecamer duplex with site-specific placement of cDPCP at the N7 position of the central deoxyguanosine residue and characterized it by X-ray crystallography. The sequence of the DNA was similar to that used in previous studies of platinum–DNA duplexes (5–7) but modified to contain only one platinum binding site.

A site-specifically platinated DNA duplex having the platinated strand 5'-CCTCTCG*TCTCC-3' (where G* indicates the Pt site) was synthesized and crystallized and its X-ray structure determined at 2.17 Å resolution as described (8). Phases for the structure (depicted in Fig. 2a) were obtained by single-wavelength anomalous diffraction data arising from the platinum atom. Crystals belonged to the orthorhombic space group $C222_1$ with unit cell dimensions $a = 46.4$ Å, $b = 66.0$ Å, and $c = 56.1$ Å, one molecule in the asymmetric unit, and a solvent content of 56%.

Two predominant packing interactions organize the platinated DNA molecules within the unit cell (see Fig. 3). End-to-end packing, which is commonly encountered in B-DNA structures, is facilitated by hydrogen bonding of deoxyribose moieties of C1 and C12, and similarly of G13 with G24, in neighboring duplexes, creating a pseudo-continuous double helix throughout the crystal. Groove-to-groove packing also occurs between molecules, aided in part by hydrogen-bonding interactions between an ammine ligand on platinum of one duplex and the phosphate backbone on G16 of an adjacent molecule. Sixteen water molecules were located, with the most ordered ones being located in the major groove between two adjacent duplexes.

The duplex maintains linear, B-form DNA conformation despite the coordination of platinum to the central dG residue (see Fig. 2), and all Watson–Crick hydrogen-bond base pairing throughout the dodecamer is conserved. The double helix is unwound by ~8° in the vicinity of the platination site, in agreement with previous NMR spectroscopic results of a DNA duplex modified with the 4-Me-pyridine analog of cDPCP (9), but no other distortion of the global nucleic acid structure is observed.

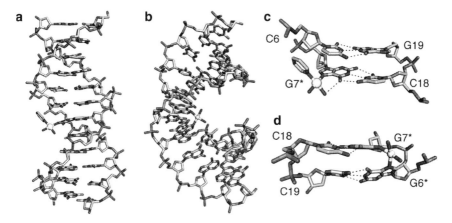

Fig. 2 The structures of (**a**) cDPCP- and (**b**) cDDP-damaged DNA duplexes. Close-up views of the platinum binding sites for cDPCP and cDDP are shown in (**c**) and (**d**), respectively. Asterisks indicate platinum binding sites. (**a**) and (**c**), PDB accession code 3CO3; (**b**) and (**d**), 1AIO

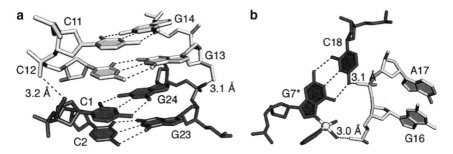

Fig. 3 End-to-end (**a**) and groove-to-groove (**b**) binding interactions between DNA molecules that contribute to crystal packing in the unit cell. Asterisks indicate platinum binding sites

The aromatic ligand of the cis-$\{Pt(NH_3)_2(py)\}^{2+}$–dG adduct is directed toward the 5′ end of the platinated strand, also in accord with previous NMR data on a DNA duplex with a bound para-substituted cDPCP analog (9). This orientation facilitates hydrogen-bond formation between the NH_3 ligand trans to pyridine and O6 on the guanosine residue (N–O distance, 2.8 Å). Interestingly, this hydrogen bond also occurs in the Pt–DNA adducts formed by oxaliplatin, (R,R)-diaminocyclohexaneoxalatoplatinum(II), but not in adducts formed by the inactive S,S-(DACH) stereoisomer (6, 10). Hydrogen-bonding interactions in cisplatin–DNA and oxaliplatin–DNA adducts have been thoroughly studied by using NMR spectroscopy and molecular dynamics simulations (10, 11), suggesting that they may be involved in differential recognition of these DNA damage sites by nuclear proteins. The precise role of these interactions in cellular processing of Pt–DNA adducts has not yet been elucidated; however, current data indicate that these hydrogen bonds are important in the mechanism of action of platinum antitumor compounds.

Compared to cisplatin, cDPCP binding only moderately distorts the structure of double helical DNA (Fig. 2a, b). Characteristics of the cisplatin 1,2-intrastrand cross-link include a roll angle of 27° between the bound guanines, global bending of 40° towards the major groove, and local unwinding of the duplex by ~25° (5). Furthermore, the platinum atom is displaced from the planes of the guanine bases by ~1 Å, causing additional strain (Fig. 2d). These distortions are hypothesized to inhibit transcription and, if the DNA damage persists, trigger cellular apoptosis (12). The monofunctional cDPCP adduct does not effect the roll or global bend angle of the DNA duplex, and it unwinds the helix by only 8°. The Pt atom of cDPCP lies within the guanine plane, as shown in Fig. 2c. DNA geometric parameters for the cDPCP–DNA and cisplatin–DNA adducts were calculated with 3DNA (13) and are compared in Table 1.

Although cDPCP and cisplatin modify nucleic acids in mono- and bifunctional manners, respectively, the resulting adducts share one common feature. Pt–DNA damage causes distortion of the base pair step on the 5' side of the lesion, regardless of the nature of binding. This base pair step, first identified by Marzilli (14), is marked by large shift and slide values; i.e., the base pair containing the platinum adduct is translocated out towards the major groove. The shift and slide values are 1.2 and 0.8 Å for the cDPCP–dG adduct, respectively, and 1.5 and 1.9 Å for the cisplatin 1,2-intrastrand cross-link, respectively. The effect, if any, of this perturbation towards cellular recognition and cytotoxicity has not yet been determined, but it is compelling to note that cDPCP and cisplatin cause a similar alteration in DNA geometry while forming fundamentally different adducts.

Both cisplatin and cDPCP bind the N7 atom of guanine bases to form stable DNA adducts, but the structural consequences to the nucleic acid double helix are significantly different. These results suggest that the two platinum antitumor compounds may destroy cancer cells through different mechanisms. We have postulated that cisplatin and cDPCP each block transcription by RNA polymerase II through unique interactions (8). It was reported from the X-ray crystal structure of the transcriptional elongation complex containing a cisplatin intrastrand adduct in the template strand that cisplatin may inhibit pol II when the Pt cross-link initially enters the active site of the enzyme because translocation and rotation of the strand are blocked by the covalently linked $Pt(NH_3)_2$–d(GpG) dinucleotide (15). We hypothesize that cDPCP would inhibit transcription via a different pathway. The mono adduct would not offer a barrier to DNA rotation because the Pt atom binds only a single base, but modeling studies suggest that the pyridine ligand may alter the position of the modified dG residue in the pol II active site by steric interactions with a nearby α-helix (8). This transformed conformation would prevent matching of the incoming ribonucleotide and inhibit RNA elongation. The trans isomer of cDPCP and $[Pt(dien)Cl]^+$, neither of which are active antitumor agents, would not provide this steric hindrance, which we take as biochemical evidence to support our hypothesis. Pol II inhibition would presumably lead to apoptosis in each case through common pathways initiated by attempted transcription-coupled repair.

Monofunctional complexes represent a class of platinum(II) compounds with known antineoplastic properties that could potentially offer a lower toxicity profile or differential tumor specificity compared to more conventional cisplatin analogs.

Table 1 Nucleic acid geometric parameters for Pt–DNA adducts (* platination sites)

Base pair	Sx	Sy	Sz	κ	ω	σ	Base	α	β	γ	δ	ε	ζ	χ
cDPCP-DNA							cDPCP-DNA: Pt strand (listed 5′–3′)							
5 T–A	-0.2	-0.1	0.1	-0.2	-18.8	-1.2	5 T	-28	161	41	147	-160	-109	-102
6 C–G*	0.2	-0.1	0.1	-4.6	-14.2	-1.0	6 C	-49	168	37	123	-165	-102	-107
7 G*–C	0.1	-0.1	-0.1	-3.9	-13.1	-0.8	7 G*	-40	167	33	143	-169	-150	-89
8 T–A	-0.1	0.1	0.1	-2.1	-15.1	-1.0	8 T	-35	167	37	147	-164	-111	-108
Cisplatin-DNA							Complementary strand (listed 3′–5′)							
5 T–A	0.6	-0.2	0.1	7.1	-3.4	3.5	20 A	-10	155	17	144	-168	-99	-99
6 G*–C	-0.1	-0.3	0.3	15.4	-18.4	-5.5	19 G	-54	157	17	161	-167	-149	-89
7 G*–C	-1.0	-0.6	0.2	-2.0	-14.5	-4.6	18 C	-66	172	42	135	-103	173	-99
8 T–A	0.5	0.2	0.2	-2.4	-22.7	6.9	17 A	-42	160	42	149	-173	-92	-107

bp step	Dx	Dy	Dz	τ	ρ	Ω	Base	α	β	γ	δ	ε	ζ	χ
cDPCP-DNA							Cisplatin-DNA: Pt strand (listed 5′–3′)							
5 TC/GA	0.4	0.3	3.5	2.2	1.3	39.4	5 T	-67	169	56	77	-173	-80	-154
6 CG*/CG	1.2	0.8	3.4	5.8	1.7	33.3	6 G*	-66	175	52	91	-144	-56	-147
7 G*T/AC	-0.9	-0.5	3.3	-2.6	2.9	31.0	7 G*	-77	164	73	82	-168	-82	-169
							8 T	-74	159	62	92	-163	-71	-154
Cisplatin-DNA							Complementary strand (listed 3′–5′)							
5 TG*/CA	-1.4	-1.4	3.2	-0.6	10.9	25.6	20 A	151	-169	173	86	-160	-71	-168
6 G*G/CC	1.5	-1.9	3.4	0.1	26.9	24.8	19 C	-71	-177	53	83	-162	-68	-157
7 G*T/AC	-0.2	-1.0	3.4	1.9	2.4	43.1	18 C	-75	176	56	86	-161	-84	-156
							17 A	-82	149	62	83	-166	-57	-159

[a] Base pair parameters are defined as follows: S_x shear (Å); S_y stretch (Å); S_z stagger (Å); κ buckle (deg); ω propeller twist (deg); σ opening (deg).

[b] Base pair step parameters are defined as follows: D_x shift (Å); D_y slide (Å); D_z rise (Å); τ tilt (deg); ρ roll (deg); Ω twist (deg).

[c] Torsion angles (deg) are defined as phos-α-o5′-β-c5′-γ-c4′-δ-c3′-ε-o3′-ζ-phos. χ is the glycosyl torsion angle

Here we describe the X-ray structural characterization of *cis*-diammine(pyridine)-chloroplatinum(II), a potent member of this group, bound to duplex DNA, and propose how this compound may act differently from cisplatin to destroy tumor cells. The information obtained from this structure can be utilized to design new monofunctional Pt compounds and provide a paradigm to expand the platform of "rule breakers" in the platinum antitumor compound family.

References

1. Jamieson ER, Lippard SJ. Structure, recognition, and processing of cisplatin-DNA adducts. Chem Rev 1999;99:2467–98.
2. Hollis LS, Amundsen AR, Stern EW. Chemical and biological properties of a new series of *cis*-diammineplatinum(II) antitumor agents containing three nitrogen donors: *cis*-[Pt(NH$_3$)$_2$(N-donor)Cl]$^+$. J Med Chem 1989;32:128–36.
3. Payet D, Leng M. DNA, *cis*-platinum and heterocyclic amines: catalytic activity of the DNA double helix. In: Sarma RH, Sarma MH, eds. Structural biology: the state of the art. Albany: Adenine Press, 1994:325–33.
4. Hollis LS, Sundquist WI, Burstyn JN, et al. Mechanistic studies of a novel class of trisubstituted platinum(II) antitumor agents. Cancer Res 1991;51:1866–75.
5. Takahara PM, Frederick CA, Lippard SJ. Crystal structure of the anticancer drug cisplatin bound to duplex DNA. J Am Chem Soc 1996;118:12309–21.
6. Spingler B, Whittington DA, Lippard SJ. 2.4 Å crystal structure of an oxaliplatin 1,2-d(GpG) intrastrand cross-link in a DNA dodecamer duplex. Inorg Chem 2001;40:5596–602.
7. Silverman AP, Bu W, Cohen SM, Lippard SJ. 2.4 Å crystal structure of the asymmetric platinum complex {Pt(ammine)(cyclohexylamine)}$^{2+}$ bound to a dodecamer DNA duplex. J Biol Chem 2002;277:49743–9.
8. Lovejoy KS, Todd RC, Zhang S, et al. *cis*-Diammine(pyridine)chloroplatinum(II), a monofunctional platinum(II) antitumor agent: uptake, structure, function, and prospects. Proc Nat Acad Sci USA 2008;105:8902–7.
9. Bauer C, Peleg-Shulman T, Gibson D, Wang AH-J. Monofunctional platinum amine complexes destabilize DNA significantly. Eur J Biochem 1998;256:253–60.
10. Wu Y, Bhattacharyya D, King CL, et al. Solution structures of a DNA dodecamer duplex with and without a cisplatin 1,2-d(GG) intrastrand cross-link: comparison with the same DNA duplex containing an oxaliplatin 1,2-d(GG) intrastrand cross-link. Biochemistry 2007;46:6477–87.
11. Sharma S, Gong P, Temple B, Bhattacharyya D, Dokholyan NV, Chaney SG. Molecular dynamic simulations of cisplatin- and oxaliplatin-d(GG) intrastrand cross-links reveal differences in their conformational dynamics. J Mol Biol 2007;373:1123–40.
12. Wang D, Lippard SJ. Cellular processing of platinum anticancer drugs. Nat Rev Drug Discovery 2005;4:307–20.
13. Lu X-J, Olson WK. 3DNA: a software package for the analysis, rebuilding, and visualization of three-dimensional nucleic acid structures. Nucleic Acids Res 2003;31:5108–21.
14. Marzilli LG, Saad JS, Kuklenyik Z, Keating KA, Xu Y. Relationship of solution and protein-bound structures of DNA duplexes with the major intrastrand cross-link lesions formed on cisplatin binding to DNA. J Am Chem Soc 2001;123:2764–70.
15. Damsma GE, Alt A, Brueckner F, Carell T, Cramer P. Mechanism of transcriptional stalling at cisplatin-damaged DNA. Nat Struct Mol Biol 2007;14:1127–33.

Osmium Arenes: A New Class of Potential Anti-cancer Agents

Sabine H. van Rijt, Anna F.A. Peacock, and Peter J. Sadler

Abstract Our studies of half-sandwich osmium(II) arene complexes of the type [(η^6-arene)Os(XY)Z] show that hydrolysis of the Os–Z (Z = Cl) bond and degree of formation of biologically inactive hydroxo-bridged dimers can be controlled by the choice of the chelated ligand XY. The chemistry and cancer-cell cytotoxicity of complexes containing N,N-, N,O-, or O,O-chelating ligands are compared and contrasted. The wide kinetic timescales of the reactions of these osmium complexes are notable and promising for the design of novel anti-cancer agents.

Keywords Organometallic; Osmium; Arene; Anti-cancer; Hydrolysis

The only non-platinum anti-cancer transition-metal compounds currently in clinical trials are two ruthenium(III) compounds, [ImH][*trans*-RuCl$_4$(DMSO)Im] (NAMI-A) (1) and [InH][*trans*-RuCl$_4$In$_2$] (KP1019) (2), where Im = imidazole, In = indazole. This use has stimulated much interest in the medical properties of ruthenium, and in particular in ruthenium(II) arene anti-cancer complexes (3). Certain Ru^{II} arene complexes exhibit both *in vitro* and *in vivo* activity, in some cases with activity comparable to that of cisplatin and carboplatin (4). Yet the pharmacological potential of the heavier congener osmium has been little explored. In general, as a third-row transition metal, osmium is considered to be relatively inert compared to the second-row transition metal ruthenium. The advantages in using transition metals other than platinum, such as ruthenium and osmium, include the availability of additional coordination sites, alterations in ligand affinity and substitution kinetics, but also changes in redox potentials.

S.H. van Rijt (✉), A.F.A. Peacock, and P.J. Sadler
Department of Chemistry, University of Warwick, Coventry, UK
e-mail: s.h.van-Rijt@warwick.ac.uk

A. Bonetti et al. (eds.), *Platinum and Other Heavy Metal Compounds in Cancer Chemotherapy*, DOI: 10.1007/978-1-60327-459-3_10,
© Humana Press, a part of Springer Science + Business Media, LLC 2009

Structure of Osmium(II) Arene Compounds

A typical structure of a half-sandwich "piano-stool" osmium(II) arene complex (i.e., $[(\eta^6\text{-arene})Os(X)(Y)(Z)]^{n+}$) allows variation of the three main building blocks to optimize drug design: the arene, the X and Y ligands and the monodentate leaving group Z. The nature of the arene can influence cell uptake of the complex, as well as interact with potential biological targets. The lability of the leaving group Z, typically a chloride, can be important in controlled activation. The X and Y ligands can be linked together to form a bidentate chelating ligand (XY) and may help to control the stability and the ligand exchange rates of these complexes. Most research has focused on the effects of the bidentate ligand XY on the overall reactivity of osmium(II) arene complexes. Recent studies include a series of complexes with bidentate nitrogen (N,N) (5–7), oxygen (O,O) (5, 8) and nitrogen–oxygen (N,O) chelators (9), but bifunctional compounds with monodentate nitrogen (6) and phosphine ligands (10) have also been explored. Figure 1 shows the general structure of osmium(II) arene complexes with selected examples of bidentate chelators used in recent studies.

Aqueous Reactivity and Cytotoxic Activity

The lack of understanding of the aqueous chemistry of organometallic complexes under biologically relevant conditions poses an obstacle in current attempts to design anti-cancer drugs. Knowledge of the aqueous chemistry of these types of complexes may eventually lead to the control of their pharmacological properties, including cell uptake, distribution, DNA binding, metabolism and toxic side effects. It is hypothesized that one route for the activation of these types of complexes *in vivo* involves aquation of the chlorido complexes. This may be followed by DNA

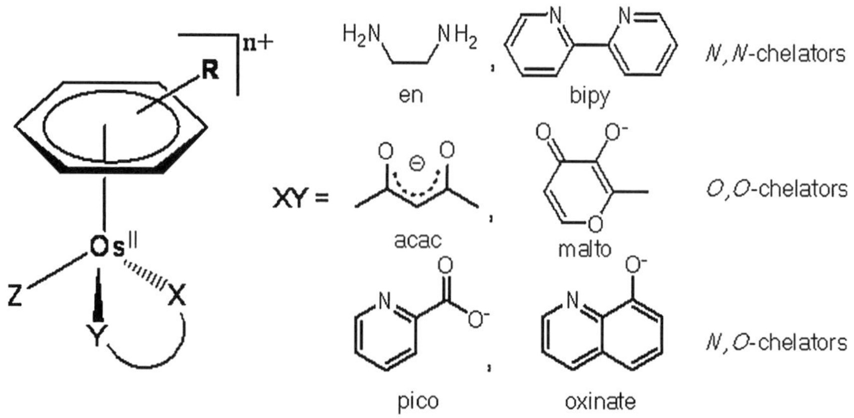

Fig. 1 Typical structure of osmium(II) half-sandwich complexes and selected examples of chelating ligands, XY

binding, resulting in the formation of monofunctional adducts with high affinity for the N7 of guanine (G) bases in the case of chelators bound by NH groups.

Studies of the rate of hydrolysis, i.e., exchange of the chlorido ligand for water, for osmium(II) arene complexes have revealed that their aqueous reactivity is greatly dependent on the nature of the chelating ligand (XY). For the ethylenediamine (en) complex $[(\eta^6$-biphenyl)Os(en)Cl]$^+$, hydrolysis occurs with a half-life of 6.4 h at 298 K, which is ca. 40 times slower than that of the Ru^{II} analogue. This highlights the lower reactivity of Os^{II} (5). Interestingly, despite its slow hydrolysis rate, $[(\eta^6$-biphenyl)Os(en)Cl]$^+$ still exhibited promising activity against the human ovarian cancer A2780 cell line (IC$_{50}$ = 9 μM, where IC$_{50}$ is the concentration that inhibits cell growth by 50%). The rate of hydrolysis was slowed down even further by incorporating a π-acceptor chelating ligand, such as 2,2′-bipyridine or 1,10-phenanthroline, by a factor of ca. 7 (6). Changing the ligand from the neutral N,N-chelator en to the anionic O,O-chelator acetylacetonate (acac) has a marked effect on the extent and rate of hydrolysis. The hydrolysis rate of $[(\eta^6$-arene)Os(acac)Cl] is too fast to monitor by NMR at 298 K. Density functional theory (DFT) calculations support the experimental observation of faster hydrolysis of the acac Os^{II}–arene complexes compared to analogues containing the N,N-chelator en. The calculated hydrolysis barrier of the Os^{II} acac compound is significantly lower than that of the en complex, by nearly 30 kJ mol^{-1} (8). However, hydrolysis of the acac compounds is complicated by the formation of the hydroxo-bridged dimer, $[(\eta^6$-arene)Os(μ^2-OH)$_3$Os(η^6-arene)]$^+$, with loss of the acac ligand. This hydroxo-bridged dimer is the only observed species at micromolar concentrations in solutions similar to those used in biological cell culture tests (5). The introduction of the five-membered maltolate chelate ring provides stabilisation towards hydroxo-bridged dimer formation compared to the six-membered acac complexes; however, the hydroxo-bridged dimer remained the dominant species present under biologically relevant conditions (8). On account of the formation of these hydroxo-bridged adducts, compounds containing O,O chelators are inactive towards the human ovarian (A2780) and human lung (A549) cancer cell lines.

Intermediate behaviour to that of the complexes containing N,N- and O,O-chelators is observed in aqueous solutions for complexes containing some anionic N,O-chelators. Although Os^{II} arene complexes containing aminoacidate ligands such as glycinate or L-alanine hydrolyse rapidly, are unstable towards hydroxo-bridged dimer formation and are non-toxic towards A2780 cells, complexes containing a pyridine derivative as the N-donor atom hydrolyse at an intermediate rate, are stable in aqueous solution at micromolar concentrations and are active towards both A549 and A2780 cell lines (9). Notably, complexes containing picolinate (pico) as the N,O-chelate display promising activity towards the human ovarian cancer cell line with IC$_{50}$ = 4.5 μM, a value similar to that of carboplatin (IC$_{50}$ = 6 μM) which is currently used in clinics. This enhanced stability probably results from the π-acceptor properties of the pyridine ring. This factor, in combination with the use of a more acidic chelating oxygen (carboxylate for pico), can minimize chelate ring-opening reactions through strengthening of the Os–N and Os–O bonds. The activation parameters show that aquation in these types of osmium(II) compounds occurs via an associative pathway, $\Delta S^{\ddagger}$ being negative (6, 9). The pK_a values of the resulting aqua adducts range from 5.8 to 6.3 for N,N-coordinated compounds (with the more acidic complexes containing pyridine ligands) (6). Therefore, at physiological pH (7.4) almost all of the hydrolyzed osmium complexes containing N,N chelators would be present as the less reactive hydroxo species, $[(\eta^6\text{-arene})Os(N,N\text{-chelate})(OH)]^+$. This is not the case for Os^{II} arene aqua compounds containing the anionic acac O,O-chelating ligand, for which the pK_a values range from 7.3 to 7.8 (depending on the arene) (5). For the N,O-chelators, pK_a values are intermediate between those of the N,N- and O,O-chelators (pK_a values of 7.1–7.5) (9).

The incorporation of a chelating ligand appears to be crucial for maintaining the stability of the complexes. The bifunctional osmium(II) arene complex containing the monodentate acetonitrile ligand, $[(\eta^6\text{-}p\text{-cym})Os(NCCH_3\text{-}N)Cl_2]$, is largely deactivated in water to form the inert hydroxo-bridged dimer (6). Such bridge formation was, however, not reported for a related Os^{II} arene complex containing a monodentate pta ligand (where pta is 1,3,5-triaza-7-phosphatricyclo[3.3.1.1]-decane), $[(\eta^6\text{-}p\text{-cym})Os(pta)Cl_2]$ (11). Os^{II} arene compounds containing bidentate-bound paullone-based ligands have a different type of instability in aqueous solution, with p-cymene arene loss occurring after 72 h. Even though arene loss was observed in aqueous solution, the compounds still exhibited low micromolar cytotoxicity in three human cancer cell lines (7).

Far less research has been dedicated to the effect of the arene on the overall reactivity of these types of osmium(II) complexes, although it has been shown that changing the arene from the electron-rich tetrahydroanthracene (THA) or p-cymene to the more electron-deficient biphenyl slows down the rate of hydrolysis significantly (6, 9). Such behaviour is also observed for the ruthenium analogues (12). In general, these studies demonstrate that the kinetics and thermodynamics of these types of complexes are important for their biological activity and, importantly, that these factors can be controlled by appropriate ligand design.

Interaction with Biologically Relevant Targets

Binding studies of osmium(II) arene complexes with nucleobases are of special interest since DNA is considered to be the main target for classical metal anti-cancer drugs (13) and distortions of DNA structure often correlate with anti-cancer activity (14). To gain insight into the reactivity of these types of complexes with DNA, nucleobase derivatives have been used as models (Fig. 2a). The osmium(II) biphenyl complex containing the N,N-chelator ethylenediamine (en) as chelating ligand reacts only slowly with 9-ethylguanine (9-EtG) and only to a limited extent with adenosine (Ado). In addition, no reaction is observed with the pyrimidine bases cytidine (Cyt) or thymidine (Thy) (5). The same base specificity is observed for the Ru^{II} analogue (i.e., $[(\eta^6\text{-bip})Ru(en)Cl]^+$) (15). In general, the lack of reactivity towards the pyrimidine bases is likely to be caused by steric interactions adjacent to the N3 position, making it an unfavourable binding site. The high discrimination for guanine over adenine binding in these types of

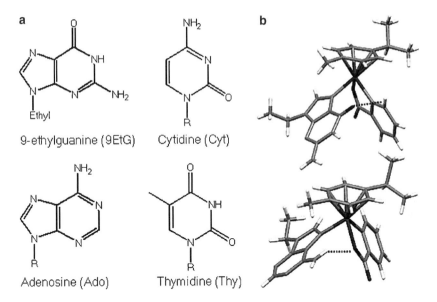

Fig. 2 (**a**) Structures of nucleobase derivatives 9-ethylguanine and mononucleosides adenosine, cytidine and thymidine (where R is deoxyribose). (**b**) X-ray structures of nucleobase adducts [(η⁶-*p*-cym)Os(pico)(9EtG)]⁺ (*top*) and [(η⁶-*p*-cym)Os(pico)(9EtA)]⁺ (*bottom*)

complexes can be rationalized in terms of favourable H-bonding for guanine and non-bonding repulsive interactions for adenine between the chelating ligand en and nucleobase substituents, in addition to the electronic properties of the various nucleobase coordination sites.

The aqua Os^{II} arene adduct containing the O,O-chelator acac or maltolate, [(η⁶-arene)Os(*O,O*-chelate)H_2O]⁺, reacts rapidly with purine bases (9-EtG and Ado) but not with pyrimidine bases (Cyt or Thy) (5). However, the hydroxo-bridged dimer, formed from the aqua Os^{II} adducts in solution by loss of the chelating O,O-ligand for both acac and maltolato complexes, is unreactive towards both purine and pyrimidine bases (5). This appears to be the key to understanding the inactivity of Os^{II} arene complexes containing O,O-chelates. The active anti-cancer compound containing picolinate (pico) as the N,O-chelate, i.e., ([(η⁶-arene)Os(pico) Cl], exhibits binding to both 9-EtG and 9-EtA, although a strong preference for 9-EtG exists when in competition. X-ray structures of the Os^{II} nucleobase adducts [(η⁶-*p*-cym)Os(pico)(9EtG)]⁺ and [(η⁶-*p*-cym)Os(pico)(9EtA)]⁺ show binding of osmium to the electronegative sterically non-hindered N7 site with the nucleobase functionality (CO for G, NH_2 for A) lying on the opposite side of the chelate for the G and A bases, respectively (Fig. 2b).

These configurations make short-range interactions possible between the functional groups on the nucleobases and the picolinate ligand, stabilizing nucleobase binding. As for the Os^{II} acac compounds, there is little or no binding of the Os^{II} pico compounds to the pyrimidine bases cytosine and thymine (9). In contrast to the base specificity observed for these Os^{II} arene complexes containing bidentate chelating ligands, non-specific binding of osmium bifunctional compounds [(η^6-*p*-cym)Os(pta)Cl$_2$] and [(η^6-*p*-cym)Os (pta-Me)Cl$_2$]$^+$ has been reported in a reactivity study towards a 14-mer oligonucleotide (11).

The first in-depth study of osmium(II) arene complexes of the type [(η^6-arene) Os(XY)Cl]$^{n+}$, where XY = N,O-chelating ligands picolinate, oxinate or N,N-chelate ethylenediamine, towards their interaction with biological target DNA in an effort to understand their mechanism of interaction has revealed some interesting results (16). All Os^{II} arene compounds tested bind to calf thymus DNA, but unlike cisplatin this binding resulted in no DNA bending. However, DNA adducts of the Os^{II} arene complexes that exhibit cancer cell cytotoxicity in the ovarian tumour cell lines show large unwinding of double-helical DNA. These data suggest that DNA binding occurs through coordination to guanine residues in addition to noncovalent interactions between the arene ligand and DNA. It is interesting to note that Os^{II} arene compounds containing en or pico ligands show similar activity in cells both sensitive and resistant to cisplatin, indicating a different mechanism of action for this class of complexes.

In conclusion, these studies show that the choice of types of ligands and coordination geometry in this novel class of anti-cancer compounds provides an ability to activate and "fine tune" the chemical reactivity of these types of compounds to obtain aqueous stability, biologically favourable ligand exchange rates and finally cytotoxic activity.

References

1. Rademaker-Lakhai JM, Van Den Bongard D, Pluim D, Beijnen JH, Schellens JHM. A phase I and pharmacological study with imidazolium-trans-DMSO-imidazole-tetrachlororuthenate, a novel ruthenium anticancer agent. Clin Cancer Res 2004;10:3717–27.
2. Jakupec MA, Arion VB, Kapitza S, et al. KP1019 (FFC14A) from bench to bedside: preclinical and early clinical development – an overview. Int J Clin Pharmacol Ther 2005;43:595–6.
3. Yan YK, Melchart M, Habtemariam A, Sadler PJ. Organometallic chemistry, biology and medicine: ruthenium arene anticancer complexes. Chem Commun 2005;(38):4764–76.
4. Aird RE, Cummings J, Ritchie AA, et al. In vitro and in vivo activity and cross resistance profiles of novel ruthenium (II) organometallic arene complexes in human ovarian cancer. Br J Cancer 2002;86:1652–7.
5. Peacock AFA, Habtemariam A, Fernandez R, et al. Tuning the reactivity of osmium(II) and ruthenium(II) arene complexes under physiological conditions. J Am Chem Soc 2006; 128:1739–48.
6. Peacock AFA, Habtemariam A, Moggach SA, Prescimone A, Parsons S, Sadler PJ. Chloro half-sandwich osmium(II) complexes: influence of chelated N,N-ligands on hydrolysis, guanine binding, and cytotoxicity. Inorg. Chem. 2007;46:4049–59.
7. Schmid WF, John RO, Arion VB, Jakupec MA, Keppler BK. Highly antiproliferative ruthenium(II) and osmium(II) arene complexes with paullone-derived ligands. Organometallics 2007;26:6643–52.
8. Peacock AFA, Melchart M, Deeth RJ, Habtemariam A, Parsons S, Sadler PJ. Osmium(II) and ruthenium(II) arene maltolato complexes: Rapid hydrolysis and nucleobase binding. Chem Eur J 2007;13:2601–13.
9. Peacock AFA, Parsons S, Sadler PJ. Tuning the hydrolytic aqueous chemistry of osmium arene complexes with N,O-chelating ligands to achieve cancer cell cytotoxicity. J Am Chem Soc 2007;129:3348–57.

10. Dorcier A, Ang WH, Bolano S, et al. In vitro evaluation of rhodium and osmium RAPTA analogues: the case for organometallic anticancer drugs not based on ruthenium. Organometallics 2006;25:4090–6.
11. Dorcier A, Dyson PJ, Gossens C, Rothlisberger U, Scopelliti R, Tavernelli I. Binding of organometallic ruthenium(II) and osmium(II) complexes to an oligonucleotide: a combined mass spectrometric and theoretical study. Organometallics 2005;24:2114–23.
12. Wang F, Chen HM, Parsons S, Oswald LDH, Davidson JE, Sadler PJ. Kinetics of aquation and anation of ruthenium(II) arene anticancer complexes, acidity and X-ray structures of aqua adducts. Chem Eur J 2003;9:5810–20.
13. Zhang CX, Lippard SJ. New metal complexes as potential therapeutics. Curr Opin Chem Biol 2003;7:481–9.
14. Brabec V, Novakova O. DNA binding mode of ruthenium complexes and relationship to tumor cell toxicity. Drug Resist Update 2006;9:111–22.
15. Fernandez R, Melchart M, Habtemariam A, Parsons S, Sadler PL. Use of chelating ligands to tune the reactive site of half-sandwich ruthenium(II)-arene anticancer complexes. Chem Eur J 2004;10:5173–9.
16. Kostrhunova H, Florian J, Novakova O, Peacock AFA, Sadler PJ, Brabec V. DNA interactions of monofunctional organometallic osmium(II) anti-tumor complexes in cell-free media. J. Med. Chem. 2008;51:3635-43.

Section B
Cellular Transport and Intracellular Trafficking of Platinum Compounds

Resistance to Cisplatin Results from Multiple Mechanisms in Cancer Cells

Michael M. Gottesman, Matthew D. Hall, Xing-Jie Liang, and Ding-Wu Shen

Abstract We have studied the development of resistance to cisplatin in cultured KB-3-1 human cervical adenocarcinoma (HeLa) cells and BEL-7404 human hepatoma cells. In a single-step selection, it is possible to develop a pleiotropic phenotype consisting of the following: (a) cross-resistance to other platinum compounds, arsenite, cadmium, methotrexate and nucleoside analogs; (b) corresponding reduced accumulation of these agents; (c) reduced receptor-mediated and fluid phase mediated endocytosis; (d) altered cytoskeleton, including disruption of actin microfilaments, filament structures, and microtubules; (e) a defect in membrane protein trafficking consisting of relocalization to intracellular vesicles of several transmembrane proteins such as the ABBC1 transporter (MRP1, GS-X pump), glucose transporter (GluT1), and folate binding protein (FBP); and (f) altered mitochondrial morphology and function. We hypothesize that this pleiotropic phenotype reflects a basic cellular defense mechanism against cytotoxic materials that are not hydrophobic enough to enter the cell by simple diffusion, but have multiple other mechanisms of cell entry including piggybacking on existing receptors and endocytosis, and speculate that a relatively simple cellular switch can actuate this pleiotropic response.

Keywords Cisplatin; Resistance; Uptake; Reduced accumulation; Pleiotropic mechanism

The development of clinical resistance to cisplatin, and subsequent analogs such as carboplatin and oxaliplatin, has prompted an extensive body of in vitro research into the cellular mechanisms by which this resistance is conferred. The commonly accepted cellular processes that contribute to resistance against the platinums are: (a) increased expression of glutathione and metallothionein, which chelate Pt drugs and deactivate them [1]; (b) improved nuclear repair mechanisms (mismatch repair, nucleotide excision repair), and tolerance of platination through lowered apoptosis signaling [2]; and

M.M. Gottesman (✉), M.D. Hall, X.-J. Liang, and D-W. Shen
Laboratory of Cell Biology, National Cancer Institute, National Institutes of Health,
Bethesda, MD, USA
e-mail: mgottesman@nih.gov

A. Bonetti et al. (eds.), *Platinum and Other Heavy Metal Compounds in Cancer Chemotherapy*, DOI: 10.1007/978-1-60327-459-3_11,
© Humana Press, a part of Springer Science + Business Media, LLC 2009

(c) reduced cellular accumulation of drug by a variety of proposed mechanisms (3). In vivo, a range of multicellular and physiological phenomena further contribute to poor clinical response (4). Understanding clinical resistance to cisplatin is further complicated since chemotherapeutic regimes usually employ a platinum drug in combination with other cytotoxic drugs such as 5-fluorouracil or paclitaxel (5), which is associated with P-glycoprotein-mediated multidrug resistance (6).

The least understood of the unicellular resistance mechanisms is the diminished cellular accumulation observed in cisplatin-resistant cell lines; most platinum-resistant tissue-culture cell lines accumulate less drug than their parental lines. Platinum drugs enter cells by a variety of mechanisms – recently reviewed by us (3) – including passive diffusion, fluid-phase endocytosis, and facilitated transport by solute carriers (SLCs) such as the organic cation transporters 1–3 (OCT1–3) and the copper transporter (CTR1). The diminished accumulation in resistant cells can be attributed to a reduction in energy-dependent drug uptake (7), while the small residual passive entry component is relatively unaffected (3). Given the multiple mechanisms of uptake available to platinum drugs, how is it possible that single-step mutants substantially reduce this uptake?

To identify cellular mechanisms of resistance, we have developed a set of cisplatin-resistant cell lines derived from the BEL-7404 human hepatoma and KB-3-1 human cervical adenocarcinoma cell lines by single-step selection by increasing concentrations of cisplatin (Fig. 1).

Characterization of these cell lines revealed increasing resistance not only to cisplatin, but to agents such as carboplatin, methotrexate, arsenite, arsenate, and *Pseudomonas* endotoxin (8); however, cross-resistance was not observed with more hydrophobic organic compounds such as doxorubicin, paclitaxel, etoposide or mitomycin C, which are substrates of the multidrug resistance efflux pump

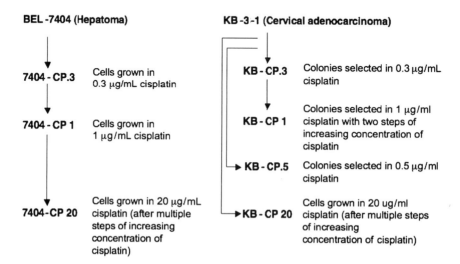

Fig. 1 Schematic showing resistant cell lines generated by stepwise exposure of BEL-7404 and KB-3-1 parental cell lines to cisplatin. Reprinted from (8) with permission from Elsevier

Table 1 Compounds that demonstrate lowered accumulation in cisplatin-resistant cells, and their known pathways of active cell entry, demonstrating the diverse array of membrane-associated transporters, and transport processes affected in the development of cisplatin resistance

Lowered accumulation	Proposed mechanism(s) of entry	Reference
Cisplatin[a]	Multiple, including copper transporter (CTR1) and organic cation transporter (OCT2)	(3)
[14C]-carboplatin	Copper transporter (CTR1)	(10)
[3H]-methotrexate	Folate-binding protein (FBP) and reduced folate carrier (RFC)	(8)
[3H]-folic acid	Folate-binding protein (FBP) and reduced folate carrier (RFC)	(11)
Arsenite, 73As(III)	Aquaporin (AQP)	(11)
Arsenate, 73As(V)	Aquaporin (AQP)	(11)
[125I]-epidermal growth factor (EGF)	EGF receptor (EGFR)	(11)
Iron, 59Fe(III)	Divalent metal transporter (DMT1)	(11)
[3H]-glucose	GluT family	(11)
Pseudomonas endotoxin	Endocytosis	(8)
[3H]-L-proline	Sodium/iminoacid transporter 1 (SIT1)	(11)

[a]Accumulation measured using AAS or ICP-OES

P-glycoprotein (9). Each of the compounds demonstrating cross-resistance is known to enter the cell via either transporters: e.g., reduced folate carrier (methotrexate), aquaporins (As compounds); or endocytosis (*Pseudomonas* endotoxin), rather than passive diffusion, suggesting that a down-regulation of importers, or mislocalization away from the plasma membrane, is occurring.

Furthermore, the increasing resistance in the selected cell lines shown in Fig. 1 is associated in each case with diminished accumulation of both cross-resistant compounds and nutrients known to enter the cell via active transport systems. Agents known to display reduced accumulation in cisplatin-resistant cells are shown in Table 1, along with their known uptake systems (3, 8, 10, 11). This reduced accumulation is not caused by P-gp, as rhodamine 123 accumulation is unaffected in cisplatin-resistant cell lines (7).

The decrease in accumulation, mediated by a broad range of transporters, takes place along with higher level cisplatin-resistant (KB-CP20) cells showing diminished uptake and altered distribution of the fluid-phase endocytosis markers horseradish peroxidase (HRPO) and Texas Red dextran-10 (12). Receptor-mediated endocytosis has also been examined using epidermal growth factor (EGF); while fewer EGF receptors were present at the cell surface (analogous to the diminished active transport described above), this was due to lowered EGF receptor expression, and the rate of internalization was unaffected, indicating that receptor-mediated endocytosis may not be directly affected. EGF degradation was observed to be slower in resistant cells, and a pH-sensitive fluorescent dye indicated increased lysosomal pH (12). When parental cells were treated with bafilomycin A₁ to increase lysosomal pH, the reduced cisplatin-uptake phenotype was induced (12). Taken together, these results suggest that the endosomal/lysosomal pathway is critical for platinum drug accumulation, either directly or through trafficking of membrane proteins.

The intracellular proteins that platinum drugs associate with were examined using photoaffinity labeling of [^{14}C]-carboplatin and the two major [^{14}C]-carboplatin-binding proteins were identified as filamin and actin, both of which are known to be involved in endocytosis and protein trafficking (13). Decreased expression of filamin and β-actin was found in the resistant KB-CP20 and 7404-CP20 compared to their respective parental cell lines, and subsequent analysis revealed that resistant lines are also deficient in other microfilament proteins such as dynamin 2 and β-tubulin. Transfection of cells with an expression vector for actin fused to enhanced green fluorescent protein (EGFP) revealed a non-filamentous actin-EGFP distribution compared with parental cells, suggesting that cytoskeletal organization is disturbed in cisplatin-resistant cells (13). In mammalian cells, an intact actin cytoskeleton is necessary for all forms of endocytosis (including endocytic recycling of membrane transporters), and the observation that cisplatin-resistant cells have lowered expression, and disrupted organization of the cytoskeleton, may provide an underpinning for the broad nature of platinum drug cross-resistance.

After endocytosis, most membrane proteins and lipids return to the cell surface, a process known as endocytic recycling. Given the defective endocytosis and disrupted cytoskeletion observed in resistant cells, it is possible that the lack of carrier-mediated accumulation described above is due to faulty endocytic recycling. Analysis of the multidrug resistance protein MRP1 in cisplatin-resistant cell lines revealed a loss of protein at the plasma membrane, but increased levels in the cytosolic fraction, and confocal imaging reveals that MRP1 and folate binding protein (FBP) are expressed mainly in the cytosol, unlike in parental lines where expression is observed at the plasma membrane (14). Biotinylation of membrane surface proteins, including MRP1, enabled tracking of MRP1 in cisplatin-sensitive and -resistant cells providing direct evidence that MRP1 gets to the cell surface in the resistant cells, but fails to recycle back once internalized (14). The transferrin receptor and its ligand transferrin are a model for endosomal recycling – after transferrin binding, the transferrin receptor is internalized to early endosomes, the iron released, and the transferrin receptor-transferrin complex returns to the cell surface via the endocytic recycling compartments (ERCs). Using fluorescently labeled transferrin, it was shown that the ERCs in cisplatin-resistant cells were abnormally distributed throughout the cell cytoplasm, and, conversely, that cell lines with defective ERCs were cross-resistant to cisplatin (15). These results confirm that it is not so much a loss of uptake transporters, as a lack of them at the plasma membrane due to faulty endocytic recycling, that contributes to lowered drug accumulation and cisplatin resistance.

The likely cause of this pleiotropic resistance is the alteration of a cellular switch that results in the disruption of membrane protein trafficking, possibly by a primary defect in cytoskeletal organization (Fig. 2). Consistent with this, it has been shown in both KB-CP20 and 7404-CP20 cells that several small GTPases that regulate crucial cellular processes such as cell cycle, gene transcription, and endocytosis are downregulated, including RhoA, rab5 and rac1 (11). It is possible that the lowered expression of genes in more highly resistant cells is due to hypermethylation, as the DNA demethylating agent 2-deoxy-5-aza-cytidine (DAC) reversed silenced genes

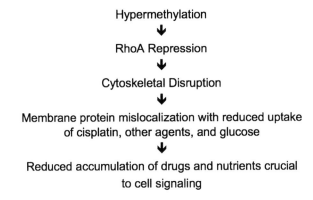

Hypermethylation
⬇
RhoA Repression
⬇
Cytoskeletal Disruption
⬇
Membrane protein mislocalization with reduced uptake
of cisplatin, other agents, and glucose
⬇
Reduced accumulation of drugs and nutrients crucial
to cell signaling

Fig. 2 The hypothetical pathway responsible for pleiotropic drug resistance in cisplatin-selected cell culture lines. Hypermethylation is associated with repression of small GTPases such as RhoA that are responsible for the regulation of crucial cell processes. The cytoskeletal disruption prevents effective endocytic recycling and the correct localization of membrane proteins, resulting in reduced drug accumulation, and disrupted cell signaling, possibly through altered mitochondrial metabolism, due to the deprivation of nutrients such as glucose

such as the folate binding protein (FBP) and partially recovered the accumulation defect for [^{14}C]-carboplatin, [^{3}H]-folic acid and [3]-methotrexate, while parental KB-3-1 lines were unaffected (11). We are currently seeking a specific molecular basis, such as altered transcription factors, to account for all or most of the downstream steps involved in this complex pleiotropic phenotype.

The robust cross-resistance of cisplatin-resistant cell lines manifests itself as diminished drug accumulation; however, the cause does not appear simply to be an alteration in the expression of specific uptake transporters. Rather, it is caused by alterations in gene methylation and expression that disrupt crucial endocytic processes and mislocalize a great many different membrane proteins. It has been demonstrated that demethylating agents can partially reverse the resistance phenotype, and demonstration of the specific molecular alterations in cisplatin-resistant cells should facilitate the development of more specific agents to overcome clinical resistance to platinum-based anti-cancer compounds.

References

1. Gately DP, Howell SB. Cellular accumulation of the anticancer agent cisplatin: a review. Br J Cancer 1993;67:1171–6.
2. Jung Y, Lippard SJ. Direct cellular responses to platinum-induced DNA damage. Chem Rev 2007;107:1387–407.
3. Hall MD, Okabe M, Shen DW, Liang XJ, Gottesman MM. The role of cellular accumulation in determining sensitivity to platinum-based chemotherapy. Annu Rev Pharmacol Toxicol 2008;48:495–535.
4. Stewart DJ. Mechanisms of resistance to cisplatin and carboplatin. Crit Rev Oncol Hematol 2007;63:12–31.

5. Kelland L. The resurgence of platinum-based cancer chemotherapy. Nat Rev Cancer 2007;7:573–84.
6. Gottesman MM, Fojo T, Bates SE. Multidrug resistance in cancer: role of ATP-dependent transporters. Nat Rev Cancer 2002;2:48–58.
7. Shen D-W, Goldenberg S, Pastan I, Gottesman MM. Decreased accumulation of [^{14}C]carboplatin in human cisplatin-resistant cells results from reduced energy-dependent uptake. J Cell Physiol 2000;183:108–16.
8. Liang XJ, Shen DW, Gottesman MM. A pleiotropic defect reducing drug accumulation in cisplatin-resistant cells. J Inorg Biochem 2004;98:1599–606.
9. Johnson SW, Shen D-W, Pastan I, Gottesman MM, Hamilton TC. Cross-resistance, cisplatin accumulation, and platinum-DNA adduct formation and removal in cisplatin-sensitive and -resistant human hepatoma cell lines. Exp Cell Res 1996;226:133–9.
10. Holzer AK, Manorek GH, Howell SB. Contribution of the major copper influx transporter CTR1 to the cellular accumulation of cisplatin, carboplatin, and oxaliplatin. Mol Pharmacol 2006;70:1390–4.
11. Shen DW, Su A, Liang XJ, Pai-Panandiker A, Gottesman MM. Reduced expression of small GTPases and hypermethylation of the folate binding protein gene in cisplatin-resistant cells. Br J Cancer 2004;91:270–6.
12. Chauhan SS, Liang XJ, Su AW, et al. Reduced endocytosis and altered lysosome function in cisplatin-resistant cell lines. Br J Cancer 2003;88:1327–34.
13. Shen DW, Liang XJ, Gawinowicz MA, Gottesman MM. Identification of cytoskeletal [^{14}C] carboplatin-binding proteins reveals reduced expression and disorganization of actin and filamin in cisplatin-resistant cell lines. Mol Pharmacol 2004;66:789–93.
14. Liang XJ, Shen DW, Garfield S, Gottesman MM. Mislocalization of membrane proteins associated with multidrug resistance in cisplatin-resistant cancer cell lines. Cancer Res 2003;63: 5909–16.
15. Liang XJ, Mukherjee S, Shen DW, Maxfield FR, Gottesman MM. Endocytic recycling compartments altered in cisplatin-resistant cancer cells. Cancer Res 2006;66:2346–53.

CTR1 as a Determinant of Platinum Drug Transport

Stephen B. Howell and Roohangiz Safaei

Abstract The copper transporter 1 (CTR1) is the major copper (Cu) influx transporter and also mediates the initial uptake of cisplatin (DDP), carboplatin (CBDCA) and oxaliplatin (L-OHP). Deletion of the gene coding for CTR1 in yeast or mouse embryonic fibroblasts substantially reduces the initial influx of all three Pt-containing drugs and renders them resistant to their cytotoxic effects. Forced over-expression of human CTR1 in the human A2780 ovarian carcinoma cells increases the uptake of DDP but appears to misdirect its distribution within the cell. DDP triggers rapid degradation of CTR1, thus reducing the level of its own influx transporter. This effect is reduced by drugs that block endocytosis or the proteosome. While CTR1 transports Cu through a pore that it forms in the plasma membrane, it transports DDP via quite a different mechanism that depends on endocytosis.

Keywords Copper homeostasis; Cisplatin; Carboplatin; Oxaliplatin; CTR1

Introduction

The three most commonly used Pt-containing drugs, cisplatin (DDP), carboplatin (CBDCA) and oxaliplatin (L-OHP) are quite polar and do not diffuse easily across the plasma membrane. Recent studies have provided evidence that the copper (Cu) transporters CTR1, ATP7A and ATP7B play a direct role in the transport of these three drugs into and out of tumor cells (1). CTR1 (SLC31A1) is an important Cu influx transporter in a wide range of species spanning yeast to humans (2). The structure and function of CTR1 is highly conserved across the species as shown by complementation studies documenting that hCTR1, yCTR1 and mCTR1

S.B. Howell (✉) and R. Safaei
Department of Medicine and the Moores Cancer Center, University of California, San Diego, La Jolla, CA, USA
e-mail: showell@ucsd.edu

A. Bonetti et al. (eds.), *Platinum and Other Heavy Metal Compounds in Cancer Chemotherapy*, DOI: 10.1007/978-1-60327-459-3_12,

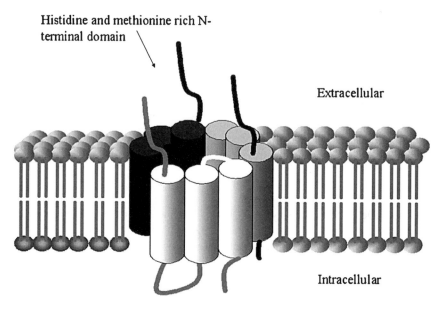

Histidine and methionine rich N-terminal domain

Extracellular

Intracellular

Fig. 1 Schematic representation of the topology of a human CTR1 trimer in the plasma membrane. Monomers are shown in black, white and gray. Each monomer has three membrane spanning domains, a histidine and methionine rich N-terminal extracellular domain, a cytosolic loop and a short C terminal tail

can rescue the phenotype produced by loss of CTR1 function in another species (3). The homology is not limited to the coding sequence but is also found in the exon–intron boundaries (4–6). CTR1 transporter Cu(I) moves across the plasma membrane following which it is chelated onto pathway-specific chaperones including the COX17, CCS and ATOX1 for transfer to mitochondria, cytosol and the secretory vesicles, respectively (7).

Deletion of both copies of the gene coding for CTR1 in mice produces embryonic lethality and developmental defects (8, 9). Human CTR1 has 190 amino acids and is rich in methionines and histidines in its extracellular N-terminal domain. Several conserved methionine residues, including the Met-Xaa-Xaa-Xaa-Met motif, methionines 150 and 154, are important to the ability of CTR1 to import Cu (10). CTR1 exists as an integral membrane trimer forming a pore that allows the transport of Cu (11, 12). The CxxxG (G4) motif in the third transmembrane domain (12) and the cysteine189 in the C terminal cytosolic domain are thought to mediate the oligomerization and stability of CTR1 respectively. (13). Figure 1 shows a schematic representation of the membrane topology of a CTR1 trimer. Like ATP7A and ATP7B, CTR1 has a large effect on the cellular pharmacology of the Pt-containing drugs (1).

Effects of Loss of CTR1 on the Regulation of Cellular Pharmacology of DDP, CBDCA, L-OHP

Studies performed in yeast, mouse and human cells demonstrate that CTR1 regulates sensitivity to DDP, CBDCA and L-OHP by controlling the influx of these drugs (14, 15). Knockout of CTR1 in yeast deficient other Cu transporters markedly reduced DDP uptake (15, 16). Accumulation of all three drugs was reduced by ~65% when embryonic fibroblasts derived from mice, in which both alleles of the gene coding for CTR1 had been knocked out, were exposed to a concentration of 2 μM of each drug for 1 h (17). In the case of DDP and CBDCA this reduction in uptake was associated with reduced sensitivity of knockout cells to the cytotoxic effect of the drug producing resistance factors of 3.2 for DDP and 2.0 for CBDCA in an assay utilizing a 72 h exposure. Loss of CTR1 had a smaller effect on sensitivity to L-OHP, producing a resistance factor of only 1.7 in this assay. When exposed to 10 μM for 1 h, the uptake of DDP and CBDCA was still reduced in the knockout cells but that of L-OHP did not suggest that L-OHP may have additional transporters that become dominant at higher drug concentrations.

Our group has examined the effect of over-expressing CTR1 on the cellular pharmacology of DDP. Ovarian carcinoma A2780 cells were stably transfected with a full length human CTR1 (hCTR1). As expected, over-expression of hCTR1 resulted in a 6.5-fold increase in the basal level of Cu in A2780 cells and enhanced their ability to accumulate ^{64}Cu when measured at various time points between 5 min and 24 h. The hCTR1-overexpressing A2780 cells accumulated substantially higher levels of DDP than controls after just an incubation involving 5 min with 2 μM DDP. Interestingly, the over-expression of hCTR1 in the A2780 cells had only a very small effect on the sensitivity of cells to Cu or DDP, suggesting that, when forcibly over-expressed, CTR1 misdirected both molecules within the cell (14).

DDP- and Cu-Induced Down Regulation of CTR1

Studies in the mouse fibroblasts (18) and human A2780 (19) and 2008 (20) ovarian carcinoma cells with digital deconvolution microscopy and western blot analysis using antibodies directed at both ends of the hCTR1 molecule, have demonstrated that exposure to clinically relevant levels of DDP (0.5–2 μM) causes down regulation of CTR1. This somewhat remarkable discovery indicates that DDP down-regulates its own major influx transporter – an observation that has important clinical implications for the use of this drug. Cu also produced this effect but only at much higher concentrations (100–300 μM) (19, 21, 22). Further studies showed that DDP-induced down regulation of CTR1 occurred very rapidly and was detectable in cell lines after just 1 min of drug exposure, and was complete by ~15 min. These studies also showed that endocytosis of CTR1 was required for the DDP- and Cu-induced down regulation of

CTR1; the endocytosis inhibitors amilioride and cytochalasin D were found to abolish the DDP- and Cu-induced down regulation of CTR1 in 2008 cells (20).

Down Regulation of CTR1 Requires Proteosomal Activity

Further studies of the mechanism by which CTR1 is degraded, documented that it was not just plasma membrane CTR1 that was disappearing but all of the detectable CTR1 — much of which was located in intracellular membranous structures (17). DDP-induced down regulation of CTR1 was shown to be mediated primarily by proteosomal rather than lysosomal digestion. The DDP-induced down-regulation of CTR1 was blocked by pre-treatment of ovarian carcinoma 2008 cells with the proteosome inhibitors lactacystin, proteosome inhibitor 1 and MG132. Western blot analysis and confocal fluorescent microscopy showed that the CTR1 has a relatively high turn over rate as indicated by rapid reappearance of CTR1 following the removal of DDP from the culture medium. The levels of hCTR1 had returned to their normal levels in 2008 cells by 30 min following the removal of DDP (17). A recent study in yeast has demonstrated that yCTR1 becomes ubiquintylated upon exposure to Cu (23); no data on ubiquintylation is yet available for hCTR1.

Conclusions

Presently available data indicates that CTR1 mediates influx of three of the most commonly used Pt-containing drugs when they are present at clinically relevant concentrations. The specificity of CTR1 for the transport of Cu is very high; it does not transport other common metal ions nor even Cu(II) (10). A study of the membrane structure of the CTR1 trimer suggests that the pore through which Cu(I) might pass is only 9 Å wide. Thus, the much larger Pt-containing drugs are unlikely to enter cells via this pore. Indeed, evidence from the study of human ovarian carcinoma and mouse fibroblast cells suggests that CTR1-mediated uptake of DDP, CBDCA and L-OHP occurs via endocytosis. This has recently been corroborated by an elegant analysis of fluorescence energy transfer (FRET) between yeast CTR1 monomers engineered to contain ECFP or EYFP domains (24). This study showed that Cu triggered a closer association between two CTR1 monomers whereas DDP did not. A mutant CTR1 defective in Cu transport retained the ability to mediate the uptake of DDP. Thus, while Cu and the Pt-containing drugs both utilize CTR1 for cell entry, the mechanism of transport appears to be quite different. The same protein functions to bring different metalloids into cells through both its ability to form a pore and its ability to undergo metalloid-induced endocytosis. It will be of interest to investigate the extent to which CTR1 serves as a sensor of toxic metalloids via their ability to trigger the endocytotic and degradative processes.

Acknowledgements This work was supported by the NIH grant CA 095298 and a grant from the Clayton Foundation for Medical Research. The production of ^{64}Cu at Washington University School of Medicine was supported by the National Cancer Institute grant R24-CA86307.

References

1. Safaei R, Howell SB. Regulation of the cellular pharmacology and cytotoxicity of cisplatin by copper transporters. In: Beverly A, Teicher PD, eds. Cancer Drug Discovery and Development. Totowa, New Jersey: Humana Press, 2006:309–27.
2. Petris MJ. The SLC31 (Ctr) copper transporter family. Pflugers Arch 2004;447:752–5.
3. Zhou B, Gitschier J. hCTR1: a human gene for copper uptake identified by complementation in yeast. Proc Natl Acad Sci USA 1997;94:7481–6.
4. Marvin ME, Williams PH, Cashmore AM. The *Candida albicans* CTR1 gene encodes a functional copper transporter. Microbiology 2003;149:1461–74.
5. Lee J, Prohaska JR, Dagenais SL, Glover TW, Thiele DJ. Isolation of a murine copper transporter gene, tissue specific expression and functional complementation of a yeast copper transport mutant. Gene 2000;254:87–96.
6. Mackenzie NC, Brito M, Reyes AE, Allende ML. Cloning, expression pattern and essentiality of the high-affinity copper transporter 1 (ctr1) gene in zebrafish. Gene 2004;328:113–20.
7. Pena MM, Lee J, Thiele DJ. A delicate balance: homeostatic control of copper uptake and distribution. J Nutr 1999;129:1251–60.
8. Kuo YM, Zhou B, Cosco D, Gitschier J. The copper transporter CTR1 provides an essential function in mammalian embryonic development. Proc Natl Acad Sci USA 2001;98:6836–41.
9. Lee J, Prohaska JR, Thiele DJ. Essential role for mammalian copper transporter Ctr1 in copper homeostasis and embryonic development. Proc Natl Acad Sci USA 2001;98:6842–7.
10. Jiang J, Nadas IA, Kim MA, Franz KJ. A Mets motif peptide found in copper transport proteins selectively binds Cu(I) with methionine-only coordination. Inorg Chem 2005;44:9787–94.
11. Nose Y, Rees EM, Thiele DJ. Structure of the Ctr1 copper trans'PORE'ter reveals novel architecture. Trends Biochem Sci 2006;31:604–7.
12. Aller SG, Unger VM. Projection structure of the human copper transporter CTR1 at 6-A resolution reveals a compact trimer with a novel channel-like architecture. Proc Natl Acad Sci U S A 2006;103:3627–32.
13. Eisses JF, Kaplan JH. Stable plasma membrane levels of hCtr1 mediate cellular copper uptake. J Biol Chem 2005; 280:9635–39.
14. Holzer AK, Samimi G, Katano K, et al. The copper influx transporter human copper transport protein 1 regulates the uptake of cisplatin in human ovarian carcinoma cells. Mol Pharmacol 2004;66:817–23.
15. Lin X, Okuda T, Holzer A, Howell SB. The copper transporter CTR1 regulates cisplatin uptake in *saccharomyces cerevisiae*. Mol Pharmacol 2002;62:1154–9.
16. Ishida S, Lee J, Thiele DJ, Herskowitz I. Uptake of the anticancer drug cisplatin mediated by the copper transporter Ctr1 in yeast and mammals. Proc Natl Acad Sci USA 2002;99:14298–302.
17. Holzer AK, Manorek GH, Howell SB. Contribution of the major copper influx transporter CTR1 to the cellular accumulation of cisplatin, carboplatin, and oxaliplatin. Mol Pharmacol 2006;70:1390–4.
18. Safaei R, Rasmussen ML, Francisco KS, Howell SB. The copper chaperone Atox1 is involved in the intracellular sequestration of cisplatin. Proc Am Assoc Cancer Res 2007;48:1330.
19. Holzer AK, Katano K, Klomp LW, Howell SB. Cisplatin rapidly down-regulates its own influx transporter hCTR1 in cultured human ovarian carcinoma cells. Clin Cancer Res 2004;10:6744–9.

20. Holzer AK, Howell SB. The internalization and degradation of human copper transporter 1 following cisplatin exposure. Cancer Res 2006;66:10944–52.
21. Petris MJ, Smith K, Lee J, Thiele DJ. Copper-stimulated endocytosis and degradation of the human copper transporter, hCtr1. J Biol Chem 2003;278:9639–46.
22. Ooi CE, Rabinovich E, Dancis A, Bonifacino JS, Klausner RD. Copper-dependent degradation of the *Saccharomyces cerevisiae* plasma membrane copper transporter Ctr1p in the apparent absence o f endocytosis. EMBO J 1996;15:3515–23.
23. Liu J, Sitaram A, Burd CG. Regulation of copper-dependent endocytosis and vacuolar degradation of the yeast copper transporter, ctr1p, by the rsp5 ubiquitin ligase. Traffic 2007;8:1375–84.
24. Sinani D, Adle DJ, Kim H, Lee J. Distinct mechanisms for CTR1-mediated copper and cisplatin transport. J Biol Chem 2007;282:26775–85.

Regulation of the Export of Platinum-Containing Drugs by the Copper Efflux Transporters ATP7A and ATP7B

Roohangiz Safaei and Stephen B. Howell

Abstract ATP7A and ATP7B are P-type ATPases that detoxifie copper (Cu) through sequestration into the secretory pathway. While ATP7A is ubiquitously expressed, the expression of ATP7B is mainly specific to the liver tissue. These transporters are up-regulated in many types of tumors refractory, to the platinum-(Pt) containing drugs. Studies on cell lines indicate that ATP7A and ATP7B mediate sequestration and efflux of cisplatin (DDP), carboplatin (CBDCA) and oxaliplatin (L-OHP). An *in vitro* transport assay system consisting of vesicles isolated from Sf9 cells that expressed either a wild type ATP7B (WT) or a mutant form of this protein (MT) was used to determine whether ATP7B plays a direct role in the transport of DDP. While both forms of ATP7B significantly enhanced the capacity of Sf9 vesicles to bind DDP in the absence of ATP, only the WT form was capable of mediating ATP-dependent accumulation of DDP and forming a transient acylphosphate inter mediate in the presence of DDP. ATP7B-mediated transport of DDP into Sf9 vesicles was similar to that for ^{64}Cu, but had a slower rate. DDP and Cu also inhibited each other's transport into the WT-expressing vesicles. These studies demonstrated that, although less effective than Cu, DDP serves as a substrate of ATP7B.

Keywords ATP7A; ATP7B; P-type ATPase; Copper homeostasis; Cisplatin

Introduction

The efflux of Pt containing drugs is an energy-requiring process and can be modulated by a number of disparate transporters and physiological conditions (1). Recent studies have identified the copper (Cu) exporters ATP7A and ATP7B as potential

---

R. Safaei (✉) and S.B. Howell
Department of Medicine and the Moores Cancer Center,
University of California, San Diego, La Jolla, CA, USA
e-mail: rsafaei@ucsd.edu

A. Bonetti et al. (eds.), *Platinum and Other Heavy Metal Compounds in Cancer Chemotherapy*, DOI: 10.1007/978-1-60327-459-3_13,
© Humana Press, a part of Springer Science + Business Media, LLC 2009

efflux transporters of cisplatin (DDP), carboplatin (CBDCA) and oxaliplatin (L-OHP) in a variety of cell culture model systems (2). While the exact mechanism by which ATP7A and ATP7B mediate the efflux of the Pt-containing drugs remains to be determined, preliminary data is consistent with a direct role of these cuproproteins in this process.

ATP7A and ATP7B are essential constituents of the Cu homeostasis system and function in coordination with several proteins, including the Cu importer CTR1 and the metallochaperones ATOX1, CCS and COX17, to deliver Cu to various cuproproteins and detoxify the excess harmful metal (3). ATP7A and ATP7B are localized to the membranes of the trans-Golgi network (TGN). They receive Cu(I) from the metallochaperone ATOX1 and translocate it across the vesicle membrane by hydrolyzing ATP. Similar to other P-type ATPases, ATP7A and ATP7B form transient acylphosphate intermediates in the process of Cu translocation (4). ATP7A is ubiquitously expressed in almost all tissues and is required for the synthesis of secretory cuproproteins such as tyrosinase, lysine oxidase and monoamine oxidase. The absence of ATP7A expression leads to severe disturbances in Cu homeostasis as evidenced by the fact that mutations that disable its function cause Menkes disease (5). ATP7B is expressed mainly in liver, and its mutations are the cause of Wilson's disease (5). Although ATP7B and ATP7A are highly similar in structure (Fig. 1) and can complement each other's function in some cases (6, 7), each serve unique roles in Cu homeostasis (8) as evidenced by the fact that they have different enzymatic activities and subcellular trafficking patterns (9). Recent data suggests that while ATP7A participates mainly in the synthesis of cuproproteins, the role of

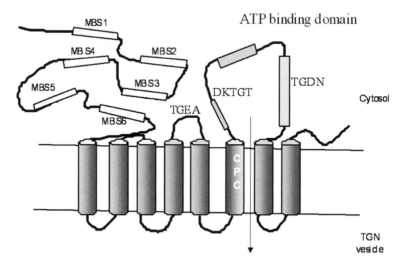

Fig. 1 Schematic drawing of the topology of ATP7A and ATP7B in the TGN. N-terminal metal binding domains are indicated by MBS1-MBS6. ATPase domain includes: TGEA, the phosphatase site; DKTGT, the phosphorylation site, with D forming the acylphosphate intermediate; and TGDN, the nucleotide binding domain

ATP7B is likely to be in the detoxification of excess Cu as well as the synthesis of holoceruloplasmin (9).

Figure 1 shows a schematic drawing of ATP7A and ATP7B structure in the TGN vesicle. These proteins interact with ATOX1 via their N-terminal domains. They receive Cu(I) from ATOX1, which they chelate to their six CxxC metal binding sequences and then transport through a pore formed by their eight transmembrane domains into the TGN utilizing the energy of the ATP hydrolysis. The conserved CPC motif in the sixth transmembrane domain is essential for translocation of Cu across the TGN membrane (4).

The increased expression of ATP7A (10–12) and ATP7B (10, 13–16) has been associated in cell culture systems with the development of resistance to DDP, CBDCA and L-OHP and an increase in intracellular sequestration or efflux of these drugs. Studies in many tumor samples have also demonstrated a correlation between the expression of ATP7B and ATP7A (12) and the outcome of therapy with Pt containing drugs (17). Together these studies have suggested that the role of ATP7A and ATP7B in the regulation of cellular pharmacology of Pt containing drugs is direct, and lies in the ability of these proteins to chelate and transport these drugs (2).

Several lines of evidence indicate that, similar to the situation for Cu, ATP7A and ATP7B have different roles in the transport of Pt-containing drugs (2). For example, while forced over-expression of ATP7B was associated with increases in the efflux of DDP (13) and CBDCA (14), the over-expression of ATP7A resulted only in increased vesicular sequestration of DDP, CBDCA, and L-OHP (10). In addition, results of studies with confocal digital microscopy also indicated distinct functions for the two proteins; it was demonstrated that DDP, like Cu, was able to stimulate trafficking of ATP7B from TGN in human ovarian carcinoma 2008 cells (15) but failed to change the TGN localization of ATP7A (10).

Analysis of the Role of ATP7B in the Transport of DDP Using ATP7B-Expressing Vesicles

The role of ATP7B in the transport of DDP was studied using vesicles isolated from Sf9 cells that were infected with baculovirus encoding, either a wild type human ATP7B (WT) or a mutant of this protein (MT), in which the sixth transmembrane CPC motif was converted into CPA (18). This mutation eliminated the ability of ATP7B to transport Cu but did not interfere with its ability to bind Cu to its N-terminal metal binding domains. Calibration of this assay system for the transport of ^{65}Cu was carried out and a pH- and ATP-dependent mode of transport was demonstrated only for the WT form of ATP7B. At pH 4.6, a K_m of 3.4 ± 0.4 (SEM) µM and a V_{max} of 0.8 ± 0.5 (SEM) nmol Cu/mg protein/min was recorded for ATP-dependent translocation of ^{64}Cu for the WT form which also showed a rapid formation of a transient acylphosphate intermediate in the presence of Cu (18).

Incubation of WT- or MT-expressing vesicles with 2-µM DDP for 10 min in the absence of ATP yielded Pt-accumulation values that were respectively 2.0 ± 0.02

(S.E.M.) – and 1.8 ± 0.01 (S.E.M.)-fold higher than the values recorded for the control vesicles that did not express any exogenous ATP7B ($p < 0.0002$ for both). Furthermore, ATP-dependent and pH-dependent transport of DDP were demonstrable only for the vesicles that expressed the WT form of the protein. The estimated K_m for ATP-dependent transport of DDP by WT-expressing vesicles at pH 4.6 was $1.2 ± 0.5$ (SEM) μM and the V_{max} was $0.03 ± 0.002$ (SEM) nmol/mg protein/min demonstrating that, like Cu, DDP was also a substrate of ATP7B. However, as indicated by the 28-fold lower V_{max} for the transport of DDP compared to Cu, DDP proved to be a much poorer substrate for this enzyme than Cu (18).

Since a hallmark of Cu transport by ATP7A and ATP7B is the formation of a transient acylphosphate intermediate in the presence of Cu and [γ-^{32}P] ATP, we sought to determine whether DDP could also stimulate the formation of this intermediate form of ATP7B. Using WT-expressing vesicles, DDP was found to induce the formation of an acylphosphate form of ATP7B but in a much slower rate than Cu indicating once again that DDP is a much poorer substrate for ATP7B than Cu (18).

Effects of Cu on the Transport of DDP and Vice Versa

Previous studies in yeast (19) and human cells (20) have demonstrated that DDP and Cu can inhibit each other's uptake and efflux. Using the WT-expressing vesicles, experiments were undertaken to determine whether Cu and DDP can influence each other's transport by ATP7B. These studies showed that DDP, even at 0.5 nM, was capable of significantly reducing ATP-dependent accumulation of 2 μM ^{64}Cu in WT-expressing Sf9 vesicles. Similarly, Cu, at concentrations as low as 100 nM inhibited ATP-dependent transport of 800 nM DDP in these vesicles, indicating that both agents reduced each other's transport (18).

Conclusions

Current data is consistent with a direct role of Cu transporters ATP7A and ATP7B in the efflux or sequestration of the three most commonly used Pt-containing drugs. Evidence is also emerging that, for Cu, the two enzymes may play different roles in the transport and intracellular sequestration of these agents. Furthermore, differences in Cu- and DDP-induced trafficking patterns, particularly in the case of ATP7A, and the inhibitory effects of these two agents on each other's transport, suggest important differences in the mechanism of transport of Cu and the Pt-containing drugs.

Acknowledgements The work reviewed in this paper was supported by the NIH grant CA78648-08 and a grant from the Clayton Medical Research Foundation. The production of ^{64}Cu at Washington University School of Medicine was supported by the National Cancer Institute grant R24-CA86307.

References

1. Hall MD, Okabe M, Shen DW, Liang XJ, Gottesman MM. The role of cellular accumulation in determining sensitivity to platinum-based chemotherapy. Annu Rev Pharmacol Toxicol 2008;48:495–535.
2. Safaei R, Howell SB. Regulation of the cellular pharmacology and cytotoxicity of cisplatin by copper transporters. In: Beverly A. Teicher PD, eds. Cancer Drug Discovery and Development. Totowa, New Jersey, US: Humana Press, 2006:309–27.
3. Pena MM, Lee J, Thiele DJ. A delicate balance: homeostatic control of copper uptake and distribution. J Nutr 1999;129:1251–60.
4. Solioz M, Vulpe C. CPx-type ATPases: a class of p-type ATPases that pump heavy metals. Trends Biochem Sci 1996;21:237–41.
5. Mercer JFB, Camakaris J. Menkes and Wilson's diseases: genetic disorders of copper transport. New York, US: Chapman and Hall, 1997.
6. Lockhart PJ, La Fontaine S, Firth SD, Greenough M, Camakaris J, Mercer JF. Correction of the copper transport defect of Menkes patient fibroblasts by expression of two forms of the sheep Wilson ATPase. Biochim Biophys Acta 2002;1588:189–94.
7. Barnes N, Tsivkovskii R, Tsivkovskaia N, Lutsenko S. The copper-transporting ATPases, Menkes and Wilson disease proteins, have distinct roles in adult and developing cerebellum. J Biol Chem 2005;280:9640–5.
8. Niciu MJ, Ma XM, El Meskini R, Pachter JS, Mains RE, Eipper BA. Altered ATP7A expression and other compensatory responses in a murine model of Menkes disease. Neurobiol Dis 2007;27:278–91.
9. Linz R, Barnes NL, Zimnicka AM, Kaplan JH, Eipper B, Lutsenko S. The intracellular targeting of copper-transporting ATPase ATP7a in a normal and ATP7$^{b–/–}$ kidney. Am J Physiol Renal Physiol 2007;294:F53–61.
10. Samimi G, Katano K, Holzer AK, Safaei R, Howell SB. Modulation of the cellular pharmacology of cisplatin and its analogs by the copper exporters ATP7A and ATP7B. Mol Pharmacol 2004; 66:25–32.
11. Samimi G, Safaei R, Katano K, et al. Increased expression of the copper efflux transporter ATP7A mediates resistance to cisplatin, carboplatin and oxaliplatin in ovarian cancer cells. Clin Cancer Res 2004;10:4661–9.
12. Samimi G, Varki NM, Wilczynski S, Safaei R, Alberts DS, Howell SB. Increase in expression of the copper transporter ATP7A during platinum drug-based treatment is associated with poor survival in ovarian cancer patients. Clin Cancer Res 2003;9:5853–9.
13. Komatsu M, Sumizawa T, Mutoh M, et al. Copper-transporting P-type adenosine triphosphatase (ATP7B) is associated with cisplatin resistance. Cancer Res 2000;60:1312–6.
14. Katano K, Safaei R, Samimi G, Holzer A, Rochdi M, Howell SB. The copper export pump ATP7B modulates the cellular pharmacology of carboplatin in ovarian carcinoma cells. Mol Pharmacol 2003;64:466–73.
15. Katano K, Safaei R, Samimi G, et al. Confocal microscopic analysis of the interaction between cisplatin and the copper transporter ATP7B in human ovarian carcinoma cells. Clin Cancer Res 2004;10:4578–88.
16. Katano K, Kondo A, Safaei R, et al. Acquisition of resistance to cisplatin is accompanied by changes in the cellular pharmacology of copper. Cancer Res 2002;62:6559–65.
17. Safaei R. Role of copper transporters in the uptake and efflux of platinum containing drugs. Cancer Lett 2006;234:34–9.
18. Safaei R, Otani S, Larson BJ, Rasmussen ML, Howell SB. Transport of cisplatin by the copper efflux transporter ATP7B. Mol Pharmacol 2007; 73:461–8.
19. Lin X, Okuda T, Holzer A, Howell SB. The copper transporter CTR1 regulates cisplatin uptake in *Saccharomyces cerevisiae*. Mol Pharmacol 2002;62:1154–9.
20. Safaei R, Katano K, Samimi G, et al. Cross-resistance to cisplatin in cells with acquired resistance to copper. Cancer Chemother Pharmacol 2004;53:239–46.

Altered Localization of Transport Proteins Associated with Cisplatin Resistance

Ganna V. Kalayda and Ulrich Jaehde

Abstract Subcellular localization of the copper homeostasis proteins ATP7A and ATP7B, which are assumed to be involved in the intracellular transport of cisplatin, has been investigated in the A2780 human ovarian carcinoma cell line and its cisplatin-resistant variant A2780cis cell line. In the sensitive cells, both proteins are localized in the trans-Golgi network, whereas they are sequestrated in more peripherally located vesicles in the resistant cells. Changes in subcellular localization of ATP7A and ATP7B may facilitate sequestration of cisplatin in vesicular structures, which may in turn prevent drug binding to genomic DNA and thereby contribute to cisplatin resistance.

Keywords Cisplatin resistance; ATP7A; ATP7B; Sequestration

Despite the success of cisplatin-based anticancer chemotherapy, its clinical application is limited because tumors often develop resistance during the treatment (1). Acquired cisplatin resistance is a net result of several resistance mechanisms operating simultaneously in a given cell. Furthermore, resistance profiles vary significantly between different cancer cell models. Due to their complexity and versatility, tumor resistance phenomena remain a challenge for scientists despite years of intensive research in this area. Much attention in investigation of cisplatin resistance has been given to the transport of the drug, because defects in cisplatin accumulation are a frequently reported feature of the cells selected for cisplatin resistance (2). Up to now, the mechanisms mediating cellular uptake, intracellular trafficking and efflux of cisplatin are not well elucidated. In the past decade, evidence that copper homeostasis proteins are involved has been accumulating. The P-type ATPases ATP7A and ATP7B, which regulate efflux of excess copper out of the cell, have been suggested to either sequester cisplatin away from its pharmacological target,

G.V. Kalayda (✉) and U. Jaehde
Department of Clinical Pharmacy, Institute of Pharmacy, University of Bonn
Bonn, Germany
e-mail: akalayda@uni-bonn.de

A. Bonetti et al. (eds.), *Platinum and Other Heavy Metal Compounds in Cancer Chemotherapy*, DOI: 10.1007/978-1-60327-459-3_14,
© Humana Press, a part of Springer Science + Business Media, LLC 2009

the nuclear DNA, or to mediate efflux of the drug (3). Increased expression of ATP7A and ATP7B has been associated with acquired cisplatin resistance (3, 4). However, the subcellular localization of these proteins in cisplatin-resistant cells has not been investigated so far.

Previously, we studied the relevance of copper transporters for cisplatin sensitivity in the A2780 human ovarian carcinoma cell line and its cisplatin-resistant variant A2780cis cell line (5). For this purpose, the cell lines were characterized regarding cisplatin uptake and efflux, DNA platination as well as expression of ATP7A and ATP7B. Cisplatin accumulation was found to be 2.5-fold reduced in the resistant cells as compared to their sensitive counterparts, while no difference in the rate of drug efflux between the sensitive and resistant cell line was observed. Interestingly, the level of DNA platination was only 5.4-fold lower in A2780cis cells than in A2780 cells. ATP7A was found overexpressed in the resistant cells, which, however, did not result in increased cisplatin efflux. Expression of ATP7B was not significantly higher in A2780cis cells compared to the parent sensitive cell line. This matched well with the similar efflux rate in both cell lines but disagreed with the results of other groups, which linked cisplatin resistance with increased levels of ATP7B expression (3, 6). In order to resolve these contradictions, we investigated the intracellular localization of ATP7A and ATP7B in A2780 and A2780cis cells using confocal fluorescence microscopy after immunohistochemical staining. We aimed to assess possible relevance of subcellular localization of these transporters for acquired cisplatin resistance in ovarian carcinoma cells.

In A2780 cells, both ATP7A and ATP7B are localized in the perinuclear region as shown in Fig. 1. Both transporters were previously reported to localize in the trans-Golgi network in other cell lines (7, 8). Co-localization experiments using NBD-C$_6$-ceramide, a fluorescent marker for the Golgi complex, confirmed localization of the proteins in the trans-Golgi network of A2780 cells (images not shown). In contrast, in the cisplatin-resistant A2780cis cells ATP7A and ATP7B are distributed away from the trans-Golgi to more peripherally located vesicles in the cytosol (Fig. 1).

In the next step, we investigated the effect of cisplatin exposure on subcellular localization of ATP7A and ATP7B in the sensitive A2780 cells. Treatment of the cells with the drug for 1 h triggered relocalization of the proteins from the trans-Golgi network to the more peripherally located sites in the cytosol. Interestingly, perinuclear localization of both transporters was fully restored 1 h after removal of cisplatin from the culture medium (Fig. 2). Fast distribution of the proteins to the cell periphery following cisplatin exposure and their rapid relocalization back to the trans-Golgi upon drug withdrawal in the A2780 cell line suggests that cisplatin-induced trafficking of ATP7A and ATP7B may represent the way of drug efflux in these cells: cisplatin binding to the protein results in protein trafficking to (secretory) vesicles, followed by drug excretion and relocalization of the protein back to the trans-Golgi. In fact, both ATP7A and ATP7B undergo copper-regulated trafficking between the trans-Golgi network and the plasma membrane (ATP7A) or vesicles on the cell periphery (ATP7B) as a way to maintain copper homeostasis (7, 8). Cisplatin-triggered trafficking

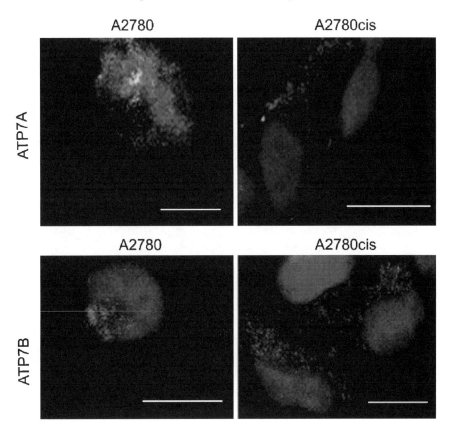

Fig. 1 Immunofluorescence localization of ATP7A and ATP7B (both *green*) in A2780 and A2780cis cells. Cell nuclei were stained with propidium iodide (*red*). Scale bar, 10 µm (*see color Plates*)

of ATP7A and ATP7B appears to be blocked in the A2780cis cell line, as the proteins are localized in peripherally located vesicular structures and not in the trans-Golgi network.

In order to investigate the role of ATP7A and ATP7B in the intracellular transport of cisplatin in A2780 and A2780cis cells, colocalization experiments using a fluorescent cisplatin analogue labeled with carboxyfluorescein-diacetate, CFDA-Pt (Fig. 3), were performed. CFDA-Pt was previously shown to be a suitable model complex for the investigation of intracellular trafficking of cisplatin. First, cellular distribution of CFDA-Pt in U2-OS human osteosarcoma cells was found to be different from that of the platinum-free fluorophore CFDA-Boc (the chemical structure is presented in Fig. 3) (9). Second, cellular accumulation of CFDA-Pt in cisplatin-resistant U2-OS/Pt osteosarcoma cells was reduced as compared to the sensitive U2-OS cells, which was in agreement with decreased cisplatin accumulation in the U2-OS/Pt cell line (10). In order to validate CFDA-Pt as a suitable model complex for cisplatin in our cell system, we compared the antitumor activity of CFDA-Pt and cisplatin against A2780 and A2780cis cells. The results are presented in Table 1. Although the cytotoxicity of the labeled complex in both cell lines was

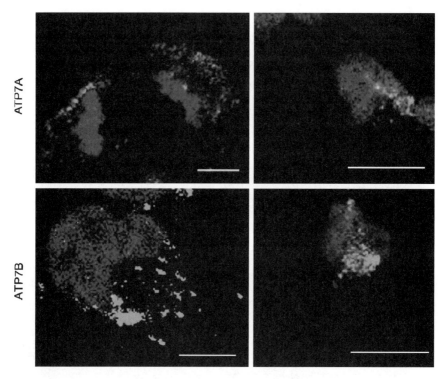

Fig. 2 Immunofluorescence localization of ATP7A and ATP7B (both *green*) in A2780 cells after cisplatin exposure for 1 h (images on the *left*) and subsequent incubation of the cells in the drug-free medium for 1 h (images on the *right*). Cell nuclei were stained with propidium iodide (*red*). Scale bar, 10 µm (*see Color Plates*)

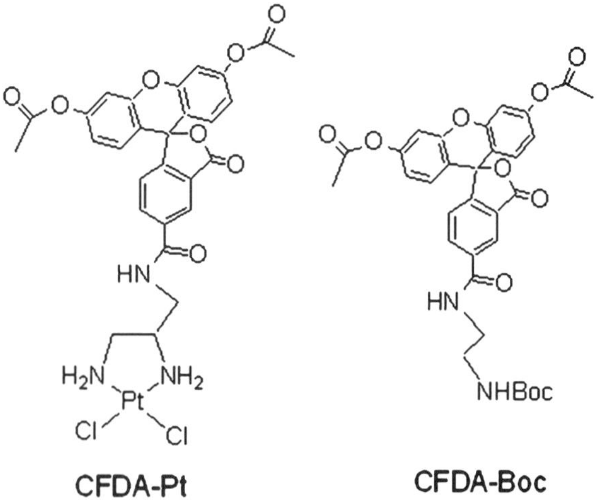

Fig. 3 Chemical structures of CFDA-Pt and the platinum-free fluorescein derivative CFDA-Boc

CFDA-Pt

CFDA-Boc

Table 1 Sensitivity of A2780 and A2780cis cells to CFDA-Pt and cisplatin. The pEC_{50} values are means ±SE of four experiments

Pt compounds	A2780		A2780cis		
	pEC_{50}	EC_{50} (µM)	pEC_{50}	EC_{50} (µM)	p
Cisplatin	5.455 ± 0.0941	3.5	4.631 ± 0.0095	23.4	<0.001
CFDA-Pt	4.445 ± 0.1524	35.9	3.856 ± 0.0711	139.3	<0.05

lower as compared to cisplatin, it retained substantial activity. CFDA-Pt was found cross-resistant with cisplatin in A2780cis cells indicating that the labeled complex is susceptible to the resistance mechanisms in this cell line. Taken together, these results suggest that CFDA-Pt represents a suitable model complex to study the intracellular trafficking of cisplatin. In A2780 cells, positive colocalization between both ATP7A and ATP7B and CFDA-Pt was observed. In the cisplatin-resistant cells, only ATP7A (and not ATP7B) colocalized with CFDA-Pt (Fig. 4).

Thus, the results presented above indicate that both ATP7A and ATP7B mediate cisplatin efflux in A2780 cells. Previous reports from the literature, however, suggested that ATP7A is involved in intracellular sequestration of the drug, whereas ATP7B indeed participates in cisplatin efflux (3, 11, 12). On the other hand, it should be noted that these studies were performed using clonal cell lines engineered to overexpress one of the ATPases, which is not the case in the A2780 cell line (11, 12). Moreover, the cell lines transfected with either ATP7A or ATP7B showed a biologically relevant degree of cisplatin resistance (11, 12) and cannot be directly compared with a drug-sensitive cell line.

In the cisplatin-resistant A2780cis cells, ATP7A appears to mediate either intracellular sequestration of cisplatin or efflux of the drug. Sequestration is more likely taking into account increased expression of the transporter in the A2780cis cell line and nonetheless similar efflux rate compared to the parent A2780 cell line (5). Given the peripheral localization of ATP7A in A2780cis cells, cisplatin may encounter this transporter immediately after it enters the cell and may get sequestrated away from its pharmacological target, nuclear DNA. This is in agreement with the previously reported results showing that cellular accumulation of cisplatin is 2.5-fold lower in the resistant cell line as compared to the sensitive cell line, whereas DNA platination is on average 5.4-fold reduced (5). Due to altered localization, ATP7B seems not to be involved in cisplatin transport. According to the previously reported data, expression of ATP7B in the resistant cell line is not significantly higher than in the sensitive cell line (5). Thus, ATP7A may dominate over ATP7B regarding cisplatin trafficking in A2780cis cells. In that way, the A2780cis cell line is similar to the clonal cell lines transfected with the ATP7A-expressing vector, in which the protein was suggested to sequester cisplatin (12).

In conclusion, the results presented here indicate that subcellular localization of transport proteins may serve as a predictive marker for the detection of clinically relevant cisplatin resistance. Early detection of resistant tumors in patients might enable individualization of the chemotherapy and thereby the achievement of the best therapeutic response.

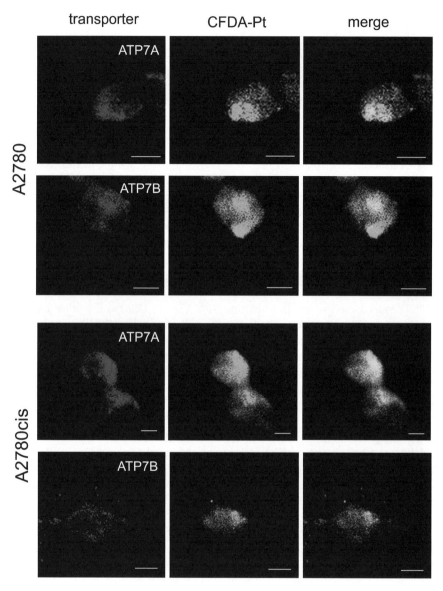

Fig. 4 Co-localization of CFDA-Pt (*green*) and fluorescent markers for ATP7A and ATP7B (both *red*) in A2780 and A2780cis cells. *Yellow*, the structure is positive for both CFDA-Pt and protein markers. Scale bar, 5 μm (*see Color Plates*)

References

1. Siddik ZH. Cisplatin: mode of cytotoxic action and molecular basis of resistance. Oncogene 2003;22:7265–79.
2. Gately DP, Howell SB. Cellular accumulation of the anticancer agent cisplatin – a review. Br J Cancer 1993;67:1171–6.

 3. Safaei R. Role of copper transporters in the uptake and efflux of platinum containing drugs. Cancer Lett 2006;234:34–9.
 4. Safaei R, Howell SB. Copper transporters regulate the cellular pharmacology and sensitivity to Pt drugs. Crit Rev Oncol Hematol 2005;53:13–23.
 5. Zisowsky J, Koegel S, Leyers S, et al. Relevance of drug uptake and efflux for cisplatin sensitivity of tumor cells. Biochem Pharmacol 2007;73:298–307.
 6. Samimi G, Katano K, Holzer AK, Safaei R, Howell SB. Modulation of the cellular pharmacology of cisplatin and its analogs by the copper exporters ATP7A and ATP7B. Mol Pharmacol 2004;66:25–32.
 7. Petris MJ, Mercer JF, Culvenor JG, Lockhart P, Gleeson PA, Camakaris J. Ligand-regulated transport of the Menkes copper P-type ATPase efflux pump from the golgi apparatus to the plasma membrane: a novel mechanism of regulated trafficking. EMBO J 1996;15:6084–95.
 8. Roelofsen H, Wolters H, Van Luyn MJ, Miura N, Kuipers F, Vonk RJ. Copper-induced apical trafficking of ATP7B in polarized hepatoma cells provides a mechanism for biliary copper excretion. Gastroenterology 2000;119:782–93.
 9. Molenaar C, Teuben JM, Heetebrij RJ, Tanke HJ, Reedijk J. New insights in the cellular processing of platinum antitumor compounds, using fluorophore-labeled platinum complexes and digital fluorescence microscopy. J Biol Inorg Chem 2000;5:655–65.
10. Kalayda GV, Zhang G, Abraham T, Tanke HJ, Reedijk J. Application of fluorescence microscopy for investigation of cellular distribution of dinuclear platinum anticancer drugs. J Med Chem 2005;48:5191–202.
11. Katano K, Safaei R, Samimi G, et al. Confocal microscopic analysis of the interaction between cisplatin and the copper transporter ATP7B in human ovarian carcinoma cells. Clin Cancer Res 2004;10:4578–88.
12. Samimi G, Safaei R, Katano K, et al. Increased expression of the copper efflux transporter ATP7A mediates resistance to cisplatin, carboplatin, and oxaliplatin in ovarian cancer cells. Clin Cancer Res 2004; 10:4661–9.

How to Overcome Cisplatin Resistance Through Proton Pump Inhibitors

Angelo De Milito, Francesca Luciani and Stefano Fais

Abstract Resistance to antitumor agents is a major cause of treatment failure in patients with cancer. Some mechanisms of tumor resistance to cytotoxic drugs may involve increased acidification of extracellular compartments. We investigated whether proton pump inhibitors (PPI), currently used in the anti-acid treatment of peptic disease, could inhibit the acidification of the tumor microenvironment and increase the sensitivity of tumor cells to cytotoxic agents.

We pretreated cell lines derived from human melanomas, adenocarcinomas, and lymphomas with the PPIs omeprazole, esomeprazole, or pantoprazole and tested their response to cytotoxic drugs in cell death assays. We also evaluated extracellular and lysosomal pH and vacuolar-ATPase (V-ATPase) expression, distribution, and activity in PPI-pretreated cells by using western immunocytochemistry and bioluminescence assays. Finally, we evaluated human melanoma and osteosarcoma growth and cisplatin sensitivity in xenografted SCID/SCID mice.

PPI pretreatment sensitized tumor cell lines to the effects of cisplatin and 5-fluorouracil, with an IC_{50} value reduction up to two logs. PPI pretreatment was associated with the inhibition of V-ATPase activity and increases in both extracellular pH and the pH of lysosomal organelles. In in vivo experiments, oral pretreatment with PPI was able to induce/increase sensitivity of human solid tumors to cisplatin.

Keywords Drug-resistance; Acidity; V-ATPase; PPI

Introduction

In classical multidrug resistance, cells exhibit resistance to a wide range of structurally and functionally unrelated compounds, including anticancer drugs such as vinca alkaloids, anthracyclines, taxoids, and other antimitotics (1, 2). The multidrug

A.D. Milito, F. Luciani and S. Fais (✉)
Department of Therapeutic Research and Medicines Evaluation, Unit of Antitumor Drugs, Drug Resistance and Experimental Therapeutic, Istituto Superiore di Sanità, Rome, Italy
e-mail: stefano.fais@iss.it

A. Bonetti et al. (eds.), *Platinum and Other Heavy Metal Compounds in Cancer Chemotherapy*, DOI: 10.1007/978-1-60327-459-3_15,
© Humana Press, a part of Springer Science + Business Media, LLC 2009

resistance (MDR) cells over-express a variety of transmembrane drug efflux pumps, belonging to the ATP binding cassette (ABC) transporters family (1). These proteins extrude against concentration gradient drug molecules from the cell to the extracellular environment and this phenomenon causes a significant decrease in intracellular drug retention. Although the increase in the expression and activity of these proteins is directly related to the in vitro generated MDR, the same relationship was not shown in the in vivo resistance of solid tumors to the various cytotoxic drugs, seriously opening severe doubts on the clinical relevance of this phenomenon (3). Another mechanism of resistance is the altered pH gradient between the extracellular environment and the cell cytoplasm and/or the pH gradient between the cell cytoplasm and lysosomal compartments observed in tumors (4). Since the mechanisms of entry of drugs into the cell are dependent on both concentration gradients and pH gradients, the reversed pH gradients of tumors may severely affect drugs entry (5). It is well known that low pH reduces the uptake of weak basic chemotherapeutic drugs and, hence, reduces their cytotoxicity preventing these weak basic drugs to reach their intracellular target (6). Agents that disrupt or normalize the pH gradient in tumors may reverse MDR and/or directly inhibit tumor growth. Lysosomotropic agents that induce pH gradient modification and alkalinization of acidic vesicles may reverse anthracycline resistance in multidrug-resistance cells (7).

Recent data suggest that vacuolar-type (V-type) H^+-ATPases, that pump protons across the plasma membrane, may have a key role in the acidification of the tumor microenvironment. Some human tumor cells are characterized by an increased V-ATPase expression and activity, and pretreatment with proton pump inhibitors – a class of H^+-ATPase inhibitors – sensitized tumor cell lines to the effects of a variety of anticancer drugs. Proton pump inhibitor pretreatment has been associated with inhibition of V-type H^+-ATPase activity and increases both in extracellular pH and pH of lysosomal organelles (10). In vivo experiments in human/mouse xenografts have shown that oral pretreatment with proton pump inhibitors is able to sensitize human solid tumors to anticancer drugs. These data suggest that tumor alkalinization may represent a key target of the future antitumor strategies.

Methods

Drugs. Omeprazole and esomeprazole (Astra-Zeneca, Sweden) sodium salts were resuspended in normal saline immediately before use. Cisplatin (Aventis) and 5-Fluorouracil (Teva Pharma) were used according to the instructions.

Cell culture. Human drug-resistant tumor cell lines, supplied by Istituto Nazionale dei Tumori, (Milan, Italy) were obtained from primary lesions. All cells were cultured in RPMI-1640 supplemented with 10% FCS and antibiotics.

Cytotoxicity Assay. The Live/Dead Viability/Cytotoxicity Assay kit (Molecular Probes, OR) was used to measure cell viability and plasma membrane integrity. The cells were run and analyzed with a FACScan cytometer. Trypan blue exclusion test was also used to assess viability.

Determination of intracellular ATP. We measured the amount of available intracellular ATP in melanoma cell lines as an indirect parameter of the activity of V-H+-ATPases. Cells were cultured for 24 h in 24-well plates at a density of 0.05×10^6 cells/well in the presence of a PPI (1 µg/mL). ATP determination was performed with an ATP Determination Kit (Molecular Probes).

Staining of acidic vesicles with a pH indicator. LysoSensor Green DND-189 (Molecular Probes) is a probe that accumulates in acidic vesicles and exhibits a pH-dependent increase in fluorescence intensity on acidification. The probe was used according to the manufacturer's indications to measure the effects of omeprazole treatment on acidic vesicles. Briefly, 5×10^5 MelM6 cells were collected after 24 h omeprazole treatment (1 µg/mL) and washed twice in PBS. Cells were then incubated for 5 min at 37°C with 500 µL previously warmed PBS containing 1 µM LysoSensor probe and analyzed by flow cytometry collecting FL1 fluorescence.

In vivo tumor growth analysis. CB.17 SCID/SCID female mice (Harlan, Italy) were used at 4–5 weeks of age and were kept under specific pathogen-free conditions. Each mouse was injected subcutaneously in the right flank with 3×10^6 human melanoma and osteosarcoma cells. Once tumors became evident, PPI (omeprazole or esomeprazole) were orally administered, by gavage, at a dose of 75 mg/kg. Cisplatin was administered by intraperitoneal injection at a dose of 5 mg/kg. Tumor weight was estimated with the formula: Tumor weight (mg) = length (mm) × width^2 (mm)/2.

Results

Effect of PPI Pretreatment on Drug-Resistant Human Tumor Cells

We examined whether PPI could reverse intrinsic resistance of human tumor cells to cytotoxic drugs. We treated human tumor cell lines of different histologies with cisplatin, 5-FU and vinblastine after a 24-h pretreatment with PPI. The results showed that PPI-pretreatment reverted the resistance of all cell lines tested to chemotherapeutics (Fig. 1). A fact to note is that PPI did not induce any change in the responsiveness of the same cells to drugs when administered simultaneously with the anti-cancer drug (not shown).

Effects of Omeprazole on Human Tumor Cells

PPI pretreatment was effective in rendering human tumor cells sensitive to the effects of basic anti-cancer drugs. We next measured the pH of the medium of human tumor cells whether treated or not with PPI and found that PPI induced an

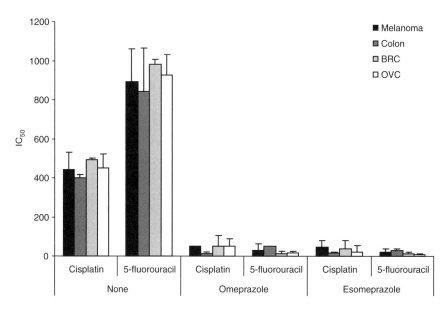

Fig. 1 The dose of cisplatin (μM) and 5-FU (μg/mL) inducing cell death in 50% of cells is shown for all tumor cells pretreated or not with PPI

increase of medium pH of 0.20 units (not shown). Consistent with inhibition of V-ATPase activity, PPI caused an increase in lysosomal pH observed by FACS and an increase in intracellular content of ATP (not shown).

PPI Effects on Sensitivity of Human Tumors to Cisplatin In vivo

To assess the potential clinical relevance of the in vitro results, we performed in vivo experiments in a xenograft model of tumor growth represented by SCID mice injected subcutaneously with human melanoma or osteosarcoma cells (MelM6 and SaOS2). Mice engrafted with human tumor cells were pretreated in groups of ten with PPI administered by gavage; 24h later they were injected intraperitoneally with cisplatin. PPI-pretreatment induced sensitization of melanoma cells to cisplatin and increased the sensitivity of osteosarcoma cells to cisplatin (Fig. 2).

Discussion

Despite major efforts of the scientific community in finding efficacious treatments for cancer, human tumors responsive to chemotherapy did not change in the last three decades (e.g., lymphomas, leukemias and some pediatric tumors), while

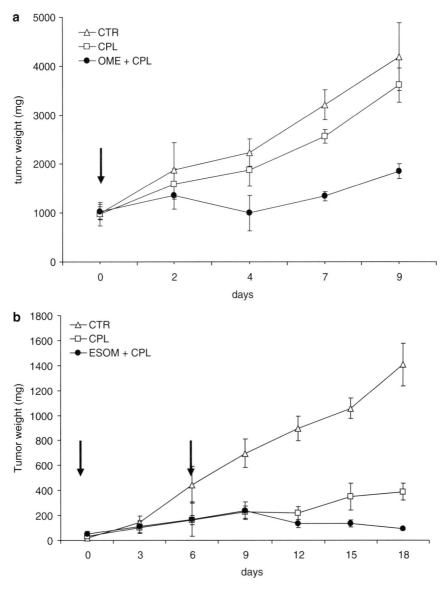

Fig. 2 The effect of PPI pretreatment on cisplatin sensitivity of melanoma (**a**) and osteosarcoma (**b**) cells is shown. The *arrows* indicate the time of treatment

others such melanomas and many carcinomas have remained unresponsive or poorly responsive. After the failure of many alternative approaches, the issue of resistance or refractoriness to chemotherapeutics has become a key problem in therapy of tumor patients. Tumor acidity being a major mechanism of tumor resistance to drugs, we tried to circumvent the problem by targeting mechanisms of pH regulation of tumor cells. To this end, we identify PPI as drugs able to "normalize" the pHi and pHe of human tumors, thus rendering tumor cells sensitive to the action of several cytotoxic drugs to which they are normally refractory. PPI are also able to increase the effect of anti-tumor drugs in sensitive cells, suggesting that PPI pretreatment may be useful in increasing the efficacy of antitumor drugs even in drug-sensitive tumors. We believe that studies aimed at investigating the major mechanisms involved in tumor acidification will provide new and useful tools in allowing an extensive, more effective and hopefully less toxic use of cytotoxic drugs. Moreover, new insights in the mechanism of tumor acidification may also provide new strategies in the treatment of human tumors based on the inhibition of their ability to live in acidic condition (8, 9).

References

1. Gottesman MM, Pastan I. Biochemistry of multidrug resistance mediated by the multidrug transporter. Annu Rev Biochem 1993;62:385–427.
2. Raghunand N, Altbach MI, Van Sluis R, et al. Plasmalemmal pH gradients in drug-sensitive and drug-resistant MCF-7 human breast carcinoma xenografts measured by 31P MR spectroscopy. Biochem Pharmacol 1999;57:309–12.
3. Leonard GD, Fojo T, Bates SE. The role of ABC transporters in clinical practice. Oncologist 2003; 8:411–24.
4. Mahoney BP, Raghunand N, Baggett B, Gillies RJ. Tumor acidity, ion trapping and chemotherapeutics. I. Acid pH affects the distribution of chemotherapeutic agents in vitro. Biochem Pharmacol 2003;66:1207–18.
5. De Milito A, Fais S. Tumor acidity, chemoresistance and proton pump inhibitors. Fut Oncol 2005;1:779–86.
6. Raghunand N, He X, van Sluis R, et al. Enhancement of chemotherapy by manipulation of tumor pH. Br J Cancer 1999;80:1005–11.
7. Ouar Z, Bens M, Vignes C, et al. Inhibitors of vacuolar H+-ATPase impair the preferential accumulation of daunomycin in lysosomes and reverse the resistance to anthracyclines in drug-resistant renal epithelial cells. Biochem J 2003;370:185–93.
8. Fais S, De Milito A, You H, Qin W. Targeting vacuolar H+-ATPases as a new strategy against cancer. Cancer Res 2007;67:10627–30.
9. Iessi E, Marino ML, Lozupone F, et al. Tumor acidity and malignancy: novel aspects in the design of anti-tumor therapy. Cancer Ther 2008;6:55–66.
10. Luciani F, Spada M, De Milito A, et al. Effect of proton pump inhibitor pretreatment on resistance of solid tumors to cytotoxic drugs. J Natl Canc Inst 2004;96:1702–13.

Cellular Resistance to Oxaliplatin and Drug Accumulation Defects

Laura Gatti and Paola Perego

Abstract Platinum drugs are employed in a wide range of solid tumors, and represent the mainstay of the first-line therapy of ovarian carcinoma. Although cisplatin has shown efficacy in the treatment of different types of tumors including ovarian carcinoma, resistance to treatment is a major limitation. At present, one of the most clinically relevant cisplatin analogues is the mononuclear compound oxaliplatin, which has shown activity and a favorable pharmacological profile in clinical therapy. In cellular models, oxaliplatin exhibits activity in some cell lines with acquired resistance to cisplatin, whereas in other models cross-resistance with cisplatin is observed. In general, oxaliplatin and cisplatin exhibit different pattern of cytotoxicity, indicating differences in drug-DNA interaction and/or cellular response or detoxification. Thus, differences in the influx or efflux mechanisms for these drugs could contribute to their unique patterns of clinical activity and at least in part to sensitivity profiles. Impaired drug accumulation has been recognized over the years as a frequent feature of cells resistant to cisplatin and more recently as an alteration of oxaliplatin-resistant models. The present chapter reviews recent studies on the molecular alterations of cells resistant to oxaliplatin, with particular reference to accumulation defects and will revisit recent literature in an attempt to describe a tentative picture of why resistant cells may display impaired accumulation.

Keywords Cisplatin; Cross-resistance; Cytotoxicity; Oxaliplatin

Introduction

Reasons for the clinical failure of chemotherapy are multiple and, although resistance of tumor cells represents a crucial determinant of the variable efficacy of antitumor therapy based on platinum drugs, additional factors such as tumor micro-environment

L. Gatti and P. Perego (✉)
Fondazione IRCCS Istituto Nazionale Tumori, Department of Experimental Oncology and Laboratories, Preclinical Chemotherapy and Pharmacology Unit, Milan, Italy
e-mail: paola.perego@istitutotumori.mi.it

A. Bonetti et al. (eds.), *Platinum and Other Heavy Metal Compounds in Cancer Chemotherapy*, DOI: 10.1007/978-1-60327-459-3_16, © Humana Press, a part of Springer Science + Business Media, LLC 2009

Table 1 Putative determinants of the variable efficacy of antitumor therapy

Players		Refs
Tumor cells	Genetic and epigenetic changes	(1)
Tumor-microenvironment interaction	Hypoxia, microvesicles	(3)
Drug characteristics	Pharmacokinetics	(1)
Patient features	Single nucleotide polymorphisms	(4)

interactions (e.g., hypoxia, microvesicles release), characteristics of the drug used for the treatment (e.g., pharmacokinetics) and specific features of the patients (i.e., genetic polymorphisms affecting drug effects) are likely to play a critical role (Table 1) (1). In fact hypoxia, that is known to induce radio-resistance, has been implicated also in chemoresistance through HIF1-mediated transcriptional activation of survival pathways (2). Sequestration of drugs in intracellular organelles and extrusion from the cells through the secretory pathway has been linked to chemoresistance and, in this context, microvesicle release could also contribute to the limited efficacy of chemotherapy (3).

Pharmacokinetics is another aspect that could contribute to the variable efficacy of antitumor treatment. In principle, as for all cytotoxic agents, inadequate intratumor concentration of platinum drugs could explain at least in part the "pharmacological" resistance to treatment, because the fraction of cells that will be reached by the drug is dependent on the total drug exposure. Several metabolism aspects will influence the drug effects i.e., conversion of pro-drugs into active metabolite, renal clearance, hepatic metabolism and tumor vascularization. Such issues have been quite widely explored for the clinically available platinum compounds, but it is conceivable that an analysis of the genetic variance among patients could provide insights to clarify the significance of specific aspects in cellular metabolism.

Due to the poor therapeutic index of antitumor drugs including Pt compounds, large variance between individuals is observed in both tumor response and toxicity after treatment (4, 5). Thus, the genetic variants associated with different responses and toxicities need to be established through genome-wide approaches as well through hypothesis-driven mechanistic studies. In this context, also a better characterization of experimental models in terms of single nucleotide polymorphisms that are likely to affect cell response to the drug could provide the rational basis for optimizing treatment and overcoming resistance.

The cellular alterations contributing to resistance to platinum compounds have been studied for several years but, in spite of the large efforts, they have not been conclusively defined. In the eighties, major attention has been paid to the study of mechanisms of drug accumulation of platinum drugs, probably because at that time the discovery of the role of *P*-glycoprotein (ABCB1, MDR1) in the multi-drug resistant phenotype (that however, does not involve cisplatin) lead to the idea that increased efflux and decreased accumulation were major components of the defense pathways activated by tumor cells to limit damage.

Studies of such a kind have been restricted at least for platinum compounds by difficulties in detection of Pt due to the poor availability of sensitive techniques and by the limited synthesis of radiolabeled cisplatin containing ^{195}Pt, characterized by a quite brief half-life. The advent of more sensitive analytical methods such as inductively coupled plasma-mass spectrometry has allowed researchers to address the role of accumulation defects in the cisplatin-resistant phenotype of tumor cells better.

This chapter will focus on recent studies about the molecular alterations of cells resistant to oxaliplatin, with particular reference to accumulation defects and will revisit recent literature in an attempt to describe a picture of why resistant cells may display impaired influx or efflux.

Cellular Resistance to Oxaliplatin
as a Multifactorial Phenomenon

Drug resistance can be regarded as a multifactorial phenomenon involving several alterations. Thus, at a cellular level, we can recognize and classify at least three major groups of alterations implicated in platinum drug resistance regarding (a) defense factors which prevent the interaction of the drug with the cellular target, (b) drug-target interaction and (c) cell response to DNA damage (Fig. 1). The first group includes influx and efflux transporters as well as factors that prevent the active form of the drug from reaching the target DNA. Indeed, cisplatin, by virtue of its electrophylic nature, can be detoxified by conjugation with glutathione through the action of glutathione-S-transferase.

Although cisplatin has been employed in the treatment of different types of tumors including ovarian carcinoma, its efficacy may be limited as a consequence of cellular resistance which is a major limitation. In an attempt to overcome resistance mechanisms, large efforts have been made over the years to generate compounds with a different mode of DNA interaction as compared with cisplatin and carboplatin. Such work has led also to the synthesis of multinuclear platinum complexes that are still an active area of research (6, 7). However, at present, the most clinically relevant cisplatin analogue appears to be the mononuclear compound oxaliplatin, which has been developed based on its activity in colorectal cancer and, more recently, has also shown activity and a favorable pharmacological profile in epithelial ovarian cancer (8, 9). The interest in understanding the cellular pharmacology of oxaliplatin has grown based on the clinical relevance of the drug, approved for clinical use in advanced colorectal cancer in 1999 in Europe and in 2004 in USA. In preclinical studies, oxaliplatin has shown activity in cell lines with acquired resistance to cisplatin and in inherently cisplatin-resistant colon cancer cell lines (10). Indeed, the differential sensitivity profile of cisplatin and oxaliplatin has been documented in a number of cisplatin-resistant models (11). In general, oxaliplatin has shown the capability to bypass cisplatin resistance in spite of the lower cytotoxic potency. This feature can be at least in part due to the fact that oxaliplatin produces fewer DNA adducts than cisplatin (12). In addition, oxaliplatin can overcome resistance to cisplatin associated with loss of DNA mismatch repair,

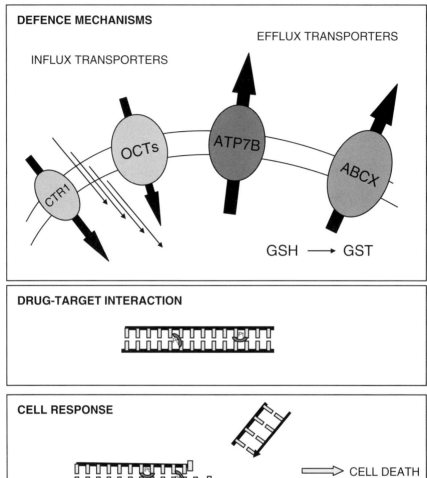

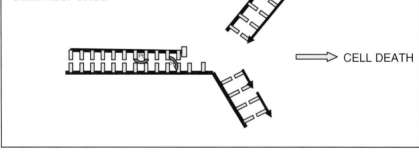

Fig. 1 Major alterations associated with cellular resistance to platinum compounds. The three groups of alterations are indicated. In the *top* group, *thin arrows* refer to passive diffusion. In the *middle* and *bottom* group, the interaction of the Pt compound with DNA is shown

a phenomenon documented by the work of different groups in several cell systems, including isogenic cell lines deficient and proficient in specific DNA mismatch repair proteins (13–16). In cellular models, oxaliplatin exhibits activity in some cisplatin-resistant cell lines with acquired resistance, whereas in other models cross-resistance with cisplatin is observed (11). In general, oxaliplatin and cisplatin exhibit different pattern of cytotoxicity indicating differences in drug-DNA interaction and/or cellular response or detoxification (12).

Cross-Resistance Between Cisplatin and Oxaliplatin and Cellular Accumulation

The mechanism of accumulation of platinum drugs may contribute to the pattern of cytotoxicity of cisplatin and oxaliplatin. Influx and efflux of the drug can in fact regulate drug accessibility to its cellular target. Impaired drug accumulation is a frequent feature of cells with acquired resistance to platinum drugs. In fact, cells with acquired resistance to cisplatin often display reduced drug accumulation that has been linked to altered expression of genes controlling copper metabolism such as the copper transporter gene 1 (CTR1) and the ATPases ATP7A and ATP7B (17–21).

Members of the ATP binding cassette (ABC) family of transporters have been implicated in accumulation defects found in cisplatin-resistant cells. Thus, resistance to cisplatin appears at least in part related to alterations at the level of both influx transporters and efflux transporters, including transporters that are ATP-dependent (i.e., ABC family) or ATP-independent (i.e., CTR1).

The precise role of such factors in resistance to oxaliplatin is less known. Holzer et al. (22) have suggested that oxaliplatin accumulation is regulated by CTR1 when cells are exposed to low concentrations ($2\,\mu M$), but not to higher concentrations. Therefore, oxaliplatin appears less dependent on CTR1 than cisplatin and carboplatin. In addition, although it has been established that cisplatin is a substrate for ATP7B, at the moment there is no evidence of transport of oxaliplatin by this ATPase. We have recently found that selected ABC transporters (i.e., ABCC1 and ABCC4) display increased levels in ovarian carcinoma cells exhibiting acquired resistance to oxaliplatin (23). Thus, it is conceivable that cisplatin and oxaliplatin share some of the influx/efflux transporters, but the molecular determinants of uptake and efflux are only in part overlapping. Indeed, several evidences have shown that cisplatin can enter the cells through passive and facilitated diffusion (24). According to this concept, platinum drugs exhibiting increased lipophilicity are expected to accumulate in the cells better than cisplatin. Indeed, platinum drug accumulation has been shown to be dependent on the physico-chemical features of the drug in the cisplatin-resistant squamous cell carcinoma subline A431/Pt, in which Pt accumulation after exposure to cisplatin, oxaliplatin or satraplatin appears correlated with drug hydrophobicity, the most lipophilic compound (satraplatin) displaying the most marked accumulation (25). In this model, oxaliplatin, endowed with intermediate hydrophobicity as compared with cisplatin and satraplatin, is capable of overcoming cisplatin resistance and to bypass the accumulation defect observed for cisplatin. Such results support the prevalent occurrence of a passive diffusion mechanism of accumulation in resistant cells and suggest that changes in the physical state of membrane lipids could participate in drug resistance as shown in cells selected for resistance to cisplatin (26).

ABC Transporters and the Platinum
Drug-Resistant Phenotype

Some lines of evidence support the involvement of specific ABC transporters in resistance to platinum drugs. Whole genome approaches have documented the existence of a wide family of ABC transporters including 50 different members that can be grouped into seven distinct classes (A-G) based on sequence similarities (27). Among them, the best known transporters mediating multidrug resistance phenotypes are ABCB1, the Multidrug resistance related proteins MRPs (ABCC1-13) and BCRP (ABCG2). Whereas it has been clearly established that ABCB1 and ABCG2 do not confer resistance to platinum compounds, selected members of the MRP family have been implicated in resistance to cisplatin.

Some components of the MRP subfamily, which include 13 members, have an established role in transporting multiple drugs, particularly glutathione (GSH)-conjugated derivatives of toxic compounds so that some members have been defined as "GS-X pumps" (28). Increased expression of MRPs may play a role in the development of drug resistance, as selected MRP transporters are induced by cytotoxic drugs (29, 30). MRPs are organic anion pumps that transport anionic drugs (i.e., methotrexate) and neutral drugs conjugated to acidic ligands, such as GSH, glucuronate, or sulfate, and in such features differ from ABCB1 which has a low affinity for such negatively charged compounds. However, ABCC1, ABCC2 and ABCC3 can also cause resistance to neutral organic drugs that are not known to be conjugated to acidic ligands by transporting these drugs together with free GSH (31).

Taken together, the available evidences do not support a precise involvement of MRPs in cisplatin resistance (32). In fact ABCC1 levels have been shown to be increased in some cisplatin-resistant sublines, but transfection of ABCC1 cDNA does not result in cisplatin resistance (33). Also, Mrp1 knock out mice are not hypersensitive to cisplatin (34). Thus, it appears that ABCC1 per se cannot confer resistance to cisplatin and this phenomenon is expected to be reproduced also in oxaliplatin-resistant cells in which we recently found increased levels of ABCC1 (23). In this context, GSH seems to be a crucial player and increased synthesis as well as conjugation to the platinum drug would be required to obtain resistance. In addition, the cisplatin-sensitive phenotype of cells transfected with ABCC1 cDNA may be due to incorrect localization of the transporter, whereas knocking out of Mrp1 in mice may produce compensatory changes in the levels of other transporters of the ABC family, thus giving a "dirty" phenotype. In fact, it has been recently shown that knocking out ABCC4 results in the up-regulation of ABCG2 in specific organs (35).

Also increased expression of ABCC2 has been related to cellular resistance to platinum drugs as a result of enhanced efflux of the glutathione-drug conjugates (32, 36, 37). A relationship between ABCC2 expression and cisplatin resistance has been documented in model systems using hammerhead ribozymes and in tumor specimens, suggesting that ABCC2 may be relevant for clinical resistance to cisplatin treatment (36, 38).

In general, altered levels of ABC transporters have been associated with reduced drug accumulation, a major feature of cellular resistance to platinum compounds (20, 39), whereas increased efflux has not always been proved. In this regard, drug sequestration in endocellular vesicles may play a role in cells in which mislocalization of ABCC1 has been implicated in reducing the uptake of cisplatin (40). Thus, although approaches of loss and gain of function have been undertaken to prove the contribution of ABC transporters to accumulation of Pt drugs, a clear correlation between anyone of the studied transporters and cellular pharmacokinetics of platinum drugs as well as sensitivity to such compounds remains to be established.

Role for Organic Cation Transporters (OCTs) as Determinants of Response to Oxaliplatin

Since the OCTs are known to mediate the cellular uptake of a broad range of structurally different organic cations with molecular weight lower than 400 Da, mononuclear platinum compounds are putative substrates. OCTs are involved in the absorption, distribution and elimination of endogenous compounds and of drugs that are positively charged at the physiological pH (41). Three human genes have been described, but although they could act as influx transporters, their specific role in relation to resistance to Pt drugs still needs to be addressed. In fact, on one hand OCTs have been recently proposed as exclusive determinants of oxaliplatin accumulation and cytotoxicity (42) – and in this perspective cisplatin should not be a substrate – whereas, on the other hand, studies in isolated human proximal tubules support that, in that experimental model, the uptake of cisplatin by renal proximal tubules is mediated by OCT2, thereby providing an interpretation of drug-induced nephrotoxicity (43).

Conclusion

Several studies have addressed the mechanisms of influx, efflux and accumulation of platinum compounds. Such studies have led to a model described by Gately and Howell (24) in the nineties, which was consistent with the concept that the accumulation of platinum drugs follows a facilitated diffusion mechanism in which the entrance of the drug into the cells occurs through diffusion as well as through a channel. After more than a decade, that model can still be considered valid because strong evidences that cisplatin influx undergoes saturation or competition by structural analogs are lacking.

Evidences relating ABC transporters to platinum drug accumulation are available, but multiple aspects are still unclear (Fig. 2). In this regard, a difficult point is the fact the ABC transporters are supposed to efflux the adduct between the drug and

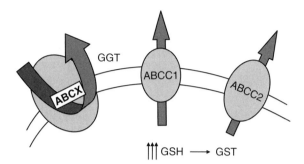

Fig. 2 ATP binding cassette transporters and resistance to Pt compounds. The major transporters that have been described as being associated with resistance to Pt compounds are shown together with enzymes of glutathione metabolism which could participated in cellular defense from Pt compounds. GST, glutathione-*S*-transferase; GGT, γ-glutamyl transferase

GSH and conjugation of GSH to platinum compounds may require some time to be formed. This aspect cannot fit with the observation of a quite early reduced accumulation in resistant cells exposed to Pt compounds. According to the model of action proposed for ABCB1 and ABCG2, ABC transporters should act very rapidly by removing toxins from the lipid bi-layer of the plasma membrane. Thus, apparently there would be no chance for platinum drugs to interact with GSH in the cell and be pumped out. However, it has been suggested that cisplatin and GSH can form adducts in the extracellular medium (44), thus providing a possible explanation for the observed accumulation defects.

In spite of the intensive efforts of scientists, several questions remain to be answered. In this context, the major goals of the future will be to understand how general some mechanisms described in specific cell systems are and to define the clinical relevance of the alterations described at a cellular level. In particular, the design of large prospective clinical trials will be required in an attempt to correlate levels of specific molecular markers in tumor samples at diagnosis with the subsequent outcome/response to treatment.

References

1. Agarwal R, Kaye SB. Ovarian cancer: strategies for overcoming resistance to chemotherapy. Nat Rev Cancer 2003;3:502–16.
2. Trédan P, Galmarini CM, Patel K, Tannock IF. Drug resistance and the solid tumor microenvironment. J Natl Cancer Inst 2007;99:1441–54.
3. Altan N, Chen Y, Schindler M, Simon SM. Defective acidification in human breast tumor cells and implications for chemotherapy. J Exp Med 1998;187:1583–98.
4. Huang RS, Duan S, Shukla SJ, et al. Identification of genetic variants contributing to cisplatin-induced cytotoxicity by use of a genomewide approach. Am J Hum Genet 2007;81:427–37.
5. Huang RS, Kistner EO, Bleibel WK, Shukla SJ, Dolan ME. Effect of population and gender on chemotherapeutic agent-induced cytotoxicity. Mol Cancer Ther 2007;6:31–6.

6. Hitt E. New platinum compound show promise. Lancet Oncol 2006;7:111.
7. Williams JW, Qu Y, Bulluss GH, Alvorado E, Farrell NP. Dinuclear platinum complexes with biological relevance based on the 1,2-diaminocyclohexane carrier ligand. Inorg Chem 2007; 46:5820–2.
8. Raymond E, Faivre S, Chaney S, Woynarowski J, Cvitkovic E. Cellular and molecular pharmacology of oxaliplatin. Mol Cancer Ther 2002;1:227–35.
9. Fu S, Kavanagh JJ, Hu W, Bast Jr RC. Clinical application of oxaliplatin in epithelial ovarian cancer. Int J Gynecol Cancer 2006; 6:1717–32.
10. Raymond E, Chaney SG, Taamma A, Cvitkovic E. Oxaliplatin: a review of preclinical and clinical studies. Ann Oncol 1998;9:1053–71.
11. Manic S, Gatti L, Carenini N, Fumagalli G, Zunino F, Perego P. Mechanisms controlling sensitivity to platinum complexes: role of p53 and DNA mismatch repair. Curr Cancer Drug Targets 2003; 3:21–9.
12. Woynarowski JM, Faivre S, Herzig MC, et al. Oxaliplatin-induced damage of cellular DNA. Mol Pharmacol 2000;58:920–7.
13. Aebi S, Kurdi-Haidar B, Gordon R, et al. Loss of DNA mismatch repair in acquired resistance to cisplatin. Cancer Res 1996;56:3087–90.
14. Vaisman A, Varchenko M, Umar A, et al. The role of hMLH1, hMSH3, and hMSH6 defects in cisplatin and oxaliplatin resistance: correlation with replicative bypass of platinum-DNA adducts. Cancer Res 1998;58:3579–85.
15. Perego P, Caserini C, Gatti L, et al. A novel trinuclear platinum complex overcomes cisplatin resistance in an osteosarcoma cell system. Mol Pharmacol 1999;55:528–34.
16. O'Brien V, Brown R. Signalling cell cycle arrest and cell death through the MMR system. Carcinogenesis 2006;27:682–92.
17. Ishida S, Lee J, Thiele DJ, Herskowitz I. Uptake of the anticancer drug cisplatin mediated by the copper transporter Ctr1 in yeast and mammals. Proc Natl Acad Sci USA 2002;99:13963–5.
18. Katano K, Kondo A, Safei R, et al. Acquisition of resistance to cisplatin is accompanied by changes in the cellular pharmacology of copper. Cancer Res 2002;62:6559–65.
19. Chauhan SS, Liang XJ, Su AW, et al. Reduced endocytosis and altered lysosome function in cisplatin-resistant cell lines. Br J Cancer 2003;88:1327–34.
20. Beretta GL, Gatti L, Tinelli S, et al. Cellular pharmacology of cisplatin in relation to the expression of human copper transporter CTR1 in different pairs of cisplatin-sensitive and -resistant cells. Biochem Pharmacol 2004;68:283–91.
21. Safaei R, Otani S, Larson BJ, Rasmussen ML, Howell SB. Transport of cisplatin by the copper efflux transporter ATP7B. Mol Pharmacol 2008;73:461–8.
22. Holzer AK, Manorek GH, Howell SB. Contribution of the major copper influx transporter CTR1 to the cellular accumulation of cisplatin, carboplatin, and oxaliplatin. Mol Pharmacol 2006;70:1390–4.
23. Beretta GL, Benedetti V, Assaraf YGA, et al. Increased level and defective glycosylation of MRP4 contribute to reduced accumulation of oxaliplatin in ovarian carcinoma cells. Proceedings of the Pharmacology and Molecular Mechanisms Group 29th Winter meeting, Palermo, Italy, 30 January—2 February 2008, p. 53.
24. Gately DP, Howell SB. Cellular accumulation of the anticancer agent cisplatin: a review. Br J Cancer 1993;67:1171–6.
25. Martelli L, Di Mario F, Ragazzi E, et al. Different accumulation of cisplatin, oxaliplatin and JM216 in sensitive and cisplatin-resistant human cervical tumour cells. Biochem Pharmacol 2006;72:693–700.
26. Huang Z, Tong Y, Wang J, Huang Y. NMR studies of the relationship between the changes of membrane lipids and the cisplatin-resistance of A549/DDP cells. Cancer Cell Int 2003;3:5.
27. Ambudkar SV, Kimchi-Sarfaty C, Sauna ZE, Gottesman MM. P-glycoprotein: from genomics to mechanism. Oncogene 2003;22:7468–85.
28. Ishikawa,T, Kuo MT, Furuta K, Suzuki M. The human multidrug resistance-associated protein (MRP) gene family: from biological function to drug molecular design. Clin Chem Lab Med. 2000;38:893–7.

29. Wielandt AM, Vollrath V, Manzano M, Miranda S, Accatino L, Chianale J. Induction of the multispecific organic anion transporter (cMoat/mrp2) gene and biliary glutathione secretion by the herbicide 2,4,5-trichlorophenoxyacetic acid in the mouse liver. Biochem J 1999; 341:105–11.
30. Oguri T, Isobe T, Suzuki T, et al. Increased expression of the MRP5 gene is associated with exposure to platinum drugs in lung cancer. Int J Cancer 2000;86:95–100.
31. Hipfner DR, Deeley RG, Cole SP. Structural, mechanistic and clinical aspects of MRP1. Biochim Biophys Acta 1999;1461:359–76.
32. Borst P, Evers R, Kool M, Wijnhold JA. A family of drug transporters: the multidrug resistance-associated proteins. J Natl Cancer Inst 2000;92:1295–1302.
33. Borst P, Kool M, Evers R. Do cMOAT (MRP2), other MRP homologues, and LRP play a role in MDR? Semin Cancer Biol 1997;8:205–13.
34. Wijnholds J, Evers R, van Leusden MR, et al. Increased sensitivity to anticancer drugs and decreased inflammatory response in mice lacking the multidrug resistance-associated protein. Nat Met 1997;3:1275–9.
35. Takenaka K, Morgan, JA, Scheffer GL, et al. Substrate overlap between Mrp4 and Abcg2/Bcrp affects purine analogue drug cytotoxicity and tissue distribution. Cancer Res 2007;67:6965–72.
36. Materna V, Holm PS, Dietel M, Lage H. Kinetic characterization of ribozymes directed against the cisplatin resistance-associated ABC transporter cMOAT/MRP2/ABCC2. Cancer Gene Ther 2001;8:176–84.
37. Cui Y, Konig J, Buchholz JK, Spring H, Leier I, Keppler D. Drug resistance and ATP-dependent conjugate transport mediated by the apical multidrug resistance protein, MRP2, permanently expressed in human and canine cells. Mol Pharmacol 1999;55:929–37.
38. Hinoshita E, Uchiumi T, Taguchi K, et al. Increased expression of an ATP-binding cassette superfamily transporter, multidrug resistance protein 2, in human colorectal carcinomas. Clin Cancer Res 2000;6:2401–7.
39. Lanzi C, Perego P, Supino R, et al. Decreased drug accumulation and increased tolerance to DNA damage in tumor cells with a low level of cisplatin resistance. Biochem Pharmacol 1998;55:1247–54.
40. Liang XJ, Shen DW, Garfield S, Gottesman MM. Mislocalization of membrane proteins associated with multidrug resistance in cisplatin-resistant cancer cell lines. Cancer Res 2003; 63:5909–16.
41. Hayer-Zillgen M, Bruss M, Bonisch H. Expression and pharmacological profile of the human organic cation transporters hOCT1, hOCT2 and hOCT3. Br J Pharmacol 2002;136:829–36.
42. Zhang S, Levejoy KS, Shima JE, et al. Organic cation transporters are determinants of oxaliplatin cytotoxicity. Cancer Res 2006;66:8847–57.
43. Ciarimboli G, Ludwig T, Lang D, et al. Cisplatin nephrotoxicity is critically mediated via the human organic cation transporter 2. Am. J. Pathol. 2005;167:1477–84.
44. Daubeuf S, Leroy P, Paolicchi A, et al. Enhanced resistance of HeLa cells to cisplatin by overexpression of γ-glutamyltransferase. Biochem Pharmacol 2002;64:207–16.

Possible Incorporation of Free *N7*-Platinated Guanines in DNA by DNA Polymerases, Relevance for the Cisplatin Mechanism of Action

Michele Benedetti, Cosimo Ducani, Danilo Migoni, Daniela Antonucci, Vita M. Vecchio, Alessandro Romano, Tiziano Verri, and Francesco P. Fanizzi

Abstract Cisplatin, *cis*-diamminedichloroplatinum (II), is one of the most widely used anticancer drugs. The main cellular target of cisplatin is DNA, where the platinum atom is able to form covalent bonds with the *N7* of purines. It is commonly accepted that there is a direct attack of cisplatin on DNA. But it should be noted that, inside cells, free purine bases, which can react with cisplatin, are also available. Free bases have many functional roles, not least the constitution of building blocks for the synthesis of new DNA and RNA molecules. For this reason, under physiological conditions, the erroneous insertion of platinated bases in the synthesized nucleic acids could compete with direct DNA/RNA platination. Moreover, due to the lower sterical hindrance offered by single nucleobases with respect to nucleic acids, platination is expected to be even easier for free purines with respect to DNA and RNA. We have recently shown, for the first time, that platinated DNA can be formed in vitro by Taq DNA polymerase promoted incorporation of platinated purines. Cytotoxicity tests with [Pt(dien)(*N7*-G)], dien = diethylenetriamine, G = 5'-dGTP, 5'-dGDP, 5'-GMP, 5'-dGMP, GUO, dGUO, complexes on HeLa cancer cells support this hypothesis of the relative cytotoxicity of [Pt(dien)(*N7*-G)] derivatives being clearly related to their bioavailability. In vivo platination of free purines before their incorporation in nucleic acids therefore opens new perspectives in platinum based antitumour drugs, for a better understanding of both the action mechanism and the new molecular design.

Keywords Cisplatin; Platinum; Purine base; DNA; RNA; Cancer; Antitumor drug

Cisplatin and other platinum-based drugs have a central role in cancer chemotherapy (1–9), especially for testicular and ovarian cancer (9, 10). However, the cisplatin

M. Benedetti, C. Ducani, D. Migoni, D. Antonucci, V.M. Vecchio,
A.Romano, T. Verri, and F.P. Fanizzi (✉)
Department of Biotechnology and Environmental Science, University of Salento,
Lecce, Italy
e-mail: fp.fanizzi@unile.it

A. Bonetti et al. (eds.), *Platinum and Other Heavy Metal Compounds in Cancer Chemotherapy*, DOI: 10.1007/978-1-60327-459-3_17,
© Humana Press, a part of Springer Science + Business Media, LLC 2009

Fig. 1 Schematic representation of cisplatin, carboplatin and oxaliplatin molecular structures

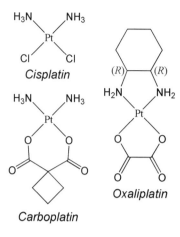

Cisplatin

Carboplatin

Oxaliplatin

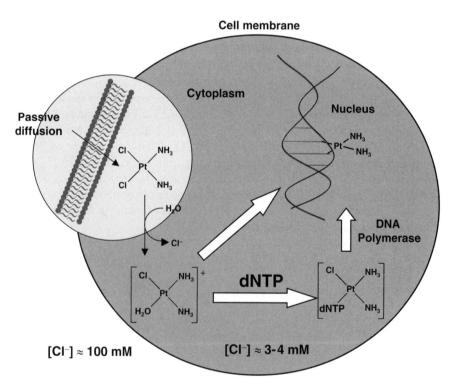

Fig. 2 Schematic representation of the mechanism of action of the cisplatin antitumor drug. Both, the mechanism of direct platination of DNA by cisplatin aquated species cis-[Pt(NH$_3$)$_2$Cl(H$_2$O)]$^+$ and the newly proposed mechanism of DNA platination, mediated by platinated nucleotides and DNA polymerases, are schematized

chemotherapic use is strongly limited by serious side effects, e.g., nephrotoxicity, emetogenesis and neurotoxicity and/or acquired or intrinsic tumor resistance. In order to overcome these problems, research activity has pointed, in the last decades, to the synthesis of thousands of novel platinum compounds as potential antitumor drugs alternative to cisplatin. Unfortunately, only a few were approved for clinical use and just one, oxaliplatin, [(*R,R*)-1,2-diaminocyclohexane(oxalato-*O,O'*)platinum(II)] (Fig. 1), was found able to overcome resistance of some tumors to cisplatin (11).

Since the beginning of cisplatin related research, strong efforts have been made to rationalize the mechanism of action and the drug design. Early studies suggested that cisplatin crosses the cell membrane mainly by passive diffusion (12) and that once inside the cell, it undergoes aquation to form *cis*-[Pt(NH$_3$)$_2$Cl(H$_2$O)]$^+$ because of the low (~3 mM) intracellular chloride concentration. The reactive aquated species could interact with DNA, which was recognized to be the primary biological target for the drug (6–8, 10, 13–22). Adducts formed with DNA are considered to be responsible for the pharmacological activity of the drug (Fig. 2).

It is known that inside the cell there are free purine bases with disparate functions, not least the constitution of building blocks for the synthesis of new DNA and RNA molecules (23). Our present working hypothesis is that there could be a mechanism of action for cisplatin, according to which free purines can be targeted by the platinum drug as well as nucleic acids. In agreement with this hypothesis, aquated cisplatin, *cis*-[Pt(NH$_3$)$_2$Cl(H$_2$O)]$^+$, could form a covalent bond with the *N*7 of free nucleosides or nucleotides, with the formation of mono-adducts of the type *cis*-[Pt(NH$_3$)$_2$Cl(*N*7-Purine)]. Because of the lower sterical hindrance around *N*7, free purines platination is expected to be even easier than platination of DNA and RNA. According to this hypothesis we thought that *N*7 platinated purines could be used as a substrate for nucleic acids synthesis by DNA polymerases. If this occurs under physiological conditions, the erroneous insertion of platinated bases in the synthesized nucleic acids should compete with the direct platination process (24). Recently we demonstrated (25), for the first time, that platinated purines can be inserted into DNA, by DNA polymerases, using an in vitro synthetic process (Fig. 3).

Our experimental system was constituted by a model DNA polymerase, i.e., Taq DNA polymerase and a model platinated purine, i.e., the complex [Pt(dien) (*N*7-dGTP)] (1), dien = diethylenetriamine; dGTP = 5'-dGTP = 5'-(2'-deoxy)-guanosine triphosphate, (Fig. 4). Because of the lack of labile chloride ligands, complex 1 is unable to bind other vicinal purine nucleotides.

The competition between dGTP and [Pt(dien)(*N*7-dGTP)] (1) for incorporation into a plasmidic DNA (pUC19), by Taq DNA polymerase, was evaluated by standard PCR-based assays (25, 26). As a result we observed a lower Taq DNA polymerase efficiency in the presence of increasing amounts of complex 1, in agreement with the reported insertion of other types of *N*7 modified nucleobases (26). In fact we observed that when only complex 1 is available, the Taq DNA polymerase activity is strongly reduced but not completely quenched. Our results were also consistent with the well-known concept that platinated DNA templates are able to severely repress DNA polymerase activity (27–29). The limits for the extension of our findings to other polymerases (including eukaryotic polymerases) and various platinum complexes, bearing purine bases, have still to be defined.

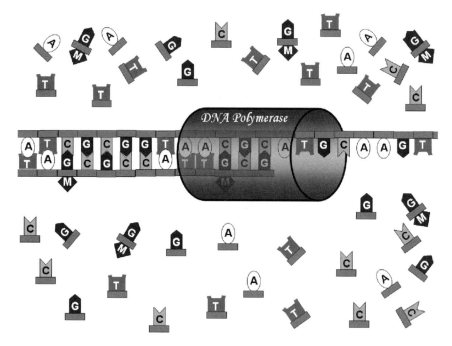

Fig. 3 Schematic representation of the insertion mechanism of platinated nucleotides operated by DNA polymerases, during the synthesis of the complementary DNA chain, in the presence of metallated guanines

We focused on the insertion of single platinated dGTP's in the newly-synthesized complementary DNA chains operated by the enzymatic activity of DNA polymerases. In this particular case, the overall yield of platination observed in *in vitro* experiments was of about 60%, showing that the insertion rate of dGTP by Taq DNA polymerase, with respect to the corresponding platinated derivative 1, is about 15 times faster. Considering that the reported minimum amount of DNA platination in human cells necessary to induce apoptosis with cisplatin, is of about 9–10 platinated nucleobases/DNA (10), even the misinsertion of very few platinated guanines could in principle, promote apoptotic pathways.

The previous findings suggested to look for a possible apoptotic pathway related to the presence of metallated primers as complex 1, in living model cells. Therefore we preliminarily evaluated the toxicological consequences of the possible incorporation of platinated purines. For this purpose, we evaluated the in vitro cytotoxicity (30), on HeLa human tumor cells, of [Pt(dien)($N7$-5'-dGTP)] (1), [Pt(dien)($N7$-5'-dGDP)] (2), [Pt(dien)($N7$-5'-GMP)] (3), [Pt(dien)($N7$-5'-dGMP)] (4), [Pt(dien)($N7$-Guo)] (5) and [Pt(dien)($N7$-dGuo)] (6) coordination compounds. Complexes 1–6 were prepared with a method similar to that previously reported (25). HeLa cells were grown in DMEM (Euroclone). The culture medium was supplemented with 10% heat-inactivated fetal bovine serum (Euroclone), 0.1 mg/mL streptomycin, 200 IU/mL penicillin. Cells were cultured routinely at 37°C and 5%

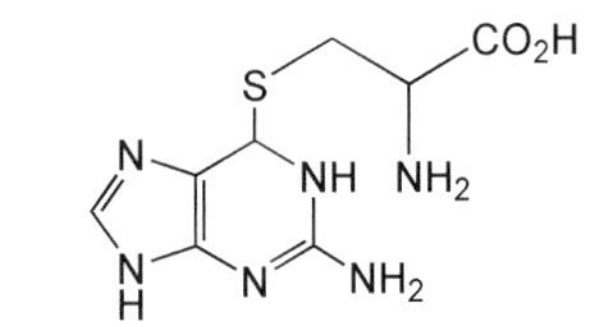

S-(guanin-6-yl)-L-cysteine (**GC**)

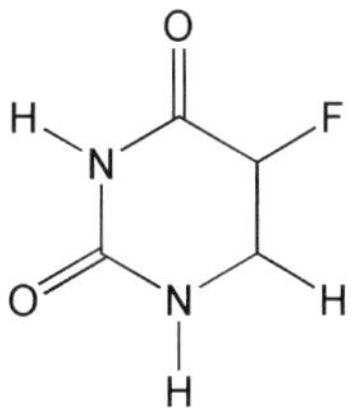

5-Fluoro-uracil (**5-FU**)

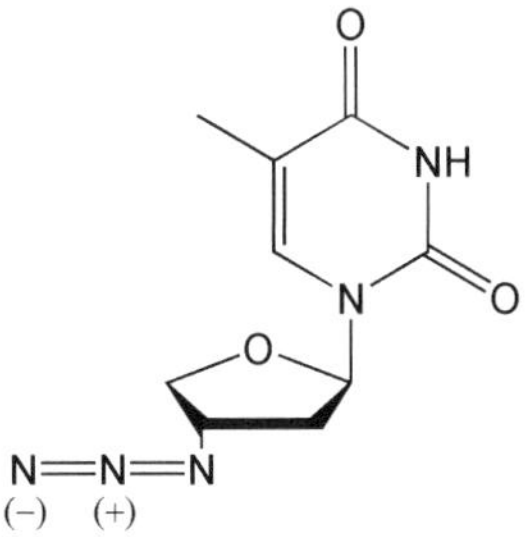

Azidotimidine (**AZT**)

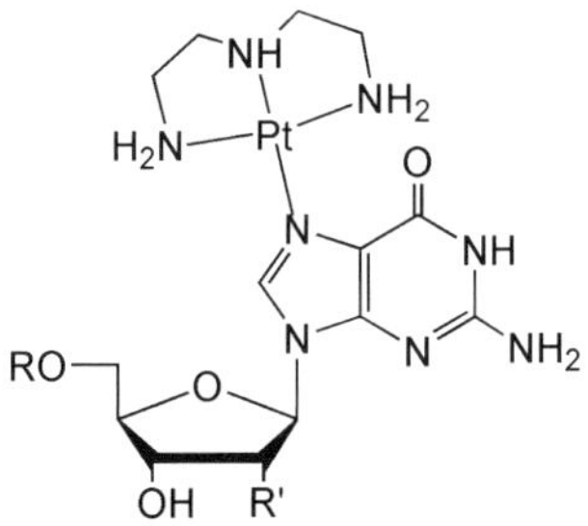

[Pt(**dien**)(*N7*-**G**)]

Fig. 4 Structure of antitumor and antiviral drugs or pro-drugs: *S*-(guanin-6-yl)-L-cysteine (GC), 5-fluoro-1*H*-pyrimidine-2,4-dione(5-fluorouracil,5-FU),3'-azido-2',3'-dideoxitimidine(Azidotimidine, AZT) and the complexes tested here, [Pt(dien)(*N7*-G)], G = 5'-dGTP, 5'-dGDP, 5'-GMP, 5'-dGMP, GUO, dGUO

CO_2 in a humidified incubator. Platinum containing compounds were administered to each well in appropriate concentrations ranging from 1 to 1,000 μM. The toxicity of these compounds was tested for 48 h of incubation. It should be pointed out that due to the lack of labile chlorides, all tested compounds (1–6), were not expected to exhibit high cisplatin cytotoxicity. Indeed the mono-adducts formed with DNA, after the insertion by DNA polymerases of a platinated guanine (complex 1), are unable to give bis-adducts lesions (including the well known 1, 2-intrastrand) generated by cisplatin, due to a lack of *cis* coordinating sites. For the latter reasons we focused on the evaluation of the relative toxicity of complexes 1–6 since differences among them could give new useful hints, although they were expected to behave differently than cisplatin. Results of the in vitro cytotoxicity tests are reported in Fig. 5. As expected, all tested complexes were less cytotoxic with respect to cisplatin. However their cytotoxicity, which could be observed only at the highest tested concentrations (500–1,000 μM), seems to be strongly related to the expected relative bioavailability. In particular, the transport across cell membranes (31, 32) of the possible GUO and dGUO derivatives and the direct incorporation of the dGTP derivatives into synthesized DNA could account for the higher cytotoxicity of complexes 1, 5 and 6 with respect to 2, 3 and 4.

In perspective, our results suggest a possible alternative mechanism for DNA platination in living cells, which may parallel the direct DNA platination process operated by cisplatin and its derivatives. Such a novel approach might open the possibility of

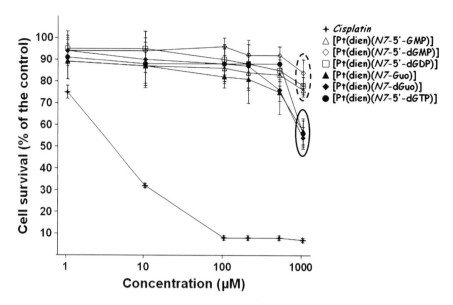

Fig. 5 HeLa cell survival measured by MTT test after 48 h of incubation. Tested complexes were administered in concentrations ranging from 1 to 1,000 μM. The data were the results of three different experiments presented as means ±*SD*

designing and developing, on a different rationale, a new generation of metal based drugs. Finally our hypothesis for the cisplatin (and analogues) mechanism of action allows the conceptual merging of these compounds (as *pro*-drugs) in the general drug/ *pro*-drug class of modified DNA and RNA nucleobases (5-fluoro-uracil, 5-FU; azidot-imidine, AZT; S-(guanin-6-yl)-L-cysteine, GC; ganciclovir, etc.) (23, 33) (see Fig. 4).

References

1. Rosenberg B, Van Camp L, Krigas T. Inhibition of cell division in Escherichia coli by elec-trolysis products from a platinum electrode. Nature 1965;205:698–9.
2. Rosenberg B, Van Camp L, Grimley EB, Thomson AJ. The inhibition of growth or cell divi-sion in *Escherichia coli* by different ionic species of platinum(IV) complexes. J Biol Chem 1967;242:1347–52.
3. Rosenberg B. Biological effects of platinum compounds. New agents for the control of tumors. Platinum Met Rev 1971;15:42–51.
4. Weiss RB, Christian MC. New cisplatin analogues in development. A review. Drugs 1993;46:360–77.
5. Wong E, Giandomenico CM. Current status of platinum-based antitumor drugs. Chem Rev 1999;99:2451–66.
6. Reedijk J. Why does cisplatin reach guanine-*N7* with competing S-donor ligands available in the cell? Chem Rev 1999;99:2499–510.
7. Wang D, Lippard SJ. Cellular processing of platinum anticancer drugs. Nat Rev Drug Disc 2005;4:307–20.

8. Lebwohl D, Canetta R. Clinical development of platinum complexes in cancer therapy: an historical perspective and an update. Eur J Cancer 1998;34:1522–34.

9. Benedetti M, Malina J, Kasparova J, Brabec V, Natile G. Chiral discrimination in platinum anticancer drugs. Environ Health Persp 2002;110:779–82.

10. Jamieson ER, Lippard SJ. Structure, recognition, and processing of cisplatin-DNA adducts. Chem Rev 1999;99:2467–98.

11. Fuertes MA, Alonso C, Pérez JM. Biochemical modulation of cisplatin mechanisms of action: enhancement of antitumor activity and circumvention of drug resistance. Chem Rev 2003;103:645–62.

12. Hromas RA, North JA, Burns CP. Decreased cisplatin uptake by resistant L1210 leukemia cells. Cancer Lett 1987;36:197–201.

13. Hambley TW. The influence of structure on the activity and toxicity of Pt anticancer drugs. Coord Chem Rev 1997;166:181–223.

14. Reedijk J. Improved understanding in platinum antitumor chemistry. Chem Commun 1996;7:801–6.

15. Ano SO, Kuklenyik Z, Marzilli LG. In: Lippert B, ed. Cisplatin: Chemistry and Biochemistry of a Leading Anticancer Drug. Weinheim, Germany: Wiley-VCH, 1999:247–91.

16. Natile G, Marzilli LG. Non-covalent interactions in adducts of platinum drugs with nucleobases in nucleotides and DNA as revealed by using chiral substrates. Coord Chem Rev 2006;250:1315–31.

17. Isab AA, Marzilli LG. Supermacrochelate complexes containing an artificial nucleic acid backbone and derived from excellent ligands formed by treating platinum anticancer agents with nucleotide triphosphates. Inorg Chem 1998;37:6558–9.

18. Brabec V, Kasparkova J. DNA interactions of platinum anticancer drugs. Recent advances and mechanisms of action. In: Pérez JM, Fuertes MA, Alonso C, eds. Metal Compounds in Cancer Chemotherapy. Trivandrum, India: Research Signpost, 2005:187–218.

19. Benedetti M, Saad JS, Marzilli LG, Natile G. Chiral discrimination in the formation reaction and at equilibrium for *N,N,N',N'*-tetramethyl-1,2-diaminocyclohexane-PtG$_2$ complexes. Dalton Trans 2003;5:872–9.

20. Benedetti M, Cini R, Tamasi G, Natile G. Crystal and molecular structure and circular dichroism of [bis-(guanosine-5'-monophosphate (−1))(*N,N,N',N'*-tetramethyl-cyclohexyl-1,2-diamine)platinum(II)] complexes with *R,R* and *S,S* configurations of the asymmetric diamine. Chem Eur J 2003;9:6122–32.

21. Benedetti M, Marzilli LG, Natile G. Rotamer stability in *cis*-[Pt(diA)G$_2$] complexes (diA = diamine derivative and G = guanine derivative) mediated by carrier-ligand amine stereochemistry as revealed by circular dichroism spectroscopy. Chem Eur J 2005;11:5302–10.

22. Benedetti M, Tamasi G, Cini R, Marzilli LG, Natile G. The first pure ΛHT rotamer of a complex with a *cis*-[Metal(nucleotide)$_2$] unit: a *cis*-[Pt(amine)$_2$(nucleotide)$_2$] ΛHT rotamer with unique molecular structural features. Chem Eur J 2007;13:3131–42.

23. Van Rompay AR, Johansson M, Karlsson A. Substrate specificity and phosphorylation of antiviral and anticancer nucleoside analogues by human deoxyribonucleoside kinases and ribonucleoside kinases. Pharmacol Ther 2003;100:119–39.

24. Seki S, Hongo A, Zhang B, Akiyama K, Sarker AH, Kudo T. Inhibition of cisplatin-mediated DNA damage in vitro by ribonucleotides. Jpn J Cancer Res 1993;84:462–7.

25. Benedetti M, Ducani C, Migoni D, et al. Experimental evidence that a DNA polymerase can incorporate *N7*-platinated guanines to give platinated DNA. Angew Chem Int Ed Engl 2008;47:507–10.

26. Tasara T, Angerer B, Damond M, et al. Incorporation of reporter molecule-labeled nucleotides by DNA polymerases. II. High-density labelling of natural DNA. Nucleic Acids Res 2003;31:2636–46.

27. Holler E, Bauer R, Bernges F. Monofunctional DNA-platinum(II) adducts block frequently DNA polymerase. Nucleic Acids Res 1992;20:2307–12.

28. Murray V, Motyka H, England PR, et al. The use of Taq DNA polymerase to determine the sequence specificity of DNA damage caused by *cis*-diamminedichloroplatinum(II),

acridine-tethered platinum(II) diammine complexes or two analogues. J Biol Chem 1992;267:18805–9.

29. Vaisman A, Warren MW, Chaney SG. The effect of DNA structure on the catalytic efficiency and fidelity of human DNA polymerase β on templates with platinum-DNA adducts. J Biol Chem 2001;276:18999–19005.

30. Mosmann T. Rapid colorimetric assay for cellular growth and survival: application to proliferation and cytotoxicity assays. J Immunol Methods 1983;65:55–63.

31. Gray JH, Owen RP, Giacomini KM. The concentrative nucleoside transporter family, SLC28. Eur J Physiol 2004;447:728–34.

32. Baldwin SA, Beal PR, Yao SYM, King AE, Cass CE, Young JD. The equilibrative nucleoside transporter family, SLC29. Eur J Physiol 2004;447:735–43.

33. Rooseboom M, Commandeur JNM, Vermeulen NPE. Enzyme-catalyzed activation of anticancer prodrugs. Pharmacol Rev 2004;56:53–102.

Section C
DNA Damage and Signal Transduction: Recognition/Repair And Cell-Respouse

Structural and Mechanistic Studies of Anticancer Platinum Drugs: Uptake, Activation, and the Cellular Response to DNA Binding

Shanta Dhar and Stephen J. Lippard

Abstract The action of platinum anticancer drugs is a multistep process involving uptake, activation, DNA binding, and cellular responses. Our research investigates these early stages of action of platinum complexes. We demonstrated that the effectiveness of oxaliplatin and *cis*-diammine(pyridine)chloroplatinum(II) (cDPCP) is a consequence of their selective delivery to cells containing organic cation transporters OCT1 and OCT2. This work inspired us to devise strategies for novel cell-targeting modalities, which include tethering receptor-binding moieties like estrogen or conjugated peptide motifs to a *cis*-diammineplatinum(II) unit, and the use of single walled carbon nanotubes as "longboat" delivery systems. Structural studies of DNA containing bound platinum complexes resulted in two significant findings. First, an X-ray structure of a site-specific monofunctional platinum-DNA dodecamer duplex containing a guanosine modified by *cis*-$\{Pt(NH_3)_2(py)\}^{2+}$ resembles that of B-DNA, differing from structures containing a 1,2- or 1,3- intrastrand cross-link. Nevertheless, certain features resemble that of the 1,2-cross-link. Second, 1,3-GTG-intrastrand *cis*-diammineplatinum(II) cross-links determine and override the natural positioning of DNA on the nucleosome core particle. Close examination of cellular responses associated with *cis*-$[Pt(NH_3)_2(py)Cl]Cl$, cDPCP, revealed the potency of this compound to be a consequence of a competition between transcription inhibition and excision repair. Photo-cross-linking studies of platinated DNA to proteins in cancer cell nuclear extracts reveal the panoply of factors that process the platinum adducts at the early stage of recognition.

Keywords Cisplatin; Uptake; Platinum(IV) compounds; Receptors; DNA binding; Cellular responses

S. Dhar and S.J. Lippard (✉)
Department of Chemistry, Massachusetts Institute of Technology, Cambridge, MA, USA
e-mail: lippard@mit.edu

A. Bonetti et al. (eds.), *Platinum and Other Heavy Metal Compounds in Cancer Chemotherapy*, DOI: 10.1007/978-1-60327-459-3_18,
© Humana Press, a part of Springer Science + Business Media, LLC 2009

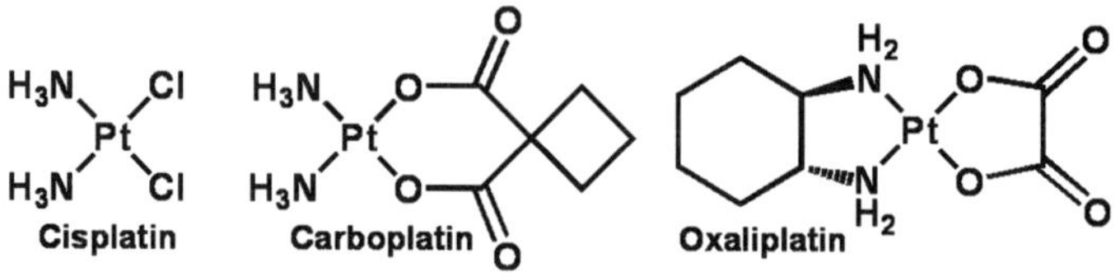

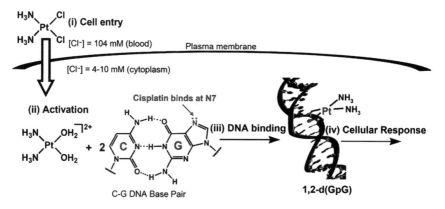

Fig. 1 FDA-approved anticancer drugs of the cisplatin family

Fig. 2 Four early stages in the cisplatin mechanism of action

Introduction

Platinum complexes are broadly applied in cancer therapy (1, 2). The widespread clinical applications of *cis*-diamminedichloroplatinum(II) or cisplatin, carboplatin, and oxaliplatin (depicted in Fig. 1) have inspired the synthesis and investigation of numerous platinum compounds as potential drug candidates (3). In particular, there is much interest in expanding the tumors that can be treated, limiting side effects, and targeting the cancer cell population. The mode of action of cisplatin is a multi-step process which includes: (i) cell entry or uptake, (ii) drug activation, (iii) DNA binding, and (iv) cellular responses to the DNA damage (see Fig. 2). A better understanding of these processes would guide the choice of new compounds for more effective therapies. Our research activities embrace all four steps of cisplatin action and the results have inspired the synthesis and evaluation of new compounds based on the insights provided.

Uptake

The mechanisms by which cisplatin is transported across the plasma membrane have not been established. Studies have implicated both passive diffusion and carrier-mediated active transport (4), but no specific membrane transporter for cisplatin has been identified that clearly leads to the formation of DNA cross-links in the nucleus. An improvement upon the current limitations of platinum-based therapy would be to deliver a biologically effective concentration of the compound to the tumor tissues with high specificity. In order to achieve this ultimate goal, new compounds can be devised that are conjugated to molecules which target plasma membrane receptors overexpressed on cancer cells.

The success of oxaliplatin for treating colorectal cancer has recently been linked to targeted uptake of the drug as mediated by organic cation transporters (OCTs) (5). This work identified the organic cation transporters OCT1 and OCT2 as mediators of oxaliplatin entry into cells. Subsequently, in evaluating a broad range of cationic platinum complexes, we discovered that *cis*-diammine(pyridine)chloroplatinum(II), cDPCP, is a strong candidate for treating colorectal cancer (6). The anticancer activity of cDPCP has been known for years (7), but unlike cisplatin it forms monofunctional rather than bifunctional cross-links with nuclear DNA. We discovered the cellular growth inhibition of cDPCP to be significantly better than that of oxaliplatin (see Fig. 3) in colon cancer cells bearing the OCT1/OCT2 receptors.

Breast cancer, the most common malignancy in women, is associated with the steroid hormone estrogen (8). The discovery of the estrogen receptor (ER) provided an efficient target for the treatment of hormone-dependent breast cancer. Our recent work showed that estrogen receptor positive or ER(+) cells treated with estrogen are sensitized towards cisplatin. Estrogen also induces overexpression of HMGB1 (Fig. 4), a protein that shields cisplatin DNA lesions from nucleotide excision repair (NER) (9). Recently, we were able to synthesize a series of 17β-estradiol-platinum(IV) complexes by connecting the 17-hydroxyl group to the terminal carboxylates of *c,c,t*-diamminedichlorodisuccinatoplatinum(IV) using polymethylene chains of varying lengths (10). Intracellular reduction of these estrogen-tethered Pt(IV) complexes delivers one molecule of cisplatin and two molecules of linker-modified estrogen derivative (Fig. 4).

Tumor cell survival, growth, and metastasis are driven by unregulated angiogenesis, the process by which new blood vessels are formed (11). Tumor blood vessels

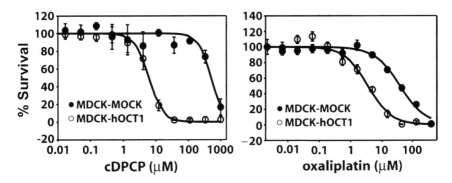

Fig. 3 Cell growth inhibition by MTT assays for cDPCP (*left*) and oxaliplatin (*right*) in MDCK cells with and without hOCT1. Modified based on Fig. 2 of (6)

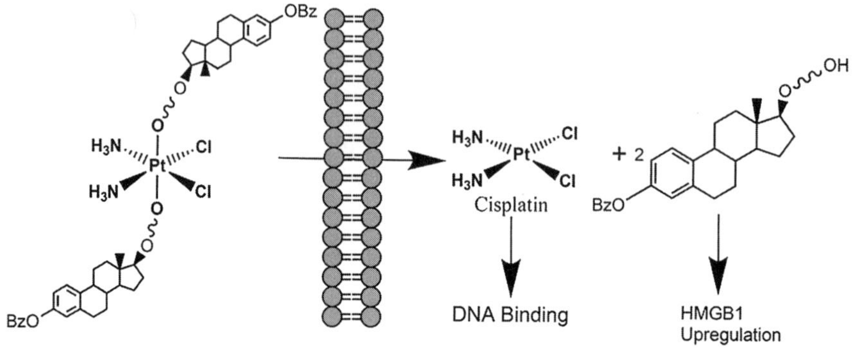

Fig. 4 Activation of estrogen-tethered Pt(IV) complexes in the reducing environment of the cell

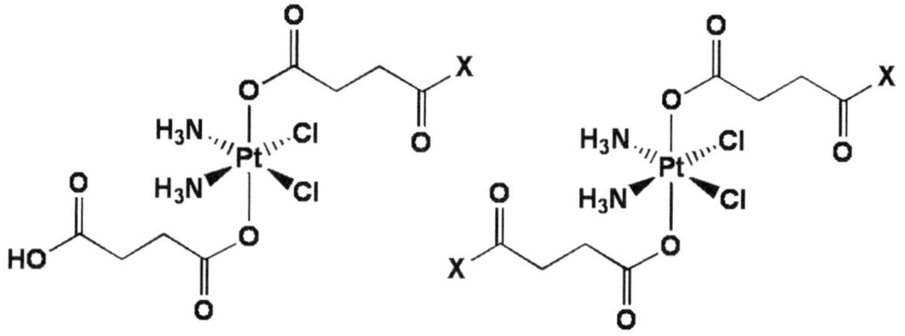

X = RDG, NGR, AGR, (CRGDC)c, (RGDfK)c

Fig. 5 Structure of Pt(IV) complexes containing tethered RGD or NGR peptides

are a major target for cancer treatment because they can be selectively recognized without affecting normal tissue. Integrins are heterodimeric cell-adhesion receptors that facilitate communication between a cell and its surroundings. Phage library screening experiments have identified three peptide motifs, RGD (Arg-Gly-Asp), NGR (Asn-Gly-Arg), and GSL (Gly-Ser-Leu), that are capable of homing into the tumor vasculature (12). We recently developed a strategy to prepare platinum(IV) anticancer drug candidates (see Fig. 5) in which the conjugated peptide motif, containing either RGD or NGR, would serve as a "tumor-targeting device" and selectively kill angiogenic tumor endothelial cells (13). As targeting moieties, we used the RGD and NGR linear tripeptides; an RGD-containing disulfide-bridged cyclic pentapeptide, (CRGDC)c; and the cyclic pentapeptide, and (RGDfK)c. The latter were chosen because cyclic peptides target angiogenic endothelial cells more efficiently compared to their linear counterparts. We discovered that RGD-tethered Pt(IV) complexes are efficient inhibitors of cellular proliferation when compared to both non-targeting platinum(IV) compounds and to the unconjugated targeting RGD tri- and pentapeptide moieties.

Recently, single-walled carbon nanotubes (SWNTs) have been investigated for their ability to interact with living systems (14). SWNTs internalize various cargoes

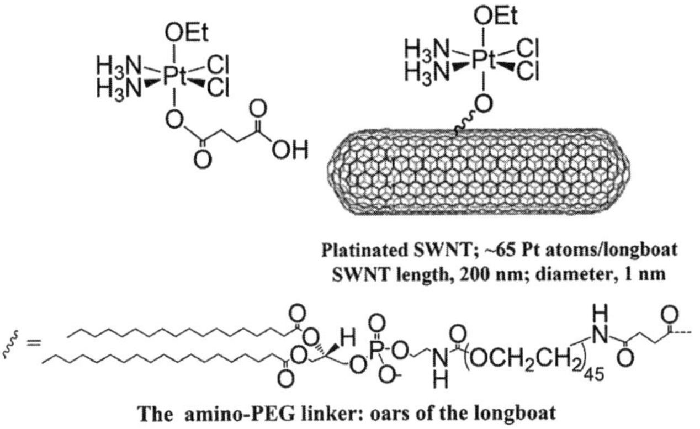

Fig. 6 An unsymmetrial Pt(IV) compound tethered to a SWNT. Modified based on Fig. 1 of (18)

into cells, including fluoresceins, plasmid DNA, proteins and other materials that would not have been able to be taken into a cell by themselves, with no apparent side effects (15, 16). The low solubility of SWNTs can be overcome by surface functionalization through the attachment of solubilizing side-chains for dispersing the SWNTs in solution. Once solubilized, the SWNTs can efficiently cross the cell membrane via endocytosis (17). We are currently using SWNTs as "longboat" delivery vehicles, named by analogy to the Viking longboats, for the intracellular delivery of platinum complexes. We recently described an asymmetrical Pt(IV) compound containing alkoxy and succinate ligands at the axial positions (Fig. 6), which was successfully delivered to human testicular NTera-2 cancer cells (18). The activity of the SWNT tethered compound was much greater than that of the untethered Pt(IV) compound. We developed a method to track the intracellular location of the SWNTs and platinum by following the movement of fluorescently labeled SWNTs and measuring the platinum content in nuclear and the cytosolic extracts. The construct employed in this study had a fluoroscein derivative co-tethered to the SWNT-Pt(IV) conjugates. With the use of fluorescence microscopy, the fluorescent SWNTs were readily detected in small vesicles within the cell, confirming the expectation that SWNTs enter through endocytosis.

Knowledge of the mechanism of platinum uptake, the role of various receptors overexpressed on cancer cell surfaces, and the use of new delivery systems significantly expands the horizon of platinum anticancer drug candidates having improved efficacy and diminished toxic side effects.

Activation

Once in the body, the high chloride ion concentrations in blood and the extracellular fluid (>100 mM) maintain the integrity of electroneutral platinum complexes like cisplatin and retard premature activation or undesired direct ligand substitution

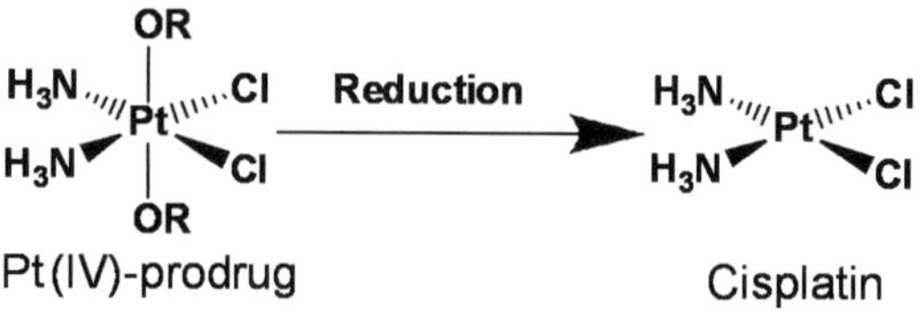

Fig. 7 Generation of active Pt(II)
species from Pt(IV) compounds

reactions. Once cisplatin enters cancer cells, the relatively low chloride ion concentration of the cytosol favors the formation of activated aqua species that react
further with intracellular nucleophiles like the DNA bases.

In the case of Pt(IV) complexes, activation is significantly different. Platinum(IV)
compounds are substitutionally more inert and less likely to be deactivated in vivo
prior to crossing the cancer cell membrane. These tetravalent platinum complexes
are prodrugs, because the first step of their activation involves in vivo reduction
with concomitant loss of the axial ligands, generating platinum(II) center that binds
to DNA (see Fig. 7). The axial ligands are ideal for altering properties such as
lipophilicity, reduction potential, stability, and biological targeting without changing the activity of the reduced, biologically active complex generated in the cancer
cell (19). Recently, we directed a significant portion of our research efforts toward
the design, synthesis, and evaluation of new Pt(IV) complexes for the conjugation
to delivery systems like SWNTs (18) and for incorporation of targeting moieties
like estrogen (10) or cancer cell-specific peptides (13), as mentioned above.

DNA Binding

The potency of cisplatin is directly related to its ability to form bifunctional intrastrand cross-links on DNA (20, 21). The platinum-DNA lesions disrupt such cellular
processes as transcription and replication, leading to apoptosis. In order to generate
1,2-intrastrand cross-links responsible for the activity of cisplatin, most platinum(II)
complexes have been based on square-planar coordination and the presence of two
labile leaving groups in a *cis* configuration. However, the discovery of many polynuclear and *trans*-platinum complexes that violate this classical rule has opened up a
new arena of non-classical platinum complexes with considerable potential for use in
clinical medicine (22). Studying the interaction of platinum compounds with DNA
is one of the most important aspects in biological investigations aimed at discover-
ing and developing such molecules. As an example, we recently focused our efforts
on the non-classical, cationic, monofunctional platinum(II) complex, cDPCP (6).
This compound has only one leaving group and is expected to form a DNA adduct
fundamentally different from that of cisplatin. This expectation was confirmed by a
2.17 Å resolution X-ray crystal structure of cDPCP bound in a monofunctional fash-
ion to deoxyguanosine in a DNA dodecamer duplex (see Fig. 8) (6). A comparison
of the geometry of cDPCP-damaged DNA with that of DNA containing a cisplatin
1,2-d(GpG) intrastrand cross-link revealed the structures to be quite different. Rather

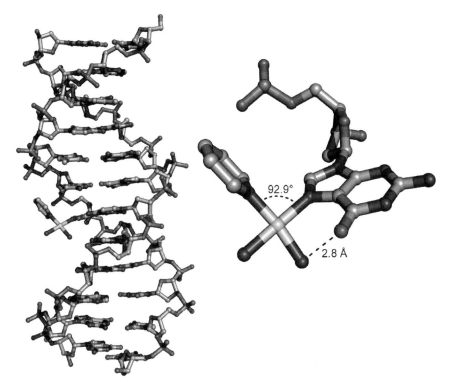

Fig. 8 The structure of cDPCP-damaged DNA duplex (*see Color Plates*)

than the duplex bent by ~40° toward the major groove at the site of cisplatin adduct, the monofunctional cDPCP adduct causes no significant bending of the double helix. However, both cisplatin and cDPCP cause a distorted base pair step to the 5' side of the platinum site that may be correlated to its ability to destroy cancer cells.

Until recently, our knowledge about the structure of platinated DNA was limited to synthetic duplexes. Since DNA is packaged in the nucleus of cancer cells as highly condensed chromatin, the building block of which is the nucleosome core particle (23), a better understanding of the interaction of cisplatin with DNA at the level of the nucleosome is desired to assist in the development of chemotherapeutic drugs with improved efficacy. Cisplatin reacts with nucleosomal DNA as well as with free DNA (24). We therefore devised an experimental system involving chromatin reconstituted from chemically synthesized (24) DNA bearing a site-specific cisplatin adduct (25, 26). We constructed two site-specifically modified nucleosomes containing intrastrand cis-$\{Pt(NH_3)_2\}^{2+}$ 1,3-d(GpTpG) cross-links positioned half a helical turn apart. Histones from HeLa-S3 cancer cells were transferred onto these synthetic DNA duplexes, which had nucleosome positioning sequences. The structures of these complexes were studied by using hydroxyl radical footprinting. Employing nucleosome positioning sequences allowed us to quantify the structural

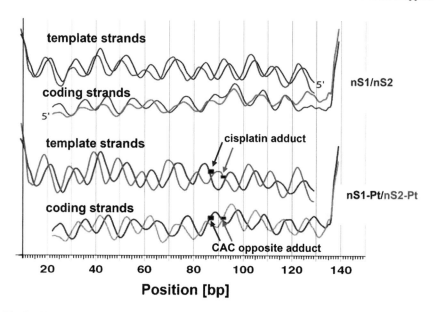

Fig. 9 Cisplatin damage overrides the predefined rotational setting pattern of nucleosomes. Blue/green – unplatinated nucleosomes, nS1 (*blue*) and nS2 (*green*) are identical sequences, but d(GpTpG) is shifted by 5 bp; the corresponding cleavage curves are out of phase by 1–2 bp. Red/orange-platinated nucleosomes, nS1-Pt (*red*) and nS2-Pt (*orange*) have identical sequences except for the fact that the 1,3-d(GpTpG) cisplatin adduct (*black rectangle*) is shifted by 5 bp. The corresponding cleavage curves are out of phase by 3–5 bp. The phasing difference is ~180° in the vicinity of the cisplatin adduct. Modified based on Fig. 3 of (25) (*see Color Plates*)

deviations induced by the cisplatin adduct. Our studies showed that a platinum cross-link locally overrides the rotational setting in the nucleosome positioning sequence (Fig. 9) such that the lesion faces toward the histone core (Fig. 10). We were also able to use the quantitative data to determine that cisplatin unwinds nucleosomal DNA by ~24°. The intrastrand cis-$\{Pt(NH_3)_2\}^{2+}$ 1,3-d(GpTpG) crosslinks are located in an area of the nucleosome that contains locally overwound DNA in undamaged reference nucleosomes. The changes in nucleosomal organization upon platinum binding could play a significant role in the disruption of transcription by cisplatin.

Cellular Responses

The anticancer drug cisplatin provokes a complex series of cellular responses. A lethal dose of platinum drugs can kill cells primarily by forming DNA adducts, causing arrest at the G2 phase of the cell cycle, and triggering apoptosis. Cisplatin–DNA adducts are recognized by several cellular proteins, including some that enhance the survival of the cell by mediating DNA repair and others that hasten death by conferring sensitivity to the drug. We have been actively studying these different cellular processes with several types of platinum complexes.

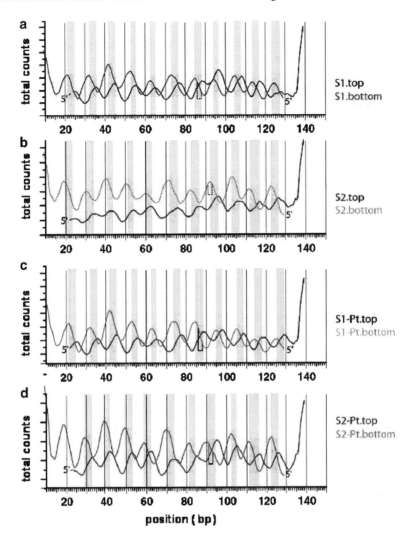

Fig. 10 Cisplatin adduct faces toward histone core. Gray bars represent areas in which the minor grove is exposed to the solvent (and the major grove faces inwards to the nucleosome). (**a**) The major grove of the unplatinated d(GpTpG) site of S1 trinucleotide faces inwards, (**b**) the major grove of the unplatinated d(GpTpG) site of S2 faces to the side, (**c, d**), the major grove of the platinated d(GpTpG) sites face in both cases inwards. Modified based on Fig. 4 of (25) (*see Color Plates*)

We discovered two notable cellular responses to cDPCP that were not anticipated based on earlier work with other monofunctional compounds such as [Pt(dien)Cl]⁺ (27). This compound blocks transcription, a mechanistic feature shared by cisplatin, while largely evading repair by the mammalian excinuclease.

Among the proteins and protein complexes that encounter cisplatin–DNA adducts, RNA polymerases are greatly affected by the lesions. The progression of human RNA polymerase II (Pol II) along the DNA strand is almost completely blocked by cisplatin–DNA adducts, and the arrest and subsequent ubiquitylation of Pol II initiate transcription-coupled repair as well as programmed cell death, or apoptosis. Our study showed that, like cisplatin, transcription is strongly inhibited by cDPCP both in cell extracts and in live cells (6).

Nucleotide excision repair (NER) is the pathway by which the major cisplatin-induced DNA lesion, the 1,2-intrastrand d(GpG) cross-link, is removed. An increased efficiency of excision repair leads to the removal of cisplatin adducts and upregulation of ERCC1, a key protein in the pathway (28, 29). We considered the possibility that the excellent cell-killing properties of the monofunctional OCT substrate cDPCP may derive from the formation of less recognizable DNA adducts, compared to cross-links, and that this compound might therefore evade identification by the excision repair machinery. Such a possibility would suggest the utility of this complex for the treatment of cisplatin-resistant tumors. We applied a well-developed in vitro excision repair assay to determine the rate of removal of cDPCP-DNA adducts by the mammalian excinuclease. We used three different platinum probes for this study. A repair yield of ~1% was observed with the DNA-cDPCP adduct after 1h (Fig. 11) (6). The repair product signal was highest after 60–90 min and declined thereafter due to exonucleolytic degradation of primary excision products by exonucleases in the rodent cell extracts employed in the assay. The cisplatin 1,3-intrastrand cross-link, by comparison, displays 3.5% repair in this assay after 60 min, and the [Pt(dien)Cl]Cl monofunctional adduct showed 0.3% repair. The observed repair rate of 3.5% for cisplatin adducts is significantly higher than that observed for our cDPCP compound.

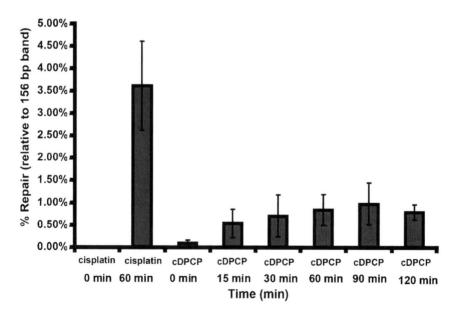

Fig. 11 Kinetics of repair for the cDPCP-DNA lesion, reported as % repair relative to the 156-mer band (CHO extracts) see ref. (6)

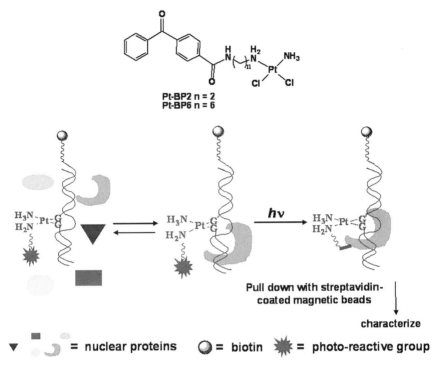

Fig. 12 Structure of the photoactive benzophenone-modified cisplatin analogue and the methodology used to identify proteins that interact with cisplatin–DNA adducts see ref. (31) (*see Color Plates*)

Platinum DNA intrastrand cross-links introduce a bend in duplex DNA and also result in unwinding. These events create recognition sites for nuclear proteins. By using a photoactive benzophenone-modified cisplatin analogue (Fig. 12) (30), 25-bp DNA duplexes containing either a 1,2-d(GpG) or a 1,3-d(GpTpG) intrastrand cross-link were synthesized. Proteins having affinity for these platinated DNAs were photo-cross-linked and identified in the nuclear extracts of several cancer cells. By using the methodology depicted in Fig. 12, a number of proteins involved in DNA repair were identified, namely RPA1, Ku70, Ku80, Msh2, DNA ligase III, PARP-1, DNA-PKcs, as well as the HMG-domain proteins HMGB1, HMGB2, HMGB3, and UBF1(31). Our studies also explored the differences in protein binding to platinated DNA for cell lines with different sensitivities to cisplatin.

Conclusions

These advances in knowledge about the chemistry of platinum anticancer drugs demonstrate significant progress in understanding their mechanism of action. They unveil a flourishing arena for future synthetic work on rationally designed platinum anticancer drug candidates. Significant progress in the development of non-classical platinum complexes, most notably monofunctional and Pt(IV) compounds, has been achieved. Systems containing new delivery vehicles, high specificity, and reduced toxicity have been developed.

Acknowledgement Our work has been supported by the National Cancer Institute under grant CA034992.

References

1. Jamieson ER, Lippard SJ. Structure, recognition, and processing of cisplatin–DNA adducts. Chem Rev 1999;99:2467–98.
2. Rosenberg B, VanCamp L, Trosko JE, Mansour VH. Platinum compounds: a new class of potent antitumour agents. Nature 1969;222:385–6.
3. Galanski M, Jakupec MA, Keppler BK. Update of the preclinical situation of anticancer platinum complexes: novel design strategies and innovative analytical approaches. Curr Med Chem 2005;12:2075–94.
4. Gately DP, Howell SB. Cellular accumulation of the anticancer agent cisplatin: a review. Br J Cancer 1993;67:1171–6.
5. Zhang S, Lovejoy KS, Shima JE, et al. Organic cation transporters are determinants of oxaliplatin cytotoxicity. Cancer Res 2006;66:8847–57.
6. Lovejoy KS, Todd RC, Zhang S, et al. *cis*-(Diammine(pyridine)chloroplatinum(II), a monofunctional platinum(II) antitumor agent: uptake, structure, function, and prospects. Proc Natl Acad Sci USA 2008;105:8902–07.
7. Hollis LS, Amundsen AR, Stern EW. Chemical and biological properties of a new series of *cis*-diammineplatinum(II) antitumor agents containing three nitrogen donors: *cis*-[Pt(NH$_3$)$_2$-(N-donor)Cl]$^+$. J Med Chem 1989;32:128–36.
8. Feigelson HS, Henderson BE. Estrogens and breast cancer. Carcinogenesis 1996;17:2279–84.
9. He Q, Liang CH, Lippard SJ. Steroid hormones induce HMG1 overexpression and sensitize breast cancer cells to cisplatin and carboplatin. Proc Natl Acad Sci USA 2000;97:5768–72.
10. Barnes KR, Kutikov A, Lippard SJ. Synthesis, characterization, and cytotoxicity of a series of estrogen-tethered platinum(IV) complexes. Chem Bio 2004;11:557–64.
11. Folkman J. Angiogenesis in cancer, vascular, rheumatoid and other disease. Nat Med 1995;1:27–31.
12. Hart SL, Knight AM, Harbottle RP, et al. Cell binding and internalization by filamentous phage displaying a cyclic arg-gly-asp-containing peptide. J Biol Chem 1994;269:12468–74.
13. Mukhopadhyay S, Barnes CM, Haskel A, Short SM, Barnes KR, Lippard SJ. Conjugated platinum(IV)-peptide complexes for targeting angiogenic tumor vasculature. Bioconjugate Chem 2008;19:39–49.
14. Kam NWS, Jessop TC, Wender PA, Dai H. Nanotube molecular transporters: internalization of carbon nanotube-protein conjugates into mammalian cells. J Am Chem Soc 2004;126:6850–1.
15. Bottini M, Cerignoli F, Dawson MI, Magrini A, Rosato N, Mustelin T. Full-length single-walled carbon nanotubes decorated with streptavidin-conjugated quantum dots as multivalent intracellular fluorescent nanoprobes. Biomacromolecules 2006;7:2259–63.
16. Liu Y, Wu D-C, Zhang W-D, et al. Polyethylenimine-grafted multiwalled carbon nanotubes for secure noncovalent immobilization and efficient delivery of DNA. Angew Chem Int Ed 2005;44:4782–5.

17. Kam NWS, Dai H. Carbon nanotubes as intracellular protein transporters: generality and biological functionality. J Am Chem Soc 2005;127:6021–6.
18. Feazell RP, Nakayama-Ratchford N, Dai H, Lippard SJ. Soluble single-walled carbon nanotubes as longboat delivery systems for platinum(IV) anticancer drug design. J Am Chem Soc 2007;129:8438–9.
19. Hambley TW, Battle AR, Deacon GB, et al. Modifying the properties of platinum(IV) complexes in order to increase biological effectiveness. J Inorg Biochem 1999;77:3–12.
20. Cohen GL, Ledner JA, Bauer WR, Ushay HM, Caravana C, Lippard SJ. Sequence dependent binding of cis-dichlorodiammineplatinum(II) to DNA. J Am Chem Soc 1980;102:2487–8.
21. Takahara PM, Frederick CA, Lippard SJ. Crystal structure of the anticancer drug cisplatin bound to duplex DNA. J Am Chem Soc 1996;118:12309–21.
22. Wong E, Giandomenico CM. Current status of platinum-based antitumor drugs. Chem Rev 1999;99:2451–66.
23. Kornberg RD, Lorch Y. Twenty-five years of the nucleosome, fundamental particle of the eukaryote chromosome. Cell 1999;98:285–94.
24. Lippard SJ, Hoeschele JD. Binding of cis- and trans-dichlorodiammineplatinum(II) to the nucleosome core. Proc Natl Acad Sci USA 1979;76:6091–5.
25. Ober M, Lippard SJ. Cisplatin damage overrides the predefined rotational setting of positioned nucleosomes. J Am Chem Soc 2007;129:6278–86.
26. Ober M, Lippard SJ. A 1,2-d(GpG) Cisplatin intrastrand cross-link influences the rotational and translational setting of DNA in nucleosomes. J Am Chem Soc 2008;130:2851–61.
27. Pinto AL, Lippard SJ. Sequence-dependent termination of in vitro DNA synthesis by cis- and trans-diamminedichloroplatinum(II). Proc Natl Acad Sci USA 1985;82:4616–9.
28. Cobo M, Isla D, Massuti B, et al. Customizing cisplatin based on quantitative excision repair cross-complementing 1 mRNA expression: a phase III trial in non-small-cell lung cancer. J Clin Oncol 2007;25:2747–54.
29. Rosell R, Cecere F, Santarpia M, Reguart N, Taron M. Predicting the outcome of chemotherapy for lung cancer. Curr Opin Pharmacol 2006;6:323–31.
30. Zhang CX, Chang PV, Lippard SJ. Identification of nuclear proteins that interact with platinum-modified DNA by photoaffinity labeling. J Am Chem Soc 2004;126:6536–7.
31. Guggenheim ER, Xu D, Zhang CX, Chang PV, Lippard SJ. Photo-affinity isolation and identification of proteins in cancer cell extracts that bind to platinum-modified DNA. 2008 ChemBioChem [in press].

Platinum Drugs and DNA Repair: Lessons from the NCI Panel and Clinical Correlates

Jacques Robert, Armelle Laurand, Delphine Meynard, and Valérie Le Morvan

Abstract To study the cellular and molecular determinants of sensitivity and resistance to the classical platinum compounds, we have mined the database of the National Cancer Institute, looking for associations between the expression of given proteins belonging to pathways involved in platinum drug processing, and in vitro sensitivity to platinum drugs. Such observations may shed light on the relative importance of different processes involved in platinum drug – induced cell death. For instance, the expression of HMGB1, which targets platinum-DNA adducts and prevents DNA repair, appears to be positively correlated with the cytotoxicity of all the platinum drugs tested. We also determined the effect of several gene polymorphisms of the DNA repair pathways on the in vitro cytotoxicity of platinum compounds. For instance, the asn118asn polymorphism in the *ERCC1* gene appears involved in the cytotoxicity of cisplatin and carboplatin, the variant cell lines being significantly less sensitive to these drugs than the wild-type cell lines or the heterozygous ones. In order to achieve better individualisation of platinum drugs prescriptions, the tracks provided by the NCI-60 panel could select the appropriate genes to be explored, at the level of either gene expression or polymorphisms. For instance, the exploration of HMGB1 expression as a predictor of drug response would be warranted.

Keywords Platinum drugs; NCI-60 panel; Gene expression profiles; Gene polymorphisms; DNA damage and repair

Introduction

The cellular processing of platinum drugs involves a great number of events, all of which may play a role in the ultimate efficiency of these drugs (1): uptake and efflux, formation of DNA adducts, recognition and repair of these adducts, transduction of DNA damage signals through various pathways, induction of cell

J. Robert (✉), A. Laurand, D. Meynard, and V.Le. Morvan
Institut Bergonié, Université Victor Segalen, Bordeaux, France
e-mail: Robert@bergonie.org

A. Bonetti et al. (eds.), *Platinum and Other Heavy Metal Compounds in Cancer Chemotherapy*, DOI: 10.1007/978-1-60327-459-3_19,
© Humana Press, a part of Springer Science + Business Media, LLC 2009

death. All these steps involve a large number of proteins, and the expression and/or intrinsic activity of these proteins may determine the level of sensitivity of a given cell line or tumour.

One of the possible models for studying the relative importance of different steps of drug processing in cell sensitivity is the NCI-60 panel, consisting of a panel of 60 human tumour cell lines that have been characterised both in terms of sensitivity to a large number of drugs and molecular characteristics such as gene expression profiles and gene polymorphisms. Data mining from the NCI-60 may lead to significant observations which can provide tracks for clinical evaluation of potential predictors of platinum drug efficacy. We have already shown that the molecular determinants of the in vitro cytotoxicity of cisplatin and oxaliplatin were considerably different, suggesting the existence of a particular mechanism of action for oxaliplatin (2). Recently, several studies have shown that differences in site-selectivity of platinum compounds could explain differences in pharmacological properties (3, 4).

In this study, we wanted to explore some of the pathways involved in recognition and repair of platinum drug-induced DNA damage, using the database of the NCI as well as personal results of single nucleotide polymorphisms (SNP) obtained on this model, combining the pharmacogenomic (gene expression profiles) to pharmacogenetic (polymorphisms) approaches.

Materials and Methods

The freely accessible database of the Developmental Therapeutic Program of the National Cancer Institute (http://dtp.nci.nih.gov) was explored at two levels: (1) for the data on cytotoxicity of five platinum compounds towards the 60-cell line panel (cisplatin, carboplatin, diaminocyclohexylplatin II, oxaliplatin, tetraplatin and iproplatin); (2) for the gene expression data of 32 genes involved in platinum transport and detoxification, DNA adduct formation, DNA repair by nucleotide excision repair and mismatch repair, and cell-cycle control.

In addition, a series of gene polymorphisms occurring in DNA repair were determined in DNA extracts of the NCI panel according to standard techniques involving PCR and restriction-fragment length polymorphisms (RFLP), as described previously (5).

The existence of correlations between platinum drug in vitro cytotoxicity and selected molecular features on gene polymorphisms and expression was sought and the results are presented below.

Results

Relationships Between Gene Expression and Platinum Cytotoxicity

Regarding platinum transport and detoxification, we have shown that, among ABC transporters, only the expression of the *ABCC1* gene (MRP1), as studied by semi-quantitative RT-PCR, was significantly negatively correlated with the cytotoxicity of the DACH platinum compounds ($p = 0.002$) but not with that of cisplatin and carboplatin. Among the copper transporters, ATP7A and ATP7B expressions did not correlate consistently with platinum drug cytotoxicity, but *SLC31A1* and *SLC31A2* gene expressions were significantly negatively correlated with the cytotoxicity of platinum drugs (Table 1).

The expressions of the glutathione-synthesising enzymes GCLC (glutamate-cysteine ligase) and GSS (glutamate-cysteine ligase) as well as those of glutathione S-transferases did not appear to be consistently related to platinum drug cytotoxicity, with the exception of GSTT2. In contrast, several metallothioneins, especially MT2A, had their expression significantly negatively correlated with the cytotoxicity of DACH platinum drugs, but not with that of cisplatin or carboplatin.

With regard to DNA adduct formation and repair, number of genes appeared to have their expression correlated with the toxicity of platinum drugs. This was the case for HMGB1, a protein targeting the platinum-DNA adducts and thereby preventing DNA repair, whose expression is positively correlated with the cytotoxicity of all the platinum drugs tested against the NCI-60 panel (Fig. 1). The same was the case for HGMB2, but only for the diaminocyclohexane-containing (DACH) platinum drugs, oxaliplatin and tetraplatin (Fig. 1).

At the level of nucleotide excision repair, the expression of ERCC1 was positively correlated with the cytotoxicity of cisplatin and carboplatin, but not the DACH platinum drugs (Fig. 2); while the expression of ERCC2 was negatively correlated with the cytotoxicity of oxaliplatin and tetraplatin, but not of cisplatin or carboplatin (Fig. 2). Expression of other proteins involved in NER (XPA, XPC, ERCC3, ERCC4, ERCC5) did not appear to play a major role in platinum drugs cytotoxicity in the NCI-60 model.

Regarding the proteins involved in mismatch repair (MMR), the expression of MSH2, and to a lesser extent MSH6, was correlated with the cytotoxicity of DACH platinum drugs, which may be related to the futile and inefficient mobilisation of these proteins to repair platinum-DNA adducts. In contrast, MLH1 expression did not present consistent significant correlations with the cytotoxicity of platinum drugs.

At the level of cell-cycle control, which has been shown to be involved in the response to platinum-induced DNA damage, it is remarkable that the expression of a number of proteins is positively correlated with platinum drug cytotoxicity, especially that of the DACH-platins. This is the case for ATR, CHK1, CHK2, RAD9A and CDC25A. This would mean that the efficiency in cell-cycle arrest could facilitate DNA repair and, therefore, enhance platinum-induced cell death.

Relationships Between Some Gene Polymorphisms and Platinum Cytotoxicity

Three polymorphisms occurring in the coding sequence of important NER genes were determined in the NCI panel: the synonymous SNP asn118asn of *ERCC1*, the non-synonymous SNPs asp312asn and lys751gln of *ERCC2* and the non-synonymous SNP asp1104his of *ERCC5*. Although there was no significant association between

Table 1 Summary of the relationships observed between the expression of genes related to platinum drug processing and the in vitro cytotoxicity of these drugs

Gene	Cisplatin carboplatin	DACH platins
ABCC1	No	Negative
ABCC2	No	No
ATPA7	No	No
ATPB7	No	No
ATOX1	No	No
SLC31A1	Negative	No
SLC31A2	Negative	Negative
SLC22A1	No	No
SLC22A2	No	No
GCLC	No	No
GSS	No	No
MT1M, MT1G	No	No
MT1H, MT1X	No	Negative
MT2A	Negative	Negative
MT3	No	No
GSTA1-A4	No	No
GSTM1-M5	No	No
GSTP1	No	No
GSTT1	No	No
GSTT2	No	Negative
GSTO1	No	No
GSTK1	No	No
GSTZ1	No	No
HMGB1	Positive	Positive
HMGB2	No	Positive
ERCC1	Positive	No
ERCC2	No	Negative
ERCC3	No	No
ERCC4	No	No
ERCC5	No	No
XPA	No	No
XPC	No	No
MLH1	No	No
MSH2	No	Positive
MSH6	No	Positive
RAG1	No	Positive
RAG2	No	No
ATR	Positive	Positive
ATM	No	No
PRKCD	No	No
CHK1	No	Positive
CHK2	No	Positive
RAD9A	No	Positive
CDC25A	Positive	Positive
CDC25B	No	No
CDC25C	No	No

No no significant expression was found between gene expression and platinum drug cytotoxicity
Positive gene expression was significantly correlated with drug sensitivity
Negative gene expression was significantly correlated with drug resistance

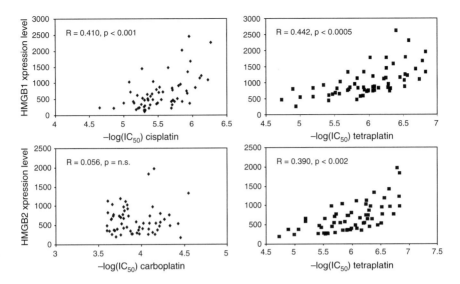

Fig. 1 Examples of relationship between cytotoxicity of platinum drugs vis-à-vis cell lines of the NCI-60 panel and expression of HMGB1 (*upper panel*) and HMGB2 (*lower panel*)

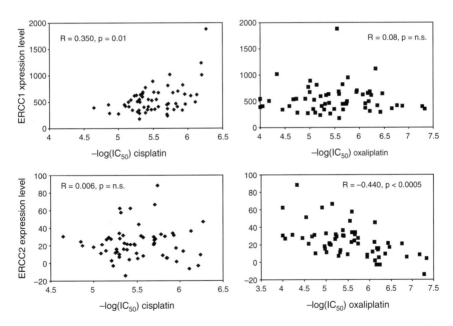

Fig. 2 Examples of relationship between cytotoxicity of platinum drugs vis-à-vis cell lines of the NCI-60 panel and expression of ERCC1 (*upper panel*) and ERCC2 (*lower panel*)

ERCC1 polymorphism and gene expression, cytotoxicity of cisplatin and carboplatin appeared higher in the homozygous variant cell lines (T/T genotype) than in the homozygous wild-type cell lines (C/C cell lines), and the heterozygous cell lines (T/C genotype) having an intermediate behaviour (Fig. 3). In the case for the DACH platinum drugs , cytotoxicity showed no association with *ERCC1* genotypes.

While the asp312asn SNP of *ERCC2* was associated with neither *ERCC2* gene expression nor platinum drugs cytotoxicity, the lys751gln SNP was associated with both *ERCC2* gene expression and platinum sensitivity: the homozygous variant cell lines (A/A genotype) presented lower gene expression and higher sensitivity to cisplatin and carboplatin than the homozygous wild-type cell lines (C/C genotype) or the heterozygous cell lines (A/C genotype). There again, the cytotoxicity of the DACH platinum drugs, in contrast, was not associated to *ERCC2* genotype. Finally, the *ERCC5* asp1104his SNP was related neither to *ERCC5* gene expression, nor to platinum drug sensitivity in the NCI-60 panel.

Discussion

Independent of the correlations that can be established in vitro between gene expression or polymorphisms and drug cytotoxicity, clinical studies have shown that several genes involved in NER played a role in patients' drug response to platinum compounds and post-treatment survival. It has been shown that the

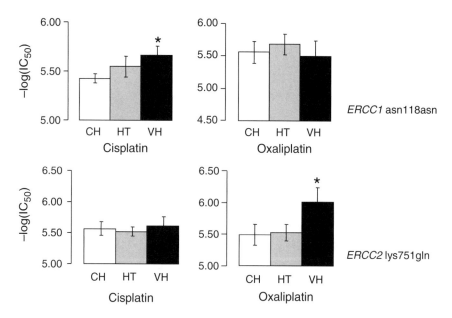

Fig. 3 Examples of relationships between cytotoxicity of platinum drugs vis-à-vis cell lines of the NCI-60 panel and polymorphims of *ERCC1* (*upper panel*) and *ERCC2* (*lower panel*). *CH* common homozygous cell lines; *HT* heterozygous cell lines; *VH* variant homozygous cell lines

expression of ERCC1 was associated with resistance to cisplatin in non-small cell lung cancer patients (6), the asn118asn SNP of *ERCC1* could be associated to oxaliplatin efficiency in colorectal cancer patients (7) to cisplatin resistance in non-small cell lung cancer patients (8), and that the lys751gln SNP of *ERCC2* was associated to the survival of colorectal patients treated with oxaliplatin (9).

Such studies are still preliminary and should be extended to larger number of patients, in a prospective setting thus firmly establishing the clinical correlations that exist between gene expression or polymorphism and drug sensitivity. In order to achieve better individualisation of prescriptions of platinum drugs, tracks provided by the NCI-60 panel could be used to select the appropriate genes to be explored, either at the level of expression or at the level of polymorphisms. For instance, the exploration of HMGB1 and HMGB2 expressions as predictors of drug response is warranted.

Differences between the processing of cisplatin- and oxaliplatin-induced DNA lesions are now considered of utmost interest for the understanding of the pharmacological and clinical differences between these two drugs, which do not share the same indications in cancer therapeutics. This is clearly corroborated in our analysis of the determinants of in vitro cytotoxicity of the two drugs. Analysis of the tumour tissue expression of the determinants of platinum drugs activity may be useful for the selection of cancer types which would be the most appropriate for clinical development.

References

1. Wang D, Lippard SJ. Cellular processing of platinum anticancer drugs. Nat Rev Drug Discov 2005;4:307–20.
2. Vekris A, Meynard D, Haaz MC, Bayssas M, Bonnet J, Robert J. Molecular determinants of the cytotoxicity of platinum compounds: the contribution of in silico research. Cancer Res 2004;64:356–62.
3. Sharma S, Gong P, Temple B, Bhattacharyya D, Dokholyan NV, Chaney SG. Molecular dynamic simulations of cisplatin- and oxaliplatin-d(GG) intrastrand cross-links reveal differences in their conformational dynamics. J Mol Biol 2007;373:1123–40.
4. Wu B, Dröge P, Davey CA. Site selectivity of platinum anticancer therapeutics. Nat Chem Biol 2008;4:110–2.
5. Le Morvan V, Bellott R, Moisan F, Mathoulin-Pélissier S, Bonnet J, Robert J. Relationships between genetic polymorphisms and anticancer drug cytotoxicity vis-à-vis the NCI-60 panel. Pharmacogenomics 2006;7:843–52.
6. Olaussen KA, Dunant A, Fouret P, et al. DNA repair by ERCC1 in non-small-cell lung cancer and cisplatin-based adjuvant chemotherapy. N Engl J Med 2006;355:983–91.
7. Viguier J, Boige V, Miquel C, et al. ERCC1 codon 118 polymorphism is a predictive factor for the tumor response to oxaliplatin/5-fluorouracil combination chemotherapy in patients with advanced colorectal cancer. Clin Cancer Res 2005;11:6212–7.
8. Ryu JS, Hong YC, Han HS, et al. Association between polymorphisms of ERCC1 and XPD and survival in non-small-cell lung cancer patients treated with cisplatin combination chemotherapy. Lung Cancer 2004;44:311–6.
9. Le Morvan V, Smith D, Laurand A, et al. Determination of ERCC2 Lys751Gln and GSTP1 Ile105Val gene polymorphisms in colorectal cancer patients: relationships with treatment outcome. Pharmacogenomics 2007;8:1693–703.

Differences in Conformation and Conformational Dynamics Between Cisplatin and Oxaliplatin DNA Adducts

Stephen G. Chaney, Srinivas Ramachandran, Shantanu Sharma, Nikolay V. Dokholyan, Brenda Temple, Debadeep Bhattacharyya, Yibing Wu, and Sharon Campbell

Abstract Some DNA damage-recognition proteins, transcription factors, mismatch repair proteins and DNA polymerases discriminate between cisplatin (CP)- and oxaliplatin (OX)-GG DNA adducts, and this is thought to help explain differences in efficacy, toxicity and mutagenicity of CP and OX. In addition, differential recognition of CP- and OX-GG adducts by some proteins has been shown to be highly dependent on the sequence context of the Pt-GG adduct. We have postulated that CP- and OX-GG adducts cause differences in the conformation and/or conformational dynamics of the DNA that provide the basis for differential protein recognition of the adducts. We have determined the NMR solution structure of CP-GG adducts, OX-GG adducts and undamaged DNA in the AGGC sequence context, and of OX-GG adducts and undamaged DNA in the TGGT sequence context. We have also employed molecular dynamics (MD) simulations to investigate the conformational dynamics of CP-GG adducts, OX-GG adducts and undamaged DNA in the AGGC and TGGA sequence contexts. These studies showed clear differences in the conformation dynamics between CP- and OX-GG adducts which correlated with the average conformational differences observed in the NMR solution structures and with conformations previously reported for the CP-GG DNA·HMG1a complex. When the conformational dynamics in both sequence contexts were compared it became evident that: (a) the patterns of hydrogen bond formation between Pt-amine-hydrogens and surrounding bases of the DNA were different for CP- and OX-GG adducts; (b) patterns of hydrogen bond formation were also influenced by the DNA sequence context of the Pt-GG adducts, and (c) differences in patterns of hydrogen bond formation were highly correlated with differences in the conformational dynamics of the adduct. Thus, we postulate that patterns of hydrogen bond formation between Pt-amine hydrogens and surrounding DNA bases are different for CP- and OX-GG adducts, and that those differences in hydrogen bond patterns result in DNA conformational differences that allow selective recognition of CP- and

S.G. Chaney (✉), S. Ramachandran, S. Sharma, N.V. Dokholyan,
B.Temple, D. Bhattacharyya, Y. Wu, and S. Campbell
Department of Biochemistry and Biophysics, School of Medicine,
University of North Carolina, Chapel Hill, NC, USA
e-mail : stephen_chaney@med.unc.edu

A. Bonetti et al. (eds.), *Platinum and Other Heavy Metal Compounds in Cancer Chemotherapy*, DOI: 10.1007/978-1-60327-459-3_20,
© Humana Press, a part of Springer Science + Business Media, LLC 2009

OX-GG adducts by a number of proteins that determine the relative cytotoxicity and mutagenicity of those adducts.

Keywords Cisplatin; Oxaliplatin; DNA adducts; Conformational dynamics; DNA damage and repair

Introduction

Cisplatin [CP, *cis*-diamminedichloroplatinum(II)] and carboplatin [CBDCA, *cis*-diammine-1,1-cyclobutanedicarboxylatoplatinum(II)] are widely used in treating several types of cancers such as ovarian, testicular, head and neck tumors. However, many tumors show resistance or develop acquired resistance towards CP or CBDCA. Tumors that are resistant to these drugs are usually cross-resistant to the other drug. CP also exhibits mutagenic properties in vivo (1) which have been associated with secondary malignancies (2). Oxaliplatin [OX, *trans*-(*R,R*)-1,2-diaminocyclohexaneoxalatoplatinum(II)] is a third-generation platinum anticancer agent and has been approved for treatment of colorectal cancer and cisplatin-resistant tumors. While OX does exhibit some mutagenicity (3), it is less mutagenic than CP (4). Although the reasons for differences in tumor range and mutagenicity of OX compared to those of CP and CBDCA are not known, these differences are thought to be determined by the discriminating ability of proteins that are involved in damage recognition, damage repair, and/or damage tolerance. For example, hMSH2 and MutS bind with greater affinity to CP-GG adducts than to OX-GG adducts (5, 6), and defects in mismatch repair result in resistance to CP and CBDCA, but not to OX (5, 7–10). In addition, several transcription factors and damage recognition proteins have been shown to discriminate between CP- and OX-GG adducts (11, 12). The binding specificity has been determined for only a few of these proteins, but where it has been studied, they bind to CP-GG adducts with higher affinity than to OX-GG adducts (11–13). Moreover, translesion DNA polymerases such as pol β and pol η have been shown to bypass OX-GG adducts with higher efficiency than CP-GG adducts (14–16), which might, at least partially, explain the difference in mutagenicity of CP and OX.

We have obtained high-resolution solution NMR structures of the OX-GG adduct (17), the CP-GG adduct and undamaged DNA (18) in the AGGC sequence context and the OX-GG adduct and undamaged DNA duplex (manuscript in preparation) in the TGGT sequence context. These were the first NMR solution structures of the OX-GG adduct and the first structures of any Pt-GG adduct in a DNA sequence context with a purine on the 5′ side of the adduct. While NMR structures were useful in assessing differences in the average conformation of Pt-DNA adducts in solution, molecular dynamic (MD) simulations are needed to assess differences in the conformational dynamics of these Pt-DNA adducts. Consequently, MD simulations were performed on Pt-DNA adducts in the AGGC and TGGA sequence contexts. Data obtained from these studies permit clear distinction between the effects of the Pt-GG intrastrand adduct, the carrier ligand of the Pt-GG adduct (*cis*-diammine vs. diaminocyclohexane), and the sequence context of the adduct (A<u>GG</u>C vs T<u>GG</u>T (NMR) or T<u>GG</u>A (MD)) on both DNA conformation and conformational dynamics in the vicinity of the adducts.

NMR Solution Structures

Conformational Flexibility on the 5′ Side of the Adduct

Previous studies in our laboratory (17, 18) (manuscript in preparation) and other laboratories (17–20) have shown that imino proton resonance of the 5′G of a Pt-<u>GG</u> adduct is more solvent accessible than that of the 3′G. This data suggests that the DNA may be more distorted and/or flexible on the 5′ side of the adduct.

In addition to the higher solvent exchange rate exhibited by the <u>G</u>6 and <u>G</u>7 imino protons, the T5 imino proton in the T<u>GG</u>T sequence context also possesses a fast exchange rate, which is comparable to that shown by the <u>G</u>6 imino proton (manuscript in preparation). We hypothesize that the distortion and flexibility observed on the 5′-side of the Pt-GG adduct is extended to the 5′-flanking residue base pair, corresponding to the T5·A20 base pair for the OX-<u>GG</u> adduct in the T<u>GG</u>T sequence context. This feature was not observed for undamaged DNA or reported previously for CP-<u>GG</u> adducts in the C<u>GG</u>C sequence context (20) or for either CP- and OX-<u>GG</u> adducts in the A<u>GG</u>C sequence context (17). While those 5′ flanking bases do not possess imino proton signals, their complementary bases (G and T) in the opposing strand do possess imino signals; and no solvent accessibility was observed for those imino protons. This data suggests that the 5′-flanking residue of Pt-<u>GG</u> adducts in the T<u>GG</u>T sequence context may exhibit greater flexibility than that of the C<u>GG</u>C or A<u>GG</u>C sequence contexts. This is best understood in terms of the molecular dynamics studies reported below.

DNA Helical Parameters Common to All Pt-<u>GG</u> Adducts

The CP-<u>GG</u> and OX-<u>GG</u> adducts that we have studied (17, 18) (manuscript in preparation) are similar to all other Pt-<u>GG</u> structures reported to date in that they display an increase in roll at the <u>G</u>6-<u>G</u>7 base-pair step, <u>G</u>6-<u>G</u>7 dihedral angle and overall bend angle compared to undamaged DNA (19–23). We hypothesize that these common conformational features of Pt-<u>GG</u> adducts, which are centered around the <u>G</u>6-<u>G</u>7 base-pair step, are important for recognition of both CP- and OX-<u>GG</u> adducts by DNA-binding proteins. It is logical that the <u>G</u>6-<u>G</u>7 base-pair step would be crucial for the recognition of Pt-<u>GG</u> adducts by DNA-binding proteins. Both mismatch-repair proteins and HMG-domain proteins bend the DNA in the direction of the major groove in part, by inserting an amino acid residue between the base pairs at the center of the bend (which in this case would be the <u>G</u>6-<u>G</u>7 base-pair step) (24–27).

Marzilli et al. (20) reported that all structures of Pt-<u>GG</u> adducts available at that time were characterized by a large positive slide and shift for the base-pair step on the 5′ side of the adduct (which would correspond to the A5-<u>G</u>6 base-pair step for the A<u>GG</u>C sequence and the T5-<u>G</u>6 base-pair step for the T<u>GG</u>T sequence) and concluded that should also be considered as a characteristic of all Pt-<u>GG</u> adducts. Our structures of the CP- and OX-<u>GG</u> adducts in the A<u>GG</u>C sequence context (17, 18) were the first of Pt-<u>GG</u> adducts with a purine on the 5′ side of the adduct, and we did not observe a large positive slide and shift at the A5-<u>G</u>6 base-pair step of those adducts. Furthermore, for the T5-<u>G</u>6 base-pair step of the OX-T<u>GG</u>T adduct we observed a large positive slide, but a slightly negative shift. Thus, while all Pt-<u>GG</u> adducts appear to have significant distortions on the 5′ side of the adduct, the exact nature of these distortions is dependent on both sequence context and the nature of the carrier ligand.

DNA Helical Parameters that Distinguish Between CP and OX-<u>GG</u> Adducts

Comparison of DNA helical parameters of the CP-<u>GG</u> adduct in the A<u>GG</u>C sequence context with the DNA helical parameters of the OX-<u>GG</u> adducts in both the A<u>GG</u>C and T<u>GG</u>T sequenced contexts has also allowed us to identify conformational differences between CP-<u>GG</u> and OX-<u>GG</u> adducts that may be relatively independent of sequence context. Specifically, the CP-<u>GG</u> adduct in the A<u>GG</u>C sequence context differs from both OX-<u>GG</u> adducts in slide, twist, and roll at the <u>G</u>6·C19-<u>G</u>7·C18 base-pair step, shift and slide at the <u>G</u>7·C18-C8·G17 base-pair step, opening for the <u>G</u>7·C18 base pair and <u>G</u>6<u>G</u>7 dihedral angle (Table 1). While structures of Pt-GG adducts in more sequence contexts will need to be examined under the same experimental conditions to confirm that these conformational differences of CP- and OX-<u>GG</u> adducts are independent of sequence contexts, we hypothesize that these differences are important for the sequence-independent, differential recognition of CP- and OX-<u>GG</u>

Table 1 Comparison of DNA helical parameters for CP-DNA and OX-DNA in the A<u>GG</u>C and T<u>GG</u>T sequence contexts

Parameters	CP-A<u>GG</u>C	OX-A<u>GG</u>C	OX-T<u>GG</u>T
<u>G</u>6·C19-<u>G</u>7·C18			
Slide (Å)	−0.55 ± 0.10	−1.36 ± 0.30	−0.95 ± 0.07
Twist (°)	18.4 ± 1.4	25.2 ± 2.0	24.99 ± 2.78
Roll (°)	36.3 ± 3.2	28.3 ± 3.2	46.6 ± 2.3
<u>G</u>7·C18-C/T8·G/A17			
Shift (Å)	−0.99 ± 0.17	−1.24 ± 0.10	−0.44 ± 0.25
Slide (Å)	−0.33 ± 0.13	0.93 ± 0.10	−1.02 ± 0.76
<u>G</u>7·C18			
Opening (°)	−1.24 ± 0.93	5.73 ± 0.53	5.91 ± 1.86
<u>G</u>6-<u>G</u>7			
Dihedral Angle (°)	42.7 ± 3.1	35.6 ± 2.8	38.2 ± 3.1

Table 2 Comparison of DNA helical parameters for
OX-DNA in the A<u>GG</u>C and T<u>GG</u>T sequence contexts

Parameters	OX-A<u>GG</u>C	OX-T<u>GG</u>T
A/T5·T/A20-<u>G</u>6·C19		
Shift (Å)	0.17 ± 0.04	−0.31 ± 0.36
Slide (Å)	−0.89 ± 0.10	1.67 ± 0.31
Twist (°)	22.1 ± 1.3	36.7 ± 4.5
<u>G</u>6·C19-<u>G</u>7·C18		
Roll (°)	28.3 ± 3.2	46.6 ± 2.3
<u>G</u>7·C18-C/T8·G/A17		
Shift (Å)	−1.24 ± 0.10	−0.44 ± 0.25
Slide (Å)	0.93 ± 0.10	−1.02 ± 0.08
<u>G</u>6·C19		
Buckle (°)	12.6 ± 2.4	6.8 ± 1.0

adducts by DNA-binding proteins. Most of these conformational differences lie on the 3′ side of the adduct, which is consistent with the observation that the damage-recognition protein HMG1a binds primarily to the 3′ side of the adduct (24).

Finally, comparison of DNA helical parameters between OX-<u>GG</u> adducts in the T<u>GG</u>T and A<u>GG</u>C (17) sequence contexts has allowed us to identify some of the conformational features of the OX-<u>GG</u> adduct that are affected by sequence context. This comparison showed significant differences in the shift, slide, and twist at the A/T5·T/A20-<u>G</u>6·C19 base-pair step, roll at the <u>G</u>6·C19-<u>G</u>7·C18 base-pair step, shift and slide at the <u>G</u>7·C18-C/T8·G/A17 base-pair step, and buckle of the <u>G</u>6·C19 base pair (Table 2). We hypothesize that some of these conformational distortions, which are found on both the 5′ and 3′ side of CP- and OX-<u>GG</u> adducts, influence the affinity of DNA-binding for the Pt-<u>GG</u> adducts and are likely to explain the influence of sequence context on the ability of the DNA-binding proteins to discriminate between CP-<u>GG</u> and OX-<u>GG</u> adducts.

MD Simulations and Differences in Conformational Dynamics

The Effect of the Diaminocyclohexane Ring on N–Pt–N Bond Angles

We then used molecular dynamics simulations to explore differences in the conformational dynamics between OX-<u>GG</u>, CP-<u>GG</u> and undamaged DNA in the A<u>GG</u>C (28) and T<u>GG</u>A sequence contexts. In theoretical terms, the most obvious effects of the diaminocyclohexane ring of oxaliplatin are to constrain the bond angle between the Pt and the two amines of diaminocyclohexane. This can be clearly seen when one compares the conformational range of the four possible N–Pt–N bond angles of CP-<u>GG</u> and OX-<u>GG</u> adducts (Fig. 1). The conformational

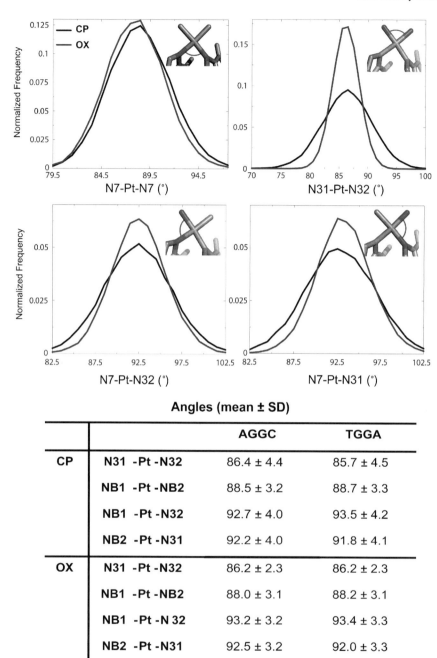

Fig. 1 Frequency distribution of platinum bond angles in the A<u>GG</u>C and T<u>GG</u>A sequence contexts. The *upper panel* shows frequency distribution of platinum bond angles in the A<u>GG</u>C sequence contexts. Table compares mean ± standard deviation for the same bond angles in the A<u>GG</u>C and T<u>GG</u>A sequence contexts

dynamics of the NB1(G6N7)–Pt–NB2(G7N7) bond angles are essentially identical for CP- and OX-GG adducts because that bond angle is primarily constrained by the DNA backbone. However, the cyclohexane ring of the OX-GG adduct strongly restricts the conformational range of N31–Pt–N32 bond angle and places modest constraints on the NB1–Pt–N32 and NB2–Pt–N31 bond angles compared to the CP-GG adduct. While the figure only shows bond angles for CP-GG and OX-GG adducts in the AGGC sequence context, these effects were essentially independent of sequence context.

The Effect of N–Pt–N Bond Flexibility and Sequence Context on Hydrogen Bond Occupancy

We next looked at hydrogen bond occupancy (the percentage of time that various hydrogen bonds formed during the simulation). As might be expected, we observed close to 100% occupancy for most of the Watson-Crick hydrogen bonds except for the ones involving the G•C base pairs containing the Pt-GG adduct (G6 and G7). However, we also observed significant formation of hydrogen bonds between the Pt-amines and the surrounding bases. The pattern of hydrogen bond formation was highly dependent on the sequence context of the Pt-GG adduct, and the occupancy of those hydrogen bonds was different for CP-GG and OX-GG adducts. For example, in the AGGC sequence context, the CP-GG adduct preferentially formed hydrogen bonds between the 5′ Pt-amine and A5N7, while the OX-GG adduct preferentially formed hydrogen bonds between the 3′ Pt-amine and G7O6 (Fig. 2). In the TGGA sequence context, the CP-GG adduct preferentially formed hydrogen bonds with A8N7 and the OX-GG adduct with G7O6 and T17O4 (Fig. 3). This data suggests that the greater conformational flexibility of the CP-GG adduct allows it to form hydrogen bonds with the adjacent bases on the same strand of the DNA, while conformation of the OX-GG adduct allows hydrogen bond formation with a 3′ base on the opposite strand of DNA. The obvious question then is how these differences in the pattern of hydrogen bond formation influence DNA conformation.

The Effect of Hydrogen Bond Occupancy on Flexibility on the 5′ side of Pt-GG Adducts

While this difference in conformational flexibility of a 5′ flanking T residue relative to a 5′ flanking A residue in the NMR experiments described earlier is difficult to explain in terms of standard Watson-Crick hydrogen bonds, it is fully consistent with the hydrogen bond occupancy between Pt-amines and the adjacent base pairs

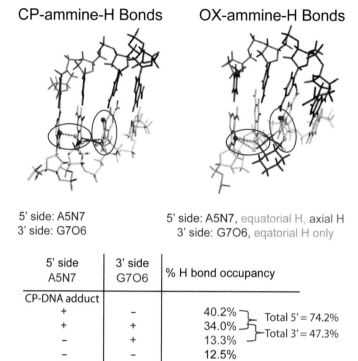

CP-ammine-H Bonds   OX-ammine-H Bonds

5' side: A5N7   5' side: A5N7, equatorial H, axial H
3' side: G7O6   3' side: G7O6, eqatorial H only

5' side A5N7	3' side G7O6	% H bond occupancy
CP-DNA adduct		
+	–	40.2% ⎤ Total 5' = 74.2%
+	+	34.0% ⎦
–	+	13.3% ⎤ Total 3' = 47.3%
–	–	12.5% ⎦
OX-DNA adduct		
+ (ax)	–	7.7% ⎤
+ (eq)	–	6.0% ⎥ Total 5' = 58.1%
+ (ax)	+	3.5% ⎥
+ (eq)	+	40.9% ⎦ ⎤ Total 3' = 78.7%
–	+	34.3% ⎦
–	–	7.6%

Fig. 2 Hydrogen bonds between Pt-amine hydrogens and surrounding bases in the A<u>GG</u>C sequence context. Structures illustrating observed hydrogen bond formation are shown in the *upper panel.* Table indicates the percent hydrogen bond occupancy (the % of time that the hydrogen bond is observed during the trajectory) for each of those hydrogen bonds (*see Color Plates*)

observed in molecular dynamic simulations. In the Pt-A<u>GG</u>C simulations, hydrogen bond formation between the Pt-amine hydrogens on the 5′ side of the adduct and the N7 of the 5′A residue was observed between 58% (OX-A<u>GG</u>C adduct) and 74% (CP-A<u>GG</u>C adduct) of the time (28). The formation of this hydrogen bond might be expected to significantly decrease the conformational flexibility of the 5′ A. In contrast, almost no hydrogen bond formation was seen between the 5′ Pt-amine hydrogens and the 5′ T residue for either CP-<u>GG</u> or OX-<u>GG</u> adducts in the T<u>GG</u>A sequence context.

Fig. 3 Hydrogen bonds between Pt-amine hydrogens and surrounding bases in the TGGA sequence context. Structures illustrating observed hydrogen bond formation are shown in the *upper panel*. Table indicates the percent hydrogen bond occupancy (the % of time that the hydrogen bond is observed during the trajectory) for each of those hydrogen bonds (*see Color Plates*)

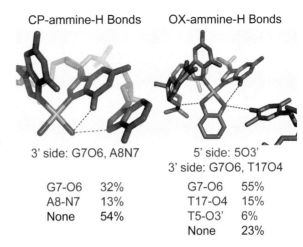

CP-ammine-H Bonds   OX-ammine-H Bonds

3' side: G7O6, A8N7   5' side: 5O3'
                            3' side: G7O6, T17O4

G7-O6	32%		G7-O6	55%
A8-N7	13%		T17-O4	15%
None	54%		T5-O3'	6%
			None	23%

The Effect of Patterns of Hydrogen Bond Occupancy on DNA Conformation

When we examined the conformational dynamics of DNA helical parameters in the vicinity of the Pt-GG adducts, it was evident that there were some significant differences between CP-GG and OX-GG adducts. For example, in the AGGC sequence context, CP-GG adducts differed from OX-GG adducts in terms of G6·C19 buckle, G6·C19 propeller twist, G7·C18 propeller twist, C8·G17 buckle, A5·T20-G6·C19 slide, G6·C19-G7·C18 slide and G7·C16-C8·G17 slide and shift (28).

To determine whether the conformational dynamics of CP- and OX-DNA adducts might be influenced by the formation of the hydrogen bonds between the Pt-amines and surrounding bases, the trajectory data for DNA helical parameters for the central four base pairs were separated according to patterns of hydrogen bond formation. When this was done, there was clear association between the pattern of hydrogen bond formation for each Pt-GG adduct and the conformational dynamics of the DNA in the vicinity of the adduct. For example, the conformational dynamics of G6·C19 and G7·C18 propeller twist are shown in Fig. 4. When the overall frequency distributions of these parameters are compared (Fig. 4a), one observes subtle differences in the conformational dynamics for CP- and OX-GG adducts. When the frequency distributions of these DNA helical parameters are segregated according to hydrogen bond pattern for the CP-GG adduct (Fig. 4b), the conformation range is clearly different for the A5N7 hydrogen bond on the 5′ side of the adduct compared to the G7O6 hydrogen bond on the 3′ side of the adduct. Similar segregation according to hydrogen bond pattern is observed for the OX-GG adduct (Fig. 4c). Finally, the frequency distributions associated with the most abundant hydrogen bond patterns (A5N7 plus both 5′ and 3′ account for 74.2% of

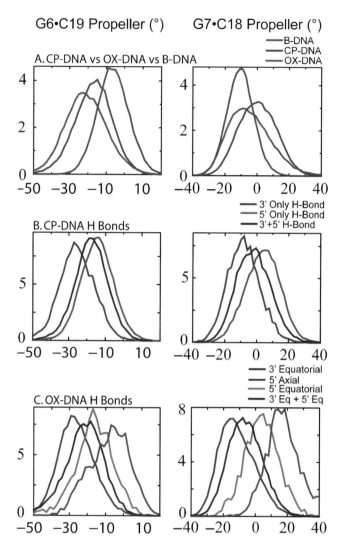

Fig. 4 Effect of patterns of hydrogen bond formation on the frequency distribution of G6·C19 and G7·C18 propeller twist for CP- and OX-<u>GG</u> adducts in the A<u>GG</u>C sequence context. (**a**) Overall frequency distribution for CP-<u>GG</u> (*green*), OX-<u>GG</u> (*red*) and undamaged DNA (*blue*). (**b**) Effect of hydrogen bond pattern on the frequency distribution for CP-<u>GG</u> adducts (5′ A5N7 = *blue*, 3′ <u>G</u>7O6 = *red* & both 5′ and 3′ = *purple*). (**c**) Effect of hydrogen bond pattern on the frequency distribution for OX-<u>GG</u> adducts (5′ axial A5N7 = *blue*, 5′ equatorial A5N7 = *cyan*, 3′ equatorial <u>G</u>7O6 = *red* & both 5′ equatorial and 3′ equatorial = *purple*) (*see Color Plates*)

hydrogen bond occupancy for CP-<u>GG</u>, and G7O6 plus both 5′ and 3′ account for 78.7% of hydrogen bond occupancy for OX-<u>GG</u>) are closely correlated with the overall differences observed in those DNA helical parameters for CP- and OX-<u>GG</u> adducts (Fig. 5).

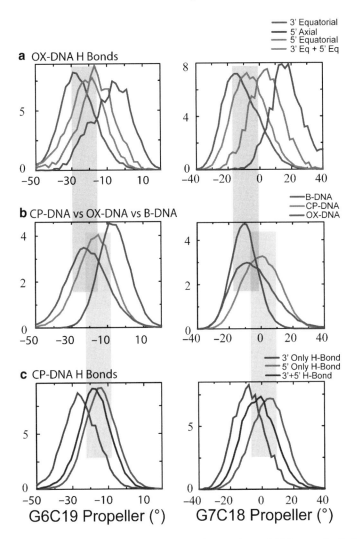

Fig. 5 Correlation between patterns of hydrogen bond formation and differences in the frequency distribution of G6·C19 and G7·C18 propeller twist for CP- and OX-<u>GG</u> adducts in the A<u>GG</u>C sequence context. (**a**) Effect of hydrogen bond pattern on the frequency distribution for OX-<u>GG</u> adducts (5′ axial A5N7 = *blue*, 5′ equatorial A5N7 = *cyan*, 3′ equatorial <u>G</u>7O6 = *red* & both 5′ equatorial and 3′ equatorial = *green*). (**b**) Overall frequency distribution for CP-<u>GG</u> (*green*), OX-<u>GG</u> (*red*) and undamaged DNA (*blue*). (**c**) Effect of hydrogen bond pattern on the frequency distribution for CP-<u>GG</u> adducts (5′ A5N7 = *blue*, 3′ <u>G</u>7O6 = *red* & both 5′ and 3′ = *purple*). *Blue rectangle* indicates correlation between the frequency distribution associated with the most frequently formed hydrogen bonds for OX-<u>GG</u> (total hydrogen bond occupancy for 3′ equatorial plus 3′ and 5′ = 78.7%) and the overall frequency distribution for OX-<u>GG</u> adducts. *Green rectangle* indicates correlation between the frequency distribution associated with the most frequently formed hydrogen bonds for CP-<u>GG</u> (total hydrogen bond occupancy for 5′ A5N7 plus 5′ and 3′ = 74.2%) and the overall frequency distribution for CP-<u>GG</u> adducts (*see Color Plates*)

Conformational Dynamics and the Differential Recognition of CP- and OX-<u>GG</u> Adducts by Damage Recognition Proteins

Data from molecular dynamics simulations suggest a hypothetical model for the differential recognition of CP- and OX-<u>GG</u> adducts by damage recognition proteins and the effect of DNA sequence context on that recognition. We propose that:

1. CP-<u>GG</u> adducts have a greater flexibility with respect to both Pt-amine bond angles and Pt-amine dihedral angles than OX-<u>GG</u> adducts because of constraints imposed by the diaminocyclohexane ring of the OX-<u>GG</u> adduct.
2. This greater flexibility allows the CP-<u>GG</u> adduct to more readily form Pt-amine hydrogen bonds with adjacent bases on the same strand of DNA than OX-<u>GG</u> adducts. At the same time the OX-<u>GG</u> adducts have some unique conformational features that allow them to form Pt-amine hydrogen bonds with bases on the opposite strand than CP-<u>GG</u> adducts.
3. These differences in the patterns of hydrogen bond formation correlate with differences in conformational dynamics that may be important for Pt-DNA adduct recognition by damage recognition proteins.

References

1. Greene MH. Is cisplatin a human carcinogen? J Nat Cancer Inst 1992;84:306–12.
2. Travis LB, Curtis RE, Storm H, et al. Risk of second malignant neoplasms among long-term survivors of testicular cancer. J Natl Cancer Inst 1997;89:1429–39.
3. Silva MJ, Costa P, Dias A, Valente M, Louro H, Boavida MG. Comparative analysis of the mutagenic activity of oxaliplatin and cisplatin in the *Hprt* gene of CHO cells. Environ Mol Mutagen 2005;46:104–15.
4. Bassett E, King NM, Bryant MF, et al. The role of DNA polymerase eta in translesion synthesis past platinum-DNA adducts in human fibroblasts. Cancer Res 2004;64:6469–75.
5. Zdraveski ZZ, Mello JA, Farinelli CK, Essigmann JM, Marinus MG. MutS preferentially recognizes cisplatin- over oxaliplatin-modified DNA. J Biol Chem 2002;277:1255–60.
6. Fink D, Nebel S, Aebi S, et al. The role of mismatch repair in platinum drug resistance. Cancer Res 1996;56:4881–6.
7. Aebi S, Kurdi-Haidar B, Zheng H, et al. Loss of DNA mismatch repair in acquired resistance to cisplatin. Cancer Res 37;3087–90.
8. Fink D, Zheng H, Nebel S, et al. In vitro and in vivo resistance to cisplatin in cells that have lost DNA mismatch repair. Cancer Res 1997;57:1841–5.
9. Vaisman A, Varchenko M, Umar A, et al. The role of hMLH1, hMSH3, and hMSH6 defects in cisplatin and oxaliplatin resistance: correlation with replicative bypass of platinum-DNA adducts. Cancer Res 1998;58:3579–85.
10. Brown R, Hirst GL, Gallagher WM, et al. hMLH1 expression and cellular responses of ovarian tumour cells to treatment with cytotoxic anticancer agents. Oncogene 1997;15:45–52.
11. Wei M, Cohen SM, Silverman AP, Lippard SJ. Effects of spectator ligands on the specific recognition of intrastrand platinum-DNA cross-links by high mobility group box and TATA-binding proteins. J Biol Chem 2001;276:38774–80.

12. Zhai X, Beckmann H, Jantzen H-M, Essigmann JM. Cisplatin-DNA adducts inhibit ribosomal RNA synthesis by hijacking the transcription factor human upstream binding factor. Biochemistry 1998;37:16307–15.

13. Coin F, Frit P, Viollet B, Salles B, Egly JM. TATA binding protein discriminates between different lesions on DNA, resulting in a transcription decrease. Mol Cell Biol 1998;18:3907–14.

14. Vaisman A, Lim SE, Patrick SM, et al. Effect of DNA polymerases and high mobility group protein 1 on the carrier ligand specificity for translesion synthesis past platinum-DNA adducts. Biochemistry 1999;38:11026–39.

15. Vaisman A, Chaney SG. The efficiency and fidelity of translesion synthesis past cisplatin and oxaliplatin GpG adducts by human DNA polymerase beta. J Biol Chem 2000;27:13017–25.

16. Vaisman A, Masutani C, Hanaoka F, Chaney SG. Efficient translesion replication past oxaliplatin and cisplatin GpG adducts by human DNA polymerase eta. Biochemistry 2000;39:4575–80.

17. Wu Y, Pradhan P, Havener J, et al. NMR solution structure of an oxaliplatin 1,2-d(GG) intrastrand cross-link in a DNA dodecamer duplex. J Mol Biol 2004;341:1251–69.

18. Wu Y, Bhattacharyya D, King CL, et al. Solution structures of a DNA dodecamer duplex with and without a cisplatin 1,2-d(GG) intrastrand cross-link: comparison with the same DNA duplex containing an oxaliplatin 1,2-d(GG) intrastrand cross-link. Biochemistry 2007;46:6477–87

19. Yang D, van Bloom SSGE, Reedijk J, van Bloom JH, Wang AHJ. Structure and isomerization of an intrastrand cisplatin-cross-linked octamer DNA duplex by NMR analysis. Biochemistry 1995;34:12912–20.

20. Marzilli LG, Saad JS, Kuklenyik Z, Keating KA, Xu Y. Relationship of solution and protein-bound structures of DNA duplexes with the major intrastrand cross-link lesions formed on cisplatin binding to DNA. J Am Chem Soc 2001;123:2764–70.

21. Herman F, Kozelka J, Stoven V, et al. A d(GpG)-platinated decanucleotide duplex is kinked an extended NMR and molecular mechanics study. Eur J Biochem 1990;194:119–33.

22. Gelasco A, Lippard SJ. NMR solution structure of a DNA dodecamer duplex containing a cis-diammineplatinum(II) dGpG intrastrand cross-link, the major adduct of the anticancer drug cisplatin. Biochemistry 1998;37:9230–9.

23. Takahara PM, Frederick CA, Lippard SJ. Crystal structure of the anticancer drug cisplatin bound to duplex DNA. J Am Chem Soc 1996;118:12309–21.

24. Ohndorf UM, Rould MA, He Q, Pabo CO, Lippard SJ. Basis for recognition of cisplatin-modified DNA by high-mobility-group proteins. Nature 1999;399:708–12.

25. Love JJ, Li X, Case DA, Giese K, Grosschedl R, Wright PE. Structural basis for DNA bending by the architectural transcription factor LEF-1. Nature 1995;376:791–5.

26. Werner MH, Huth JR, Gronenborn AM, Clore GM. Molecular basis of human 46X,Y sex reversal revealed from the three-dimensional solution structure of the human SRY-DNA complex. Cell 1995;81:705–14.

27. Murphy EC, Zhurkin VB, Louis JM, Cornilescu G, Clore GM. Structural basis for SRY-dependent 46-X,Y sex reversal: modulation of DNA bending by a naturally occurring point mutation. J Mol Biol 2001;312:481–99.

28. Sharma S, Gong P, Temple B, Bhattacharyya D, Dokholyan NV, Chaney SG. Molecular dynamic simulations of cisplatin- and oxaliplatin-d(GG) intrastrand cross-links reveal differences in their conformational dynamics. J Mol Biol 2007;373:1123–40.

Regrowth Resistance: Low-Level Platinum Resistance Mediated by Rapid Recovery from Platinum-Induced Cell-Cycle Arrest

Britta Stordal and Ross Davey

Abstract The H69CIS200 and H69OX400 cell lines are novel models of low-level platinum drug resistance developed from H69 human small-cell lung cancer cells with eight 4-day treatments of 200 ng/ml cisplatin and 400 ng/ml oxaliplatin, respectively. A recovery period was given between treatments to emulate the cycles of chemotherapy given in the clinic. The resistant cell lines were approximately twofold resistant to cisplatin and oxaliplatin, and were cross-resistant to both drugs. Platinum resistance was not associated with increased cellular glutathione, decreased accumulation of platinum or increased DNA repair capacity. The H69 platinum sensitive cells entered a lengthy 3-week growth arrest in response to low-level cisplatin or oxaliplatin treatment. This is an example of the coordinated response between the cell cycle and DNA repair. In contrast, the H69CIS200 and H69OX400 cells have an alteration in the cell cycle allowing them to rapidly proliferate post drug treatment. The resistant cell lines also have many chromosomal rearrangements most of which are not associated with the resistant phenotype, suggesting an increase in the genomic instability in the resistant cell lines. We hypothesized that there was a lack of coordination between the cell cycle and DNA repair in the resistant cell lines allowing proliferation in the presence of DNA damage which has created an increase in genomic instability. The H69 cells and resistant cell lines have mutant p53 and consequently decrease the expression of p21 in response to platinum drug treatment; promoting progression of the cell cycle instead of increasing p21 to maintain the arrest. A decrease in ERCC1 protein expression and an increase in RAD51B foci activity were observed with the platinum-induced cell-cycle arrest and did not correlate with resistance or altered DNA repair capacity. These changes may, in part, be mediating and maintaining the cell-cycle arrest in place of p21.The rapidly proliferating resistant cells have restored the levels of both these proteins to their levels in untreated cells. We use the term "regrowth resistance" to describe this low-level platinum resistance where cells survive treatment through increased proliferation. Regrowth resistance may play a role in the onset of clinical resistance.

B. Stordal (✉) and R. Davey
Bill Walsh Cancer Research Laboratories, Department of Medical Oncology, Royal North Shore Hospital and the University of Sydney, Australia
e-mail : bstordal@med.usyd.edu.au or britta.stordal@dcu.ie

A. Bonetti et al. (eds.), *Platinum and Other Heavy Metal Compounds in Cancer Chemotherapy*, DOI: 10.1007/978-1-60327-459-3_21,
© Humana Press, a part of Springer Science + Business Media, LLC 2009

Keywords H69CIS200 cell line; H69OX400 cell line; DNA repair; Regrowth resistance

The H69CIS200 cisplatin-resistant and H69OX400 oxaliplatin-resistant small-cell lung cancer cell lines are novel models of low-level platinum resistance (1). The H69CIS200 and H69OX400 cell lines were developed from parental H69 small-cell lung cancer cells with eight 4-day treatments of 200 ng/ml cisplatin and 400 ng/ml oxaliplatin, respectively with a recovery period between treatments to emulate the cycles of chemotherapy given in the clinic. These cell lines are approximately two-fold resistant to cisplatin and oxaliplatin and are cross-resistant to both the drugs. The resistance is not associated with increased cellular glutathione or decreased accumulation of platinum which are common mechanisms of platinum resistance. The H69 platinum sensitive cells enter a lengthy 3 week growth arrest in response to low-level cisplatin and oxaliplatin treatment (Fig. 1a). This is an example of the coordinated response between the cell cycle and DNA repair. In contrast, the H69CIS200 and H69OX400 cells have an alteration in the cell cycle allowing them to rapidly proliferate post drug treatment (Fig. 1b). We use the term "regrowth resistance" to describe this low-level platinum resistance where cells survive treatment through increased proliferation. Regrowth resistance may play a role in the onset of clinical resistance.

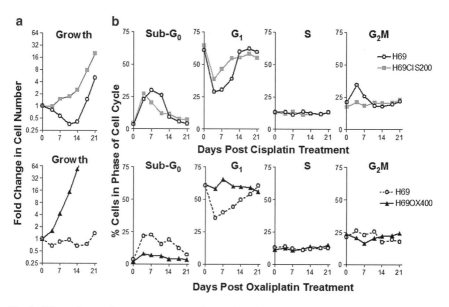

Fig. 1 Effect of acute drug treatment on cell growth and cell cycle. Cells were treated with either 1,000 ng/ml cisplatin or 2,000 ng/ml oxaliplatin for 2 h as indicated. (**a**) The number of cells that exclude trypan blue were counted and the fold change in the growth was plotted. (**b**) The proportion of cells in each phase of the cell cycle was determined by the propidium iodide/flow cytometry (1)

The resistant cell lines also have many chromosomal rearrangements most of which are not associated with the resistant phenotype, suggesting an increase in genomic instability in the resistant cell lines (2). The H69 cells and resistant cell lines have mutant p53 and consequently decrease the expression of p21 in response to platinum drug treatment, promoting progression of the cell cycle instead of increasing p21 to maintain the arrest (3). We hypothesized that there was a lack of coordination between the cell cycle and DNA repair in the resistant cell lines allowing proliferation in the presence of DNA damage which has created an increase in genomic instability. Increased DNA repair is a common mechanism of platinum resistance. However, H69CIS200 and H69OX400 cells showed no change in DNA repair capacity as measured by a repair of a platinated plasmid and expression of DNA repair marker γH2AX (3).

Despite no change in DNA repair capacity in the resistant cell lines, we found alterations in the expression and activity of two DNA repair proteins. ERCC1 is involved in the nucleotide excision repair removal of platinum adducts from DNA; increased ERCC1 mRNA and protein expression has been associated with cisplatin resistance (3). In contrast, we observed decreases in ERCC1 protein expression (Fig. 2a), which were associated with the formation of a lower molecular weight band of ~26 kDa (marked with arrow in Fig. 2a). We believe this to be an alternative spliced variant of ERCC1 associated with decreased repair activity (4). The samples in cell-cycle arrest (grey background) had a significant decrease in ERCC1 protein expression compared to the untreated control cells (Fig. 2b). This suggests that ERCC1 expression is more related to the cell-cycle state than to the resistance. The samples in the recovery from cell-cycle arrest were not significantly different from the untreated control cells, but had lower levels of mRNA and protein suggesting that part of restoring normal cell-cycle activity was associated with restoring normal ERCC1 levels.

Homologous recombination repair is mediated, in part, by the RAD51 proteins (5). An increase in homologous recombineation could mediate platinum resistance by increasing the repair of platinum-induced double-strand DNA breaks. We chose to examine RAD51B as it is linked to both cell-cycle control and DNA repair (6). We observed no change in the RAD51B protein expression. However, activity, as measured by the presence of nuclear RAD51 foci, did change. RAD51B foci were examined by immunocytochemistry in the H69, H69CIS200 and H69OX400 cell lines (Fig. 2c). The parental H69 cells had higher levels of RAD51B foci in response to oxaliplatin drug treatment than the H69OX400 cells. This is just the opposite of what would be expected, since the resistant cells would be expected to have a higher level of repair than the sensitive parental cells. RAD51B activity was increased significantly in the arrested cells compared to the nonarrested controls, suggesting that its expression and activity are related more to the cell cycle than to platinum resistance. The samples in cell-cycle recovery had no change in RAD51B foci from the untreated cells suggesting that part of the restoring normal cell cycle activity was restoring the normal RAD51B foci activity.

The changes in ERCC1 and RAD51B are associated with cell-cycle arrest rather than resistance, suggesting that they are being modulated for reasons other than

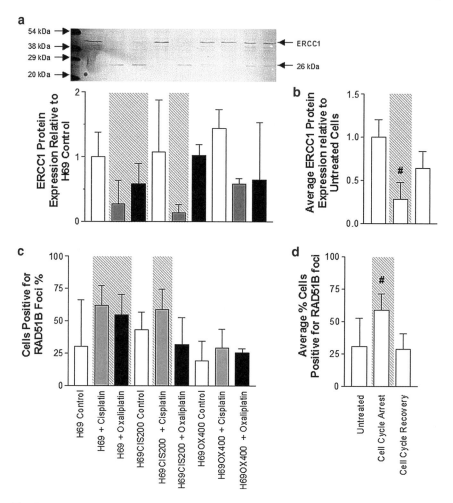

Fig. 2 Analysis of ERCC1 protein expression and RAD51B activity in H69, H69CIS200 and H69OX400 cells after a 4-day exposure to either 200 ng/ml cisplatin or 400 ng/ml oxaliplatin. Samples in cell-cycle arrest are indicated with a *gray background*. (**a**) ERCC1 protein expression determined by Western Blot and (**b**) analysis in reference to the cell cycle. (**c**) RAD51B activity determined by immunocytochemistry and (**d**) analysis in reference to the cell cycle. Means and standard deviations are presented from pooled data from parts (**a**) and (**c**). Untreated is the control cells, cell-cycle arrest is the drug-treated samples in cell arrest indicated with *gray background* shading, and cell-cycle recovery is the drug-treated cells not in the cell-cycle arrest. # indicates a significant difference compared to the untreated samples

DNA repair and are potentially participating in the regrowth resistance mechanism of cell-cycle arrest and recovery. There is some evidence to suggest that ERCC1 and RAD51B could mediate a cell-cycle arrest (7). Hepatocytes from ERCC1 knockout mice are arrested in the G_2 phase of the cell cycle (8). The expression of full-length ERCC1 decreases in association with the cell-cycle arrest; however, this is associated with the formation of an ERCC1 splice variant which has been previously reported to have reduced DNA repair activity (4). It is possible that this splice variant may have an increased role in the process of cell-cycle arrest. Fibroblasts from ERCC1 knockout mice also show a decreased rate of cell growth and disruptions in cell cycle (9), suggesting that the decrease in ERCC1 may contribute to the lengthy growth arrest in the sensitive cells. Transfection of RAD51B into CHO cells induces a cell cycle G_1 delay similar to what was observed in the H69 cells in response to platinum treatment (10). Transfection of RAD51 into human and rat fibroblasts also induces a G_1 arrest (7).

Resistance in the H69CIS200 and H69OX400 cells is dependent on a rapid cell-cycle progression after drug treatment (Fig. 1b). The regrowth resistance arrest is the same in all the cells; however, the resistant cell lines quickly exit this cell-cycle arrest and continue to cycle despite the presence of DNA damage. Therefore, the resistant cells have a decrease in DNA repair in response to platinum drug treatment, not because of a downregulation of a DNA repair pathway but because of the reduced time in cell-cycle arrest where the repair occurs. Decreases in ERCC1 (11) and increases in RAD51 (12) have also been associated with increased genomic instability which correlate with the large amount of chromosomal aberrations found in the resistant cell lines (2).

The normal exit from the cell-cycle arrest after the successful completion of DNA repair is termed checkpoint recovery. Normal checkpoint recovery in the H69 parental cells is the 3-week growth arrest (Fig. 1a). Checkpoint adaptation is related to checkpoint recovery and promotes cell-cycle reentry even when unrepairable DNA damage is present (13). The H69CIS200 and H69OX400 cells appear to have the checkpoint adaptation phenotype, the cell cycle continuing despite the presence of DNA damage. The H69OX400 cells exit the cell-cycle arrest faster than the H69CIS200 cells and this correlates with the greater amount of chromosomal aberrations in the H69OX400 cell line (2).

Conclusions

Resistance in the H69CIS200 and H69OX400 cells is associated with the speed of the recovery from the cell-cycle arrest, termed "regrowth resistance", which may involve modulation of ERCC1 and RAD51B.

References

1. Stordal BK, Davey MW, Davey RA. Oxaliplatin induces drug resistance more rapidly than cisplatin in H69 small cell lung cancer cells. Cancer Chemother Pharmacol 2006;58:256–65.
2. Stordal B, Peters G, Davey R. Similar chromosomal changes in cisplatin and oxaliplatin-resistant sublines of the H69 SCLC cell line are not associated with platinum resistance. Genes Chromosomes Cancer 2006;45:1094–105.

3. Stordal B, Davey R. ERCC1 expression and RAD51B activity correlate with cell cycle response to platinum drug treatment not DNA repair. Cancer Chemother Pharmacol DOI: 10.1007/300280-008-0783X.

4. Altaha R, Liang X, Yu JJ, Reed E. Excision repair cross complementing-group 1: gene expression and platinum resistance. Int J Mol Med 2004;14:959–70.

5. Yu JJ, Mu C, Dabholkar M, Guo Y, Bostick-Bruton F, Reed E. Alternative splicing of ERCC1 and cisplatin-DNA adduct repair in human tumor cell lines. Int J Mol Med 1998;1:617–20.

6. Sancar A, Lindsey-Boltz LA, Unsal-Kacmaz K, Linn S. Molecular mechanisms of mammalian DNA repair and the DNA damage checkpoints. Annu Rev Biochem 2004;73:39–85.

7. Havre PA, Rice M, Ramos R, Kmiec EB. HsRec2/Rad51L1, a protein influencing cell cycle progression, has protein kinase activity. Exp Cell Res 2000;254:33–44.

8. Raderschall E, Bazarov A, Cao J, et al. Formation of higher-order nuclear Rad51 structures is functionally linked to p21 expression and protection from DNA damage-induced apoptosis. J Cell Sci 2002;115(Pt 1):153–64.

9. Nunez F, Chipchase MD, Clarke AR, Melton DW. Nucleotide excision repair gene (ERCC1) deficiency causes G2 arrest in hepatocytes and a reduction in liver binucleation: the role of p53 and p21. FASEB J 2000;14:1073–82.

10. Weeda G, Donker I, de Wit J, et al. Disruption of mouse ERCC1 results in a novel repair syndrome with growth failure, nuclear abnormalities and senescence. Curr Biol 1997;7:427–39.

11. Havre PA, Rice MC, Noe M, Kmiec EB. The human REC2/RAD51B gene acts as a DNA damage sensor by inducing G1 delay and hypersensitivity to ultraviolet irradiation. Cancer Res 1998;58:4733–9.

12. Sargent RG, Meservy JL, Perkins BD, et al. Role of the nucleotide excision repair gene ERCC1 in formation of recombination-dependent rearrangements in mammalian cells. Nucleic Acids Res 2000;28:3771–8.

13. Richardson C, Stark JM, Ommundsen M, Jasin M. Rad51 overexpression promotes alternative double-strand break repair pathways and genome instability. Oncogene 2004;23:546–53.

14. Harrison JC, Haber JE. Surviving the breakup: the DNA damage checkpoint. Annu Rev Genet 2006; 40:209–235.

Targeting Nucleotide Excision Repair as a Mechanism to Increase Cisplatin Efficacy

John J. Turchi, Sarah C. Shuck, Emily A. Short, and Brooke J. Andrews

Abstract Tumor resistance to chemotherapeutic DNA damaging agents, such as cisplatin, is an obstacle in the treatment of many cancers, including lung and ovarian. Resistance is influenced by nucleotide excision repair (NER) catalyzed removal of cisplatin-DNA lesions. NER is the primary pathway used by the cells in the repair of helix-distorting cisplatin lesions; therefore, inhibition of NER may increase the efficacy of cisplatin treatment. More specifically, the recognition and verification of DNA damage by NER is a critical step in the pathway, making it an ideal target for inhibition. Recognition of DNA damage occurs primarily through two proteins, Xeroderma Pigmentosum Group A (XPA) and replication protein A (RPA). XPA has been shown to have a role exclusively in NER, thus making it a highly specific target for inhibition that will lead to a decrease in NER and an increase in sensitivity to cisplatin treatment. RPA is a single-stranded DNA-binding protein that has roles in NER as well as in other metabolic pathways, including DNA replication and recombination. We have developed a high-throughput (HT) assay for XPA/RPA binding to DNA and screened libraries of small molecules to identify compounds capable of interrupting the protein/DNA interaction, an effort that has lead to the identification of small molecule inhibitors of both RPA and XPA. These inhibitors have been validated in secondary in vitro screens and structure–activity relationships were determined for one class of inhibitors. Further development of this class of compounds is anticipated to display cytostatic/cytotoxic activity and sensitize cells to cisplatin therapy.

Keywords DNA repair; Cisplatin; Drug discovery; RPA; XPA; Chemotherapy

J.J. Turchi (✉), S.C. Shuck, E.A. Short, and B.J. Andrews
Departments of Medicine, Biochemistry, and Molecular Biology,
Indiana University School of Medicine, Indianapolis, IN, USA
e-mail: jturchi@iupui.edu

A. Bonetti et al. (eds.), *Platinum and Other Heavy Metal Compounds in Cancer Chemotherapy*, DOI: 10.1007/978-1-60327-459-3_22,
© Humana Press, a part of Springer Science + Business Media, LLC 2009

Background

The nucleotide excision repair pathway (NER) removes bulky DNA adducts caused by UV irradiation and chemical mutagens. The repair of DNA damage begins with a damage recognition step and assembly of a preincision complex, followed by excision of the damaged strand and gap-filling DNA synthesis. NER uses two mechanisms for recognition of DNA damage. One mechanism is global genomic NER (GG-NER), which relies on proteins that have a greater affinity for damaged DNA compared to undamaged DNA. These proteins include XPC/RAD23B, RPA, XPA, and the damaged DNA-binding protein, DDB (1). We have extensively characterized the interaction of RPA and XPA with cisplatin-damaged DNA (2–6). Based on these studies and studies of others, we proposed a model for the interaction of RPA and XPA with cisplatin-damaged DNA that we more recently expanded to include XPC-RAD23B (5, 7).

RPA, a heterotrimer composed of 70-, 34-, and 14-kDa subunits, is a single-stranded DNA-binding protein that has several roles in the cell; including DNA replication, recombination, and repair. RPA is required early in the NER process, specifically for DNA binding and complex formation with XPA (8). Furthermore, RPA forms a high-affinity interaction with the undamaged strand of a cisplatin-damaged duplex DNA (4, 6). XPA, a 40-kDa zinc metalloprotein, is another protein involved in the recognition step. However, unlike RPA, XPA's only known role in the cell is its involvement in NER. XPA interacts with several of the core repair factors in NER and without XPA no stable preincision complex can form, therefore, NER cannot occur. We have demonstrated that XPA contacts both strands of a duplex-damaged DNA, which positions XPA at the single-strand/double-strand DNA junction (5). This is also consistent with other data from our laboratory demonstrating that XPA inhibits the strand separation activity of RPA to stabilize the RPA–XPA complex on duplex-damaged DNA (4). XPC-RAD23B and DDB also contribute to damage recognition in the GG-NER pathway, though their interactions are subpathway and damage-specific in many cases (7).

The second pathway for DNA damage recognition by NER, transcription-coupled repair (TC-NER), involves coupling the recognition process to transcription (9). In this process, a transcribing RNA polymerase II encounters damage on the template strand and stalls. The stalled polymerase, along with transcription factor IIH (TFIIH), initiates the repair process. TFIIH is an essential factor for both TC-NER and GG-NER and is a complex of at least nine polypeptides (10). TC-NER-mediated recognition of cisplatin-DNA damage requires RPA and XPA while the XPC/RAD23B protein complex is not required in this pathway. Interestingly, recent evidence measuring the response of a series of matched cell lines deficient or proficient for the NER subpathways to cisplatin treatment revealed that TC-NER is a major determinant of sensitivity (11). Our collaborative analysis of TC-NER recognition of cisplatin-DNA damage was the first report describing how the eukaryotic TC-NER machinery responds to cisplatin lesions (12). Importantly, RPA and XPA are required for both pathways of NER.

Fig. 1 Central role of RPA in repair of Pt-DNA lesions and in chromosomal DNA replication. RPA is depicted as the *green heterotrimer*. In the NER complex, the nucleases are *shaded yellow*, TFIIH *orange*, XPA *red*, and the Pt-lesion as the *white circle*. The DNA polymerase and helicase are *shaded purple* and *blue* in the replication complex (*see Color Plates*)

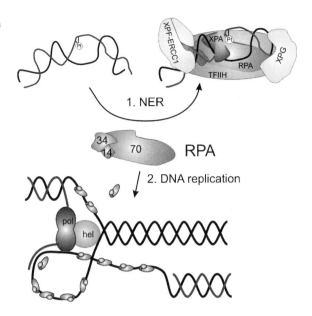

RPA and XPA are attractive targets for cancer chemotherapy because of their roles in DNA metabolism (Fig. 1). The vital role of both RPA and XPA in NER coupled with clear data demonstrating that there is an up-regulation of NER in cisplatin-resistant ovarian cancers provides the rationale for targeting NER as a mechanism to increase cisplatin efficacy. Activation of the Jun kinase pathway, which is involved in repair signaling, has been shown to up-regulate NER and contribute to cisplatin resistance in recurrent cancers (13–15). Therefore, targeting RPA and XPA in this capacity holds the potential to reverse cisplatin resistance. Increased cisplatin efficacy has been observed by targeting other NER proteins with antisense technology (16, 17). In addition to its role in NER, RPA is also required for DNA replication and S-phase progression, which suggests that RPA inhibitors may display cytostatic or antiproliferative activity as single agents. While RPA has been observed to be overexpressed in a limited number of cancers, its activity is upregulated in rapidly dividing cells, including cancer cells. This differential may allow for an increased therapeutic window in which cancer cells can be targeted more specifically. XPA's exclusive role in NER presents it as an interesting target for inhibition due to an increase in cisplatin efficacy that coincides with NER inhibition. The role of XPA in cisplatin efficacy has been shown when examining testicular cancer cells. Testicular cancer, which after the inclusion of cisplatin into a multidrug regimen, has a cure rate of 95% (18). This extreme chemosensitivity has been attributed to decreased DNA repair capacity and specifically decreased levels of XPA (19–21). The abundance of structural and biochemical characterization coupled with an essential role in relevant DNA metabolic pathways suggests that RPA and XPA are valid targets for cancer chemotherapy.

Results

Structure–Activity Relationships for RPA Inhibitors

Our previous results revealed a molecule containing a heterobicyclic structure was effective as an inhibitor of RPA DNA binding activity in both fluorescence polarization and electrophoretic mobility shift assays (EMSA) (22). In addition, this compound was able to inhibit in vitro NER-catalyzed repair of a cisplatin lesion. We therefore selected this molecule for the analysis of structure–activity relationships of heterobicyclics. Analogs of the original heterobicyclic were purchased and additional analogs were synthesized. These analogs were then analyzed in EMSAs (Fig. 2a) to assess RPA binding. A representative binding curve is presented in Fig. 2b and demonstrates inhibition of the DNA binding activity of RPA with an IC50 value of 15 μM. The results presented in Fig. 3 reveal the IC50 values for RPA

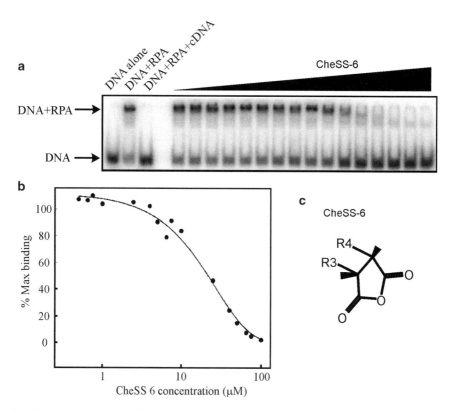

Fig. 2 CheSS6 inhibits RPA's DNA binding activity. (**a**) RPA binding to a 44-base-pair duplex cisplatin-damaged DNA was assessed in an EMSA in the presence of increasing concentrations of CheSS6. (**b**) Quantification of RPA binding as a function of CheSS6 concentration. (**c**) Structure of CheSS6

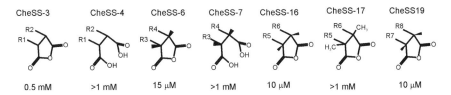

Fig. 3 CheSS Structure–Activity Relationships. Analogs to the previously identified heterobicyclic RPA inhibitor were either purchased or synthesized. These analogs were analyzed for RPA DNA binding activity via EMSA and IC50 values for each analog were determined. Analysis revealed that the anhydride functional group was fundamental to inhibition while dicarboxylic acids, chloro derivatives (R1 and R2), and methyl group additions resulted in less inhibition

inhibition for a series of analogs and identifies the anhydride functional group as a key determinant of RPA inhibition. The dicarboxylic acid analogs were considerably less active, displaying IC50 values greater than 1 mM. Chloro derivatives, R1 and R2, were also less active, partially as a result of limited solubility (data not shown). The data also demonstrate that methyl group additions to the anhydride reduce inhibitory activity.

Considering the reactive nature of the anhydride, we designed an experiment to determine if this compound was acting as an irreversible inhibitor. To test this, RPA was either incubated with an active inhibitor, or mock-treated. RPA was then dialyzed overnight to remove unreacted inhibitor. If binding of the inhibitor to RPA was reversible, dialysis would decrease the concentration of the inhibitor to a level that would not inhibit RPA binding. Analysis of the inhibitor and mock-treated RPA in an EMSA confirms that the anhydride is binding irreversibly to RPA (Fig. 4). Experiments are underway to determine the exact sites of modification by these inhibitors (named as CheSS compounds). Unfortunately, while displaying excellent in vitro activity against RPA, none of the analogs tested resulted in cellular activity as measured by cytotoxic cell-cycle perturbation or sensitization to cisplatin (data not shown).

Fluorescence Screening for RPA Inhibitors

In order to identify compounds that have the potential for in vitro and in vivo activity, we screened an additional 10,000 compounds from the NCI DTP library of pure and synthetic compounds using our previously published HT assay (22). Hits were identified and then validated in a secondary EMSA assay (Table 1). One of the validated hits was comprised of a heterobicyclic structure with a modified ester functional group. Analysis of this compound revealed weaker RPA inhibitory activity than the heterobicyclic with the anhydride functional group but significant cellular activity (data not shown). Further analyses of this compound in vitro as well as in cell-based and animal studies are underway.

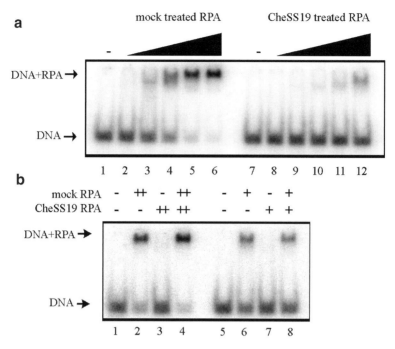

Fig. 4 Irreversible inactivation of RPA via CheSS 19. (**a**) EMSA analysis of mock- or CheSS 19 treated RPA binding cisplatin-damaged duplex DNA. (**b**) Mock-treated or Chess 19 treated RPA were mixed as indicated in the figure and DNA binding activity determined by EMSA

Table 1 RPA screen of the NCI library of pure and synthetic compounds

		Compounds screened	No. of hits	Percent
Diversity set	HTS	2,000	79	3.95
	EMSA	79	9	11.39
Large scale	HTS	10,000	415	4.15
	EMSA	338	135	39.94

Screening was performed using our published assay for RPA DNA binding activity (22). Hits were identified, validated and confirmed in EMSA experiments

High-Throughput Fluorescence Polarization Assays

To further expand these analyses to include the XPA protein and to obtain a more robust assay, we established a fluorescence polarization (FP) assay for DNA binding and converted this to a high-throughput format. The basis for this assay is that the fluorescently labelled DNA exhibits a low polarization as a free DNA molecule. Upon binding to a protein, increased polarization is observed (Fig. 5a,c).

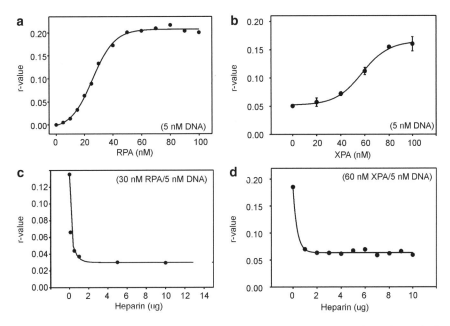

Fig. 5 FP-assay for DNA binding. (**a**) 5 nM F-DNA was mixed in 50 μL reactions with the indicated concentration of XPA and polarization determined as described previously (2). (**b**) 5 nM DNA and 60 nM XPA were incubated with the indicated concentration of heparin inhibitor and polarization was determined as in (**a**). (**c**) 5 nM F-DNA was mixed in 50 μL reactions with the indicated concentration of RPA and polarization was determined. (**d**) 5 nM DNA and 30 nM RPA were incubated with the indicated concentration of heparin inhibitor and polarization was determined as described in (**a**)

Independent FP assays have been established for RPA and XPA DNA binding activity and the results of these assay development efforts are presented in Fig. 5. The data demonstrate that in a 384-well format in 50 μL reactions, an excellent dynamic range is observed for both XPA and RPA. Titration of heparin to inhibit the binding and hence the polarization was used to simulate the effect of an inhibitor. These results demonstrate efficient inhibition in binding and reduction in FP (Fig. 5b, d). Analysis of the RPA assay yielded a Z-score of 0.80 indicating an "excellent assay" according to the criteria established by Zhang et al. (23) for analysis of HTS. This Z-score is significantly better than that obtained from our original assay (~0.4), which is largely a result of a greater dynamic range compared to the initial fluorescence stimulation assay (22). Analysis of the XPA screening assay yielded a Z-score of 0.60, again indicating an "excellent assay".

FP-Based HTS for RPA and XPA Inhibitors

We have screened nearly 38,000 compounds from the ChemDiv library for RPA and XPA independently. The results of this screen are presented in Table 2. Hits

Table 2 RPA and XPA screen of the ChemDiv library

Target protein	Compounds screened	No. of hits	Percent
RPA	42,400	54	0.13
XPA	35,200	58	0.16

Screening of the ChemDiv library of drug-like molecules was performed using the methods developed in Fig. 5. Screening was performed in collaboration with the IUSM Chemical Genetic core facility

that were identified in both the screens were not pursued as they could represent molecules that bind DNA or have characteristics that are not compatible with the optical fluorescence based screen. RPA hits segregated into a few different classes. The most active class contained a 4,5-dihydro-1*H*-pyrazole scaffold with substitutions at position 1, 3 and 5. This class of compounds, along with hits from previous screens, is currently being investigated for in vitro and in vivo activity. XPA inhibitors are also being validated and confirmed in secondary screens.

Discussion

The ability to inhibit NER via disrupting RPA- and XPA-catalyzed recognition of damaged DNA has significant implications for cancer therapy, as many chemotherapeutics impart their efficacy via inducing DNA damage. Thus, inhibiting the repair of these lesions, including cisplatin–DNA adducts, holds the potential to increase the steady-state level of DNA damage without increasing the treatment doses. In addition, targeting RPA's role in DNA replication could prove useful in treating various types of cancer.

The two mechanisms of the NER pathway, GG-NER and TC-NER, have been shown to affect cisplatin sensitivity differently. Cells that are deficient in TC-NER show increased sensitivity to cisplatin treatment compared to cells deficient in GG-NER (24). Therefore, TC-NER must play a larger role in the repair of cisplatin-induced DNA lesions compared to GG-NER, which limits the role of XPC-RAD23B as it is involved exclusively in GG-NER. By targeting RPA and XPA, both GG-NER and TC-NER can be inhibited, which is anticipated to completely abrogate NER-catalyzed repair of cisplatin lesions. While inhibition of XPA's DNA binding activity is likely to impact only NER, inhibition of the single-stranded DNA binding activity of RPA has broader implications for cancer therapy because of the many roles that RPA plays in the cell, including DNA replication, recombination and numerous repair pathways.

The DNA-binding domains of XPA and RPA are very distinct and allow for identification of small molecules that are able to interact with one or the other, but not both. RPA contains six oligosaccharide/oligonucleotide (OB) folds, four of which are used to bind DNA (25–29). RPA is one of several proteins that contain OB folds that are used to bind DNA; however, there is a lack of sequence similarity among the members of the OB-fold-containing family. This may prove to be beneficial in that the lack of similarity between these domains can be exploited to identify small-molecule inhibitors specific to the RPA OB-folds, thus limiting off-target effects. RPA has also been observed to undergo a conformational change upon binding to DNA with reorientation of the two main OB-folds in the p70 central DNA-binding domain (30). These changes may allow targeting of distinct regions of the RPA protein that influence DNA binding, resulting in greater specificity for RPA.

Though less is known regarding the role of the other OB-fold domains in RPA, RPA employs the main p70 central OB-folds for binding single-stranded DNA regardless of the pathway it is involved in. However, the potential exists that the other OB-fold domains are pathway-specific. Thus one could envision using small-molecule inhibitors to specific RPA-OB folds to discern the roles each plays in the numerous metabolic pathways in which RPA participates. This would then translate to pathway-specific inhibition which could be of clinical utility.

Considering RPA's role as the major eukaryotic single-strand DNA-binding protein, inhibiting this global activity would have widespread cellular implications. The outcome of inhibiting global RPA single-strand DNA binding activity is likely to depend on the state of the cell at any given time. A rapidly dividing cell would be expected to undergo S-Phase cell-cycle arrest when RPA's DNA binding activity is inhibited. Additionally, towing to RPA's role in repair, a cell that has undergone cisplatin treatment would be unable to repair the damage and potentially induce apoptosis as a result of abrogation of RPA's DNA binding activity. RPA is, therefore, an attractive target for inhibition because of the versatile role it plays in numerous DNA metabolic pathways. Beyond targeting RPA's DNA binding activity, the potential exists to target RPA with a small molecule to make it specific for one metabolic process. For example, binding the XPA-binding domain of RPA with a small molecule would prevent association of the two proteins and, therefore, would result in an inhibition of NER. While an inhibitor of this type would not be identified in our HTS, this would specifically target the cell to increased cisplatin sensitivity while not affecting the role of RPA in other DNA metabolic processes.

XPA binds DNA using a zinc-containing domain that is distinct from zinc-finger domains found in other DNA-binding proteins such as transcription factors (31, 32). This atypical zinc-binding domain holds the potential for increased specificity and minimal off-target effects that one would anticipate for targeting such a large class of proteins. Whether this potential is realized depends on extensive analysis of the molecules identified in our XPA screen.

Conclusion

The ability to inhibit the activity of proteins in the NER pathway, specifically XPA and RPA, represents a novel chemotherapeutic treatment to increase the efficacy of cisplatin therapy. The inhibition of RPA single-stranded DNA binding activity will also affect other DNA metabolic pathways in the cell, including replication and recombination. Therefore, inhibition of RPA affects cancer therapy both as a novel chemotherapeutic target and, like XPA, as a means of increasing cisplatin efficacy. Our laboratory has developed a high-throughput screening assay for identification of SMIs of RPA and XPA. Using this assay, we have identified small-molecule inhibitors of RPA and have confirmed this inhibition with secondary in vitro assays showing inhibition of both DNA binding and NER activity. We are also currently investigating small-molecule inhibitors of XPA and determining the effects of these compounds in both lung and ovarian cancer cell systems.

Acknowledgment This work was supported by NIH grant CA82741, Flight Attendants Medical Research Institute, and Walter Cancer Research Institute.

References

1. Batty DP, Wood RD. Damage recognition in nucleotide excision repair of DNA. Gene 2000; 241:193–204.
2. Patrick SM, Oakley GG, Dixon K, Turchi JJ. DNA damage induced hyperphosphorylation of replication protein A. 2. Characterization of DNA binding activity, protein interactions, and activity in DNA replication and repair. Biochemistry 2005;44:8438–48.
3. Nuss JE, Patrick SM, Oakley GG, et al. DNA damage induced hyperphosphorylation of replication protein A. 1. Identification of novel sites of phosphorylation in response to DNA damage. Biochemistry 2005;44:8428–37.
4. Patrick SM, Turchi JJ. Xeroderma pigmentosum complementation group A protein (XPA) modulates RPA-DNA interactions via enhanced complex stability and inhibition of strand separation activity. J Biol Chem 2002;277:16096–101.
5. Hermanson-Miller IL, Turchi JJ. Strand-specific binding of RPA and XPA to damaged duplex DNA. Biochemistry 2002;41:2402–8.
6. Patrick SM, Turchi JJ. Stopped-flow kinetic analysis of replication protein A-binding DNA – Damage recognition and affinity for single-stranded DNA reveal differential contributions of k(on) and k(off) rate constants. J Biol Chem 2001;276:22630–7.
7. Shuck SC, Short EA, Turchi JJ. Eukaryotic nucleotide excision repair: from understanding mechanisms to influencing biology. Cell Res 2008;18:64–72.
8. Lee SH, Kim DK, Drissi R. Human xeroderma pigmentosum group A protein interacts with human replication protein A and inhibits DNA replication. J Biol Chem 1995;270:21800–5.
9. Fousteri M, Mullenders LH. Transcription-coupled nucleotide excision repair in mammalian cells: molecular mechanisms and biological effects. Cell Res 2008;18:73–84.
10. Fukuda A, Yamauchi J, Wu SY, Chiang CM, Muramatsu M, Hisatake K. Reconstitution of recombinant TFIIH that can mediate activator-dependent transcription. Genes Cells 2001;6:707–19.
11. Furuta T, Ueda T, Aune G, Sarasin A, Kraemer KH, Pommier Y. Transcription-coupled nucleotide excision repair as a determinant of cisplatin sensitivity of human cells. Cancer Res 2002;62:4899–902.
12. Tornaletti S, Patrick SM, Turchi JJ, Hanawalt PC. Behavior of T7 RNA polymerase and mammalian RNA polymerase II at site-specific cisplatin adducts in the template DNA. J Biol Chem 2003;278:35791–7.
13. Hayakawa J, Depatie C, Ohmichi M, Mercola D. The activation of c-Jun NH2-terminal kinase (JNK) by DNA-damaging agents serves to promote drug resistance via activating transcription factor 2 (ATF2)-dependent enhanced DNA repair. J Biol Chem 2003;278: 20582–92.

14. Mayer F, Honecker F, Looijenga LHJ, Bokemeyer C. Towards an understanding of the biological basis of response to cisplatin-based chemotherapy in germ-cell tumors. Ann Oncol 2003;14: 825–32.
15. Hayakawa J, Mittal S, Wang Y, et al. Identification of promoters bound by c-Jun/ATF2 during rapid large-scale gene activation following genotoxic stress. Mol Cell 2004;16:521–35.
16. Selvakumaran M, Pisarcik DA, Bao R, Yeung AT, Hamilton TC. Enhanced cisplatin cytotoxicity by disturbing the nucleotide excision repair pathway in ovarian cancer cell lines. Cancer Res 2003;63:1311–6.
17. Wu XM, Fan W, Xu SW, Zhou YK. Sensitization to the cytotoxicity of cisplatin by transfection with nucleotide excision repair gene xeroderma pigmentosun group a antisense RNA in human lung adenocarcinoma cells. Clin Cancer Res 2003;9:5874–9.
18. Einhorn LH. Curing metastatic testicular cancer. Proc Natl Acad Sci USA 2002;99:4592–5.
19. Koberle B, Roginskaya V, Wood RD. XPA protein as a limiting factor for nucleotide excision repair and UV sensitivity in human cells. DNA Repair (Amst) 2006;5:641–8.
20. Welsh C, Day R, McGurk C, Masters JRW, Wood RD, Koberle B. Reduced levels of XPA, ERCC1 and XPF DNA repair proteins in testis tumor cell lines. Int J Cancer 2004;110: 352–61.
21. Köberle B, Masters JR, Hartley JA, Wood RD. Defective repair of cisplatin-induced DNA damage caused by reduced XPA protein in testicular germ cell tumours. Curr Biol 1999;9: 273–6.
22. Andrews BJ, Turchi JJ. Development of a high-throughput screen for inhibitors of replication protein A and its role in nucleotide excision repair. Mol Cancer Ther 2004;3:385–91.
23. Zhang JH, Chung TD, Oldenburg KR. A simple statistical parameter for use in evaluation and validation of high throughput screening assays. J Biomol Screen 1999;4:67–73.
24. Bulmer JT, Zacal NJ, Rainbow AJ. Human cells deficient in transcription-coupled repair show prolonged activation of the Jun N-terminal kinase and increased sensitivity following cisplatin treatment. Cancer Chemother Pharmacol 2005;56:189–98.
25. Bochkareva E, Korolev S, Lees-Miller SP, Bochkarev A. Structure of the RPA trimerization core and its role in the multistep DNA-binding mechanism of RPA. EMBO J 2002;21: 1855–63.
26. Bochkareva E, Belegu V, Korolev S, Bochkarev A. Structure of the major single-stranded DNA-binding domain of replication protein A suggests a dynamic mechanism for DNA binding. EMBO J 2001;20:612–8.
27. Mer G, Bochkarev A, Chazin WJ, Edwards AM. Three-dimensional structure and function of replication protein A. Cold Spring Harb Symp Quant Biol 2000;65:193–200.
28. Bochkarev A, Bochkareva E, Frappier L, Edwards AM. The crystal structure of the complex of replication protein A subunits RPA32 and RPA14 reveals a mechanism for single- stranded DNA binding. EMBO J 1999;18:4498–504.
29. Bochkarev A, Pfuetzner RA, Edwards AM, Frappier L. Structure of the single-stranded-DNA-binding domain of replication protein A bound to DNA. Nature 1997;385:176–81.
30. Theobald DL, Mitton-Fry RM, Wuttke DS. Nucleic acid recognition by OB-fold proteins. Annu Rev Biophys Biomol Struct 2003;32:115–33.
31. Ikegami T, Kuraoka I, Saijo M, et al. Solution structure of the DNA- and RPA-binding domain of the human repair factor XPA. Nat Struct Biol 1998;5:701–6.
32. Morita EH, Ohkubo T, Kuraoka I, Shirakawa M, Tanaka K, Morikawa K. Implications of the zinc-finger motif found in the DNA-binding domain of the human XPA protein. Genes Cells 1996;1:437–42.

CHK2 and ERCC1 in the DNA Adduct Repair Pathway that Mediates Acquired Cisplatin Resistance

Jing Jie Yu, Xiaobing Liang, Qing-Wu Yan, Eddie Reed*, Antonio Tito Fojo#, Ying Guo, Qi He, and Michael D. Mueller

Abstract Increased DNA-adduct repair is a leading mechanism of acquired cisplatin resistance. Our previous studies show that overexpression of ERCC1, the essential component of nucleotide excision repair, is associated with enhanced repair of cisplatin-induced DNA-adduct and with clinical resistance to platinum chemotherapy. Current investigations provide extensive data on the mechanism of cisplatin resistance via the DNA-adduct repair pathway. In a study of cisplatin-induced molecular signature in human ovarian cancer A2780 cells, activation of ATM, p53, Chk2, P48, and P21 were observed, with Chk2 identified as an upstream regulator of the ERCC1 recognition/repair pathway. Our data demonstrate that Chk2 is activated and regulated by p53 in wild-type p53-replete cells. We also found that activated Chk2 can be dephosphorylated by PP2A. In other words, PP2A negatively regulates Chk2 by dephosphorylating phosphorylated Chk2. Previous findings by our group suggested that ovarian cancer A2780/CP70 cells, in response to cisplatin exposure, showed an increase of ERCC1 mRNA, with increased transcription and prolonged ERCC1 mRNA half-life. Functional analysis of the ERCC1 promoter by CAT assay indicates that the region from −220 to −110 appears essential to constitutive expression of ERCC1 gene and a more forward upstream region is responsible for cisplatin-induced ERCC1 overexpression. Identification of a functional cis-element in

J.J. Yu (✉), X. Liang, Q.-W. Yan, Y. Guo, Q. He, and M.D. Mueller
Department of Biochemistry, School of Medicine,
Department of Basic Pharmaceutical Sciences, School of Pharmacy,
and Mary Babb Randolph Cancer Center, Robert C. Byrd Health Sciences Center,
West Virginia University, Morgantown, WV, USA
e-mail: jyu@hsc.wvu.edu

*E. Reed
Mitchell Cancer Institute, University of south Alabama, Mobile, Alabama, USA.

#A.T. Fojo
Center for Cancer Research, National Cancer Institute, National Institutes of Health,
Bethesda, Maryland, USA.

A. Bonetti et al. (eds.), *Platinum and Other Heavy Metal Compounds in Cancer Chemotherapy*, DOI: 10.1007/978-1-60327-459-3_23,

189

the drug-responsive region by EMSA revealed that activator AP1 and repressor MZF1 responded to cisplatin stimulation. Overexpression of MZF1 repressed the ERCC1 promoter activity in cisplatin treated cells, indicating that MZF1 is a repressor in regulation of ERCC1 transcription. After cisplatin exposure, the mRNA level of MZF1 decreased and mRNA levels of c-jun and c-fos increased, suggesting that MZF1 and AP1 coordinately mediate cisplatin-invoked gene expression in these cells. Taken together, in response to cisplatin treatment, decreased MZF1 and increased AP1 binding activities within the drug-responsive region of the ERCC1 promoter appear to be the leading mechanism of up-regulation of ERCC1 expression. In conclusion, our investigations reveal two key factors—Chk2 and ERCC1—that participate in the DNA-adduct repair pathway that mediates acquired cisplatin resistance. Down-regulation of these two critical genes may antagonize cisplatin resistance in the treatment of human ovarian cancer.

Keywords Chk2; PP2A; ERCC1; MZF1; Cisplatin resistance

Introduction

Platinum-compounds, the core treatment for a wide variety of cancers, continue to play a key role in cancer chemotherapy. However, platinum chemotherapy often results in the development of drug resistance, the main cause of treatment failure (1). Therefore, overcoming drug resistance is the key to successful treatment of cancers.

Platinum-resistance is multifactorial in nature. Increased DNA-adduct repair is one of the leading mechanisms of acquired platinum resistance (2, 3). ERCC1, the essential component of nucleotide excision repair (NER), the only known mechanism for the removal of intrastrand bulky DNA adducts, is highly conserved in nature (4). The expression of ERCC1 is elevated in tumor tissue from patients refractory to cisplatin therapy. ERCC1 expression reflects DNA repair capacity and clinical resistance (5, 6). In vitro studies suggest that overexpression of the ERCC1 gene is associated with a platinum-resistant phenotype in ovarian cancer cells (7, 8).

Chk2, the mammalian homolog of the checkpoint kinases Cds1 (*Schizosaccharomyces pombe*) and Rad53 (*Saccharomyces cerevisiae*), is a key factor among cisplatin-activated protein kinases (9). Activated Chk2 plays a pivotal role in checkpoint control activities and phosphorylates downstream substrates of cell cycle control (10–12).

Our current investigations demonstrate that cisplatin activates the DNA-adduct repair pathway, with marked Chk2 phosphorylation and ERCC1 overexpression, resulting in cell cycle arrest and increase in cisplatin resistance (Fig. 1). We have identified modulators and transcriptional factors that can downregulate and control these two critical genes.

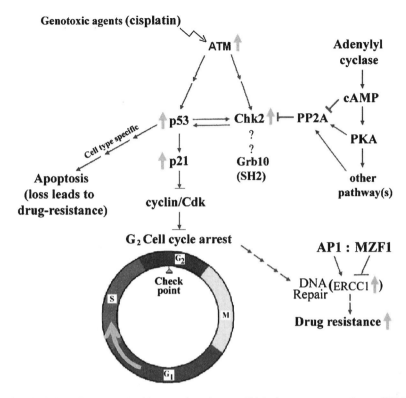

Fig. 1 Cisplatin activates DNA-adduct repair pathways. Chk2, the upstream regulator of ERCC1 is activated by p53 and dephosphorylated by PP2A. Cisplatin-induced ERCC1 overexpression contributes to an increase in cisplatin resistance. Transcriptional factors AP1 and MZF1 can modulate ERCC1 expression

Results

Cisplatin-activated Chk2 can be Negatively Regulated by PP2A Through Dephosphorylation

Exposure of A2780 (p53 wild type) cells to cisplatin for 1 hr at the IC_{50} concentration resulted in an increase in the amount of phosphorylated Chk2 at Thr-68 in a time-dependent manner (Fig. 2a). Quantitative analysis of phosphorylated Chk2 expression revealed that the amount of cisplatin-induced phosphothreonine Chk2 was doubled at 48 h compared to the control (9). The protein phosphatase 2A (PP2A) can dephosphorylate phospho-Chk2 as shown in Fig. 2b. At concentration 0.5 nM, PP2A completely depleted phospho-Chk2 (a); addition of okadaic acid (OA) prevented dephosphorylation of phospho-Chk2 (b). Treatment of cells with OA at 20 nM resulted in an augmentation of the phospho-Chk2 induced by cisplatin (Fig. 2c) indicating that PP2A is a negative regulator of phospho-Chk2. This was further demonstrated by knocking down Chk2 using an siRNA. Cells transfected with specific siRNA to PP2A and

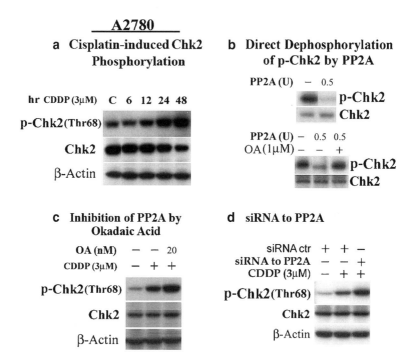

Fig. 2 PP2A effects on cisplatin-activated Chk2 Phosphorylation. (**a**) Cisplatin-induced Chk2 phosphorylation at Thr-68 determined by Western blotting. (**b**) Direct dephosphorylation of phospho-Chk2 by PP2A in vitro. (**c**). Inhibition of PP2A by okadaic acid (OA) restored phospho-Chk2. (**d**) PP2A affects on phospho-Chk2 are blocked by siRNA to PP2A

treated with cisplatin resulted in a blockage of PP2A effects on phospho-Chk2, indicating that inhibition of PP2A promoted Chk2 phosphorylation (Fig. 2d).

Cis-element MZF1 Acts as Repressor of ERCC1 Transcription upon Cisplatin Exposure

Functional analysis of ERCC1 promoter region revealed that the region from −220 to −110 appears essential to constitutive expression of the ERCC1 gene (13). A more upstream region containing AP1 and MZF1 binding sites is responsible for cisplatin-induced ERCC1 up-regulation (13). Identification of a functional cis-element in the drug-responsive region by EMSA revealed that activator AP1 and repressor MZF1 responded to cisplatin treatment. In response to cisplatin exposure, the AP1 and MZF1 sites formed DNA-protein complexes (Fig. 3a), and the binding activities of AP1 increased and binding activities of MZF1 decreased during the time course of the response. Overexpression of MZF1 by cDNA transfection repressed ERCC1 promoter activity in cisplatin treated cells (Fig. 3b). MZF1 mRNA level was affected by cisplatin and decreased nearly 75% at 48 h compared to the untreated control (Fig. 3c). These data suggest that MZF1 acts as repressor of ERCC1 transcription upon cisplatin exposure.

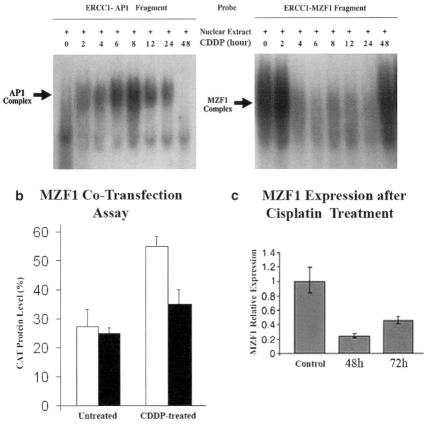

Fig. 3 MZF1 acts as repressor of ERCC1 transcription upon cisplatin exposure. (**a**) Cisplatin-induced binding activities of AP1 and MZF1 elements within the ERCC1 promoter during time course of the response as demonstrated by EMSA. (**b**) The effects of MZF1 overexpression on ERCC1 transcription activity analyzed by co-transfection CAT assay. (**c**) MZF1 mRNA expression affected by cisplatin measured by real-time quantitative PCR

Discussion

Investigation of the cisplatin-induced molecular signature in human ovarian cancer A2780 cells revealed that several kinases of the DNA damage-repair pathway become activated after 1 h of cisplatin exposure. This activation includes phosphorylation of p53 at serines 15 and 20, phosphorylation of Chk2 at threonine 68, and increased levels of ATM, p53, p48 and p21 (data not shown). Among the activated signals, we observed that Chk2 is activated and regulated by p53 in a wild-type p53 cell model. Overexpression of p53 through cDNA transfection doubled the amount of phospho-Chk2; siRNA to p53 greatly reduced Chk2 phosphorylation (data not shown).

Our previous data from A2780/CP70 cells showed a sixfold increase in ERCC1 mRNA level in response to cisplatin exposure. This increase is caused by increased transcription and by prolonged mRNA half-life (14). These cells also showed increased up-regulation of c-jun and c-fos mRNA after cisplatin treatment (14). In contrast, MZF1 mRNA decreased nearly 75% at 48h after cisplatin exposure, suggesting that MZF1 and AP1 coordinately mediate cisplatin-invoked over expression of ERCC1 (13). Taken together, in response to cisplatin treatment, decreased MZF1 and increased AP1 binding activities within the drug-responsive region of the ERCC1 promoter appear to be the leading mechanism of up-regulation of ERCC1 expression.

In conclusion, our investigations reveal two key factors—Chk2 and ERCC1—in the DNA-adduct repair pathway known to modulate sensitivity to cisplatin. Down-regulation of these two critical genes may antagonize cisplatin resistance during the treatment of human ovarian cancer.

References

1. Greenlee RT, Hill-Harmon MB, Murray T, et al. Cancer statistics, 2001. CA Cancer J Clin 2001;51:15–36.
2. Yu JJ. Unlocking the Molecular mechanisms of DNA repair and platinum drug resistance in cancer chemotherapy. Curr Drug Ther 2009;4(1): 19–28.
3. Masuda H, Ozols RF, Lai G-M, et al. Increased DNA repair as a mechanism of acquired resistance to cis-diamminedichloroplatinum (II) in human ovarian cancer cell lines. Cancer Res 1988;48:5713–16.
4. Reed E. ERCC1 Measurements in clinical oncology. N Engl J Med 2006;355:1054–5.
5. Yu JJ, Dabholkar M, Bennett WP, et al. Platinum-sensitive and platinum-resistant ovarian cancer tissues show differences in the relationships between mRNA levels of p53, ERCC1 and XPA. Intl J Oncol 1996;8:313–7.
6. Dabholkar M, Vionnet JA, Bostick-Bruton F, et al. mRNA levels of XPAC and ERCC1 in ovarian tumor tissue correlates with response to platinum containing chemotherapy. J Clin Invest 1994;94:703–8.
7. Parker RJ, Eastman A, Bostick-Bruton F, et al. Acquired cisplatin resistance in human ovarian cancer cells is associated with enhanced repair of cisplatin-DNA lesions and reduced drug accumulation. J Clin Invest 1991;87:772–7.
8. Lee KB, Parker RJ, Bohr VA, et al. Cisplatin sensitivity/resistance in UV-repair deficient Chinese hamster ovary cells of complementation groups 1 and 3. Carcinogenesis 1993;14:2177–80.
9. Liang XB, Reed E, Yu JJ. Protein phosphatase 2A interacts with Chk2 and regulates phosphorylation at Thr-68 after cisplatin treatment of human ovarian cancer cells. Intl J Mol Med 2006;17:703–8.
10. Falck J, Mailand N, Syljuasen RG, et al. The ATM-Chk2-Cdc25A checkpoint pathway guards against radioresistant DNA synthesis. Nature 2001;410:842–7.
11. Zhou BB, Elledge SJ. The DNA damage response: putting checkpoints in perspective. Nature 2000;408:433–9.
12. Matsuoka S, Huang M, Elledge SJ. Linkage of ATM to cell cycle regulation by the Chk2 protein kinase. Science 1998;282:1893–7.
13. Yan QW, Reed E, Zhong XS, et al. MZF1 possesses a repressively regulatory function in ERCC1 expression. Biochem Pharmacol 2006;71:761–71.
14. Li Q, Gardner K, Zhang L, et al. Cisplatin induction of ERCC-1 mRNA expression in A2780/CP70 human ovarian cancer cells. J Biol Chem 1998;273:23419–25.

Modulation of Survival Pathways in Ovarian Carcinoma Cells Resistant to Platinum Compounds

Paola Perego, Valentina Benedetti, Cinzia Lanzi, and Franco Zunino

Abstract Alterations of various signaling pathways implicated in cell survival or cell death may have relevance in cancer cell drug resistance. In particular, the EGF-R pathway may affect cellular response to platinum compounds, because these drugs are capable of modulating the signaling occurring through activation of EGF-R or EGF-R-mediated activation of downstream events. Recent evidence indicates that ovarian carcinoma cells selected for resistance to cisplatin and oxaliplatin exhibits decreased sensitivity to gefitinib. The effect appears not dependent on failure to inhibit the target receptor, but is associated with increased phospho-ERK1/2 levels in the resistant variants. Cells resistant to gefitinib also exhibit reduced sensitivity to MEK1/2 inhibitors. The concomitant activation of distinct mitogen-activated protein kinases, i.e., ERK1/2 and p38 appears a relevant feature of cell resistance to cisplatin.

Thus, the development of resistance to platinum drugs is associated with multiple alterations including deregulation of survival pathways activated by EGF-R resulting in a reduced cellular response to gefitinib.

Keywords Platinum drug resistance; Ovarian cancer cell lines; Epidermal growth factor receptor

Recently, the focus of cancer research in the field of therapeutics has moved from conventional cytotoxic agents to target specific agents designed to selectively hit a molecular target (1). In spite of this, conventional cytotoxic agents still represent the mainstay of antitumor treatment in most tumor types. The molecular characterization of the alterations of different tumor types is expected to provide the rationale for using tailored drugs in several settings. Thus, it will be critical to establish whether targeted therapy can provide advantages in the treatment of tumor resistance to conventional cytotoxic drugs, including platinum compounds. Activation of survival pathways is a

P. Perego (✉), V. Benedetti, C. Lanzi, and F. Zunino
Fondazione IRCCS Istituto Nazionale Tumori, Department of Experimental Oncology and Laboratories, Preclinical Chemotherapy and Pharmacology Unit, Milan, Italy
e-mail: paola.perego@istitutotumori.mi.it

A. Bonetti et al. (eds.), *Platinum and Other Heavy Metal Compounds in Cancer Chemotherapy*, DOI: 10.1007/978-1-60327-459-3_24,
© Humana Press, a part of Springer Science + Business Media, LLC 2009

common feature of cancer cells and may thus play a role in tumor drug resistance (2). In fact, protective signaling pathways are involved in the cellular stress response, including the DNA damage response. It is conceivable that alterations contributing to the platinum-drug resistant phenotype can result also in reduced sensitivity to small molecules targeting signaling pathways implicated in cell survival. Indeed, the mitogen activated protein kinase (MAPK) pathway which couples signals from cell-surface receptors to transcription factors, is frequently aberrantly expressed in many tumors. Also in ovarian carcinoma cell systems, alterations in signaling pathways mediated by the ErbB family of receptors have been documented (3, 4). Increased defence mechanisms, augmentation of DNA repair, inhibition of apoptosis (5) could influence the outcome of the cellular response after treatment with platinum compounds, which represent the first-line therapy for ovarian cancer.

In this chapter, we will briefly discuss the results that we recently obtained in ovarian carcinoma cell systems characterized by acquired resistance to cisplatin and oxaliplatin, where we found reduced sensitivity to gefitinib. Particular attention will be paid to the possible impact of alterations of such pathways on cellular sensitivity to target specific agents tailored to growth factor receptors.

Ovarian Cancer and Signaling Pathways

During tumorigenesis, multiple signaling pathways are deregulated through accumulation of genetic and epigenetic alterations. Mutation of KRAS have been found in mucinous and serous ovarian tumors, and activation of the RAS/RAF signaling pathway in the absence of RAS mutation appears a common feature of high grade ovarian cancer (6). This behavior has been linked to deregulation of upstream signalling molecules of the erbB family (7) Available evidence also supports that the epidermal growth factor receptor (EGF-R) expression is implicated in the progression of disease (8). Patients with alterations in tyrosine kinase receptors tend to have a more aggressive disease and poor prognosis (9).

Survival Pathways and Cell Response to Platinum Compounds

Although the resistant phenotype is probably the result of multiple changes acquired during tumor progression, deregulation of EGF-R signaling has been associated with the development of resistance to cisplatin in different cell lines (3). Proteins of the MAPK family are important mediators of signal transduction processes, which are involved in both growth factor and stress response, and play a complex and controversial role in determining the ultimate fate of the cells depending on cell type and molecular background (10, 11). Three major mammalian MAPK subfamilies have been described including the extracellular signal-regulated kinases (ERK), the c-Jun N-terminal kinases (JNK) and the p38 kinases. The ERK pathway plays a major role in regulating cell growth and differentiation and in ovarian cancer it has been implicated in regulation of proliferation, differentiation and survival (12).

Survival pathways, involving the MAPK or PI3-kinase/Akt cascade, activated in response to cytotoxic stresses appear to be largely shared by signaling pathways mediated by growth factor receptors, including EGF-R. The family of erbB receptors (i.e., EGF-R, erb2, erb3) has been shown to promote cell growth and invasion in ovarian cancer (13, 14). Such concepts have provided a rational basis to the use of selective inhibitors of receptor tyrosine kinases in antitumor therapy. For example, preclinical studies have documented marked antitumor activity as well as oral bioavailability and tolerability of gefitinib (15, 16), which has reached the clinical setting and has been approved for non-small cell lung cancer patients showing disease progression following one or two lines of chemotherapy.

Activation of Survival Pathways in Ovarian Carcinoma Cells with Acquired Resistance to Platinum Drugs

We have recently observed that ovarian cancer cell lines characterized by acquired resistance to cisplatin or oxaliplatin exhibit reduced sensitivity to the EGF-R inhibitor gefitinib (4). In such cell lines, the development of resistance to platinum drugs has been associated with multiple alterations including increased DNA damage tolerance and resistance to apoptosis.

In our study, we found that the observed reduced sensitivity to gefitinib was not associated with the occurrence of EGF-R gene mutations in the receptor kinase domain, quite differently from what is described in other cellular models, in which specific mutations have been related to sensitivity/resistance to treatment with the agent (17–20). The reduced sensitivity was not due to failure of the EGF-R inihibitor to interfere with the target, but was related to ERK activation (4). In fact, we found an increase in phospho-ERK1/2 levels in the platinum drug resistant variants. Such a phenotype was reminiscent of that described in another cisplatin-resistant ovarian carcinoma cell system in which increased ERK activity was documented in the absence of changes in the expression of erbB receptors (3).

The role of ERK in cisplatin response appears controversial, because ERK activation has been associated both with enhanced survival and increased cell death after cisplatin treatment (21–23). In keeping with a pro-apoptotic role of these MAP kinases, recent studies indicate that pharmacological inhibition of ERK1/2 attenuates the cytotoxicity of cisplatin in some cell types (24). However, we and others have documented that, at least in ovarian carcinoma cell lines with acquired resistance to platinum drugs, the ERK pathway provides a survival advantage (3, 4).

Thus, in different model systems diverse effects can be found. Such discrepancies may be due to the different cellular genetic background, but could also be dependent on the experimental conditions (i.e., concentrations of platinum drug used and exposure times). In this context, the duration and intensity of ERK signaling may be a crucial issue. In our platinum drug resistant sublines, we could exclude that increased levels of phospho-ERK were due to decreased expression of protein phosphatases such as MKP-1 and MKP-3, differently from what was observed in other reports (25, 26), but since MKPs are a large family (27), other dual specificity phosphatase may be implicated. Moreover, in principle, activation of ERK could be the result of high levels of activated Ras or Raf as well as of other alterations acquired during the development of resistance.

The cisplatin-resistant variant was characterized by a higher degree of resistance to gefitinib as compared to the oxaliplatin resistant one. Such phenotypes appeared dependent on a different pattern of cell response to the EGF-R inhibitor. In fact, whereas gefitinib was less effective in inhibiting ERK1/2 phosphorylation in both resistant sublines as compared with what was observed in IGROV-1, in the IGROV-1/Pt1 cells the drug produced only a marginal down-regulation of phospho-Akt levels. Such a behavior, supports that deregulation of both ERK1/2 and Akt are implicated in providing survival advantages.

The multifactorial nature of the alterations of survival pathways in drug resistant cells is further supported by the evidence of a high constitutive activation of p38. Such a feature may account for the peculiar localization of EGF-R, which is mainly internalized in the resistant sublines, and for the marginal down-regulation of phospho-Akt observed in oxaliplatin- and cisplatin-resistant cells treated with gefitinib. It has been reported, in fact, that p38 may mediate EGF-R internalization and that Akt activation is induced by cisplatin (28). The persistent activity of Akt and ERK1/2 pathways has been related to lack of sensitivity to EGF-R inhibitors also in non-small cell lung cancer (29).

Overall, our results indicate that the development of resistance to platinum drugs is associated with multiple alterations including deregulation of survival pathways activated by EGF-R resulting in a reduced cellular response to gefitinib (Fig. 1).

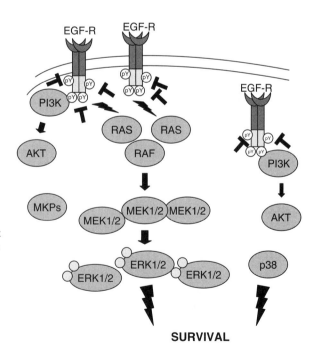

Fig. 1 Schematic representation of survival pathways activated in ovarian carcinoma cells resistant to platinum compounds. The concomitant activation of ERK1/2 and the putative mechanism as well as the possible activation of p38 by internalized EGF receptors (EGF-R) is shown. T, tyrosine kinase inhibitor; MKPs, mitogen activated protein kinase phosphatases

Conclusions

The development of cell systems characterized by acquired resistance to platinum compounds has allowed the identification of several factors that contribute to the drug-resistant phenotype. Such factors include survival pathways, whose deregulation can lead to reduced sensitivity to target-specific agents such as gefitinib. The available results support the view that deregulation of signaling pathways activated by EGF-R, which account for reduced response to gefitinib, may be implicated in the platinum drug-resistant phenotype of ovarian carcinoma cell lines, thereby contributing to cross-resistance between platinum compounds and gefitinib. Therefore, the therapeutic potential of approaches targeting EGF-R could be limited by expression or activation of protective pro-survival pathways. More generally, these observations may be relevant in the development of therapeutic approaches combining cytotoxic agents and targeted signaling inhibitors. A better understanding of the molecular defects leading to the inappropriate activation of the ERK pathway in drug-resistant cells could be useful to define novel therapeutic strategies.

It is now evident that targeting a single alteration may be not sufficient to treat solid tumors efficiently. In addition to this conceptual problem, the available evidences indicate that the development of resistance may involve not only mechanisms of cellular defence, but also alterations resulting in lack of sensitivity to targeted therapies.

References

1. Sebolt-Leopold JS, English JM. Mechanisms of drug inhibition of signalling molecules. Nature 2006;441:457–62.
2. Hanahan D, Weinberg RA. The hallmarks of cancer. Cell 2000;100:57–70.
3. Macleod K., Mullen, P, Sewell J, et al. Altered ErbB receptor signaling and gene expression in cDDP-resistant ovarian cancer. Cancer Res 2005;65:6789–800.
4. Benedetti V, Perego P, Beretta GL, et al. Modulation of survival pathways in ovarian carcinoma cell lines resistant to platinum compounds. Mol Cancer Ther 2008;7:679–87.
5. Manic S, Gatti L, Carenini N, et al 2003. Mechanisms controlling sensitivity to platinum complexes: role of p53 and DNA mismatch repair. Curr Cancer Drug Targets 2003;3:21–9.
6. Downward J. Targeting RAS signalling pathways in cancer therapy. Nat Rev Cancer 2003;3: 11–22.
7. Tanner B, Hasenclever D, Stern K, et al. ErbB-3 predicts survival in ovarian cancer. J Clin Oncol 2006;24:4317–23.
8. Zeren T, Inan S, Vatansever HS, et al. Significance of tyrosine kinase activity on malign transformation of ovarian tumors: a comparison between EGF-R and TGF-α. Acta Histochemica 2008;110:256–63.
9. Serrano-Olvera A, Duenas-Gonzalez A, Gallardo-Rincon D, Candelaria M, De La Garza-Salazar J. Prognostic, predictive and therapeutic implications of HER2 in invasive epithelial ovarian cancer. Cancer Treat Rev 2006;32:180–90.
10. Chang L, Karin M. Mammalian MAP kinase and signalling cascades. Nature 2001; 410: 37–40.
11. Yoon S, Seger R. The extracellular signal-regulated kinase: multiple substrates regulate diverse cellular functions. Growth Factors 2006;24:21–44.

12. Steinmetz R, Wagoner HA, Zeng P, et al. Mechanisms regulating the constitutive activation of the extracellular signal-regulated kinase (ERK) signalling pathway in ovarian cancer and the effect of ribonucleic acid interference for ERK1/2 on cancer cell proliferation. Mol Endocrinol 2004; 18:2570–82.

13. Morishige K, Kurachi H, Amemiya K, et al. Evidence for the involvement of transforming growth factor alpha and epidermal growth factor receptor autocrine growth mechanism in primary human ovarian cancers in vitro. Cancer Res 1991; 51:5322–8.

14. Gilmour LM, Macleod KG, McCaig A, et al. Neuregulin expression, function, and signalling in human ovarian cancer cells. Clin. Cancer Res 2002;8:3933–42.

15. Cantarini MV, McFarquhar T, Smith RP, Bailey C, Marshall AL. Relative bioavailability and safety profile of gefitinib administered as a tablet or as a dispersion preparation via drink or nasogastric tube: results of a randomized, open-label, three-period crossover study in healthy volunteers. Clin. Ther 2004;26:1530–6.

16. Wakeling AE, Guy SP, Woodburn JR, et al. ZD1839 (Iressa): an orally active inhibitor of epidermal growth factor signalling with potential for cancer therapy. Cancer Res 2002;62: 5749–54.

17. Johnson BE, and Janne PA Epidermal growth factor receptor mutations in patients with non-small cell lung cancer. Cancer Res 2005;65:7525–9.

18. Paez JG, Jannem PA, Lee JC, et al. EGFR mutations in lung cancer: correlation with clinical response to gefitinib therapy. Science 2004;304:1497–500.

19. Pao W, Miller VA, Politi KA, et al. Acquired resistance of lung adenocarcinomas to gefitinib or erlotinib is associated with a second mutation in the EGFR kinase domain. PLoS Med 2005;2:73.

20. Lynch TJ, Bell DW, Sordella R, et al. Activating mutations in the epidermal growth factor receptor underlying resposiveness of non-small-cell lung cancer to gefitinib. N. Engl J Med 2004; 350:2129–39.

21. Hayakawa J, Ohmichi M, Kurachi H, et al. Inhibition of extracellular signal-regulated protein kinase or c-Jun N-terminal protein kinase cascade, differentially activated by cisplatin, sensitizes human ovarian cancer cell line. J Biol Chem 1999;274:31648–54.

22. Wang X, Martindale JL, Holbrook NJ. Requirement for ERK activation in cisplatin-induced apoptosis. J Biol Chem 2000;275:39435–43.

23. Schweyer S, Soruri A, Meschter O, et al. Cisplatin-induced apoptosis in human malignant testicular germ cell lines depends on MEK/ERK activation. Br J Cancer 2004;91:589–98.

24. Amran D, Sancho P, Fernandez C, et al. Pharmacological inhibitors of extracellular signal-regulated protein kinases attenuate the apoptotic action of cisplatin in human myeloid leukemia cells via glutathione-independent reduction in intracellular drug accumulation. Biochim Biophys Acta 2005;743:269–79.

25. Xaus J, Comalada M, Valledor AF, et al. Molecular mechanisms involved in macrophage survival, proliferation, activation or apoptosis. Immunobiology 2001;204:543–50.

26. Camps M, Nichols A, Gillieron C, et al. 1998. Catalytic activation of the phosphatase MKP-3 by ERK2 mitogen-activated protein kinase. Science 1998;280:1262–5.

27. Wu G S. Role of mitogen-activated protein kinase phosphatases (MKPs) in cancer. Cancer Metastasis Rev 2007;26:579–85.

28. Winograd-Katz SE, Levitzki A. Cisplatin induces PKB/Akt activation and p38(MAPK) phosphorylation of the EGF receptor. Oncogene 2006;25:7381–90.

29. Janmaat ML, Kruyt FA, Rodriguez JA, Giaccone G. Response to epidermal growth factor receptor inhibitors in non-small cell lung cancer cells: limited antiproliferative effects and absence of apoptosis associated with persistent activity of extracellular signal-regulated kinase or Akt kinase pathways. Clin Cancer Res 2003;9:2316–26.

Paraptotic Cell Death Induced by the Thioxotriazole Copper Complex A0: A New Tool to Kill Apoptosis-Resistant Cancer Cells

Saverio Tardito, Claudio Isella, Enzo Medico, Luciano Marchiò, Maurizio Lanfranchi, Ovidio Bussolati, and Renata Franchi-Gazzola[*]

Abstract The copper(II) complex A0 induces non-apoptotic programmed cell death in human HT1080 fibrosarcoma cells but not in normal fibroblasts (J Med Chem, 50(8):1916–1924, 2007). While typical apoptotic features, such as caspase-3 activation or nuclear fragmentation, are evident in cisplatin-treated cells, they are absent in A0-dependent cell death. In contrast, the latter process is hallmarked by the development of huge vacuoles originating from endoplasmic reticulum (Histochem Cell Biol 126(4):473–482, 2006), a feature consistent with the newly described type of cell death named paraptosis (PNAS 97(26):14376–14381, 2000). Consistently, in a panel of human cancer cells there is no correlation between the sensitivities to A0 and cisplatin. In the same panel, paraptosis-like cell death is observed in all the A0-sensitive cell lines. Moreover, the copper complex kills cisplatin-sensitive cells (HT1080 and ovarian carcinoma 2008) as well as their cisplatin-resistant counterparts (C13[*] cells and the newly established HT1080PTR line) with comparable potencies. The different activity spectrum between A0 and cisplatin suggests distinct mechanisms of action for the two drugs. In agreement with this hypothesis, a whole-genome expression analysis, performed in HT1080 cells, showed that the transcriptional response evoked by the two drugs is poorly overlapping. A0 induces genes involved in oxidative- and endoplasmic reticulum-stress (ER stress), while cisplatin increases the expression of typical p53 targets. Moreover, A0 strongly induces metal responsive genes, as well as HSPs, chaperones and other genes involved in the Unfolded Protein Response (UPR). The validation of the microarray results by qRT PCR and Western Blot confirms that A0, but not cisplatin, activates two pathways of the UPR. In particular, IRE1 mRNA is up-regulated, resulting in the increased abundance of the spliced form of XBP1 mRNA that encodes for the active transcription factor. Moreover, the translation initiator complex subunit eIF2alpha is rapidly phosphorylated, with the consequent attenuation of protein synthesis and the concomitant preferential translation of the pro-death ER stress responsive proteins ATF4, CHOP and GADD34. In conclusion, A0 kills sensitive cancer

S. Tardito, O. Bussolati, and R. Franchi-Gazzola (✉), Dept. of Experimental Medicine
L. Marchiò, M. Lanfranchi, Dept. of General and Inorganic, Analytical, and Physical Chemistry
University of Parma, Italy
C. Isella, E. Medico, Division of Molecular Oncology,
Institute for Cancer Research and Treatment, Candiolo (TO), Italy
e-mail: renata.franchi@unipr.it

A. Bonetti et al. (eds.), *Platinum and Other Heavy Metal Compounds in Cancer Chemotherapy*, DOI: 10.1007/978-1-60327-459-3_25,
© Humana Press, a part of Springer Science + Business Media, LLC 2009

cells through the triggering of ER stress, inducing a paraptotic process. Therefore, the copper complex may constitute a novel device to overcome apoptosis resistance.

Keywords Copper complex; Non-apoptotic cell death; Paraptosis; Vacuolization; Endoplasmic reticulum stress

In recent years, experimental oncology has moved towards the design of anticancer compounds based on metals other than platinum. The goal of these new metal based anticancer compounds is to achieve a specific anticancer activity, with a particular focus for those complexes exhibiting a strong selectivity for a particular type of cancer. Thus, non-platinum complexes that do not mimic cisplatin in their mechanism of action (MOA) are being increasingly developed and some of these compounds have even reached clinical trials. Examples of these are ruthenium (1–2) gadolinium (3) and gallium (4) complexes. The need of new antineoplastic compounds endowed with a specific MOA and lower toxicity, has stimulated the research on potentially therapeutic agents based on endogenous metals, such as copper (5–6).

Indeed, due to its capacity to move between transition states, copper, together with iron, is the most abundant metal within redox enzymes and is an essential cofactor for approximately a dozen of cuproenzymes (7). The redox potential of copper provides the enzymes with their electron transfer capabilities. Paradoxically, it is the same redox potential of copper that makes it potentially toxic for the cell. Under conditions where copper is allowed to accumulate freely, the redox active metals contribute directly to cell oxidative damage. Cells have, therefore, developed sophisticated regulations and transfer systems to ensure a tight control of copper concentrations according to a "no free metal" principle (8). The two disorders of copper metabolism (Menkes and Wilson diseases) are a proof of the essential need of a tight homeostatic control of the intracellular levels of the metal. Such precise control is mediated through the coordinated action of several proteins, including the transporter CTR1, cytosolic carriers called metallochaperones, and Cu-ATPases (9). The modulation of copper reactivity by proteins with metal-chaperone activity could be considered a natural lesson to design copper complexes endowed with a biologically relevant activity. For this purpose, the ligand structure becomes crucial since through the metal coordination it modifies the reactivity of copper for biological macromolecules, modifies metal bioavailability and enhances its uptake or extrusion.

Thiosemicarbazone ligands emerged in the sixties for their antitumoral activity in vitro and in vivo through copper complexation (10–11). The peripheral parts of thiosemicarbazone ligands have been opportunely modified and Cu(II) complexes synthesized. Some of them were able to inhibit growth or to induce death of human cancer cells in vitro (12–14) and in vivo (15–17) although they never reached the standards required for an anticancer drug.

Assuming the N-S coordination of thiosemicarbazones as a model for the modulation of the copper reactivity, a new class of thioxotriazole complexes that retain the rich chemistry of N-Cu-S moieties have been designed and screened. Only a few copper complexes emerged from the screening exhibiting a significant cytotoxic effect specific for tumor cells when compared with the normal counterparts (18). In addition, neither the ligand nor the metal alone produced effects compared to those complexes, demonstrating a great synergism between the two components.

We performed an in-depth characterization of the chemical and biological properties of the most active complex, called A0 (the copper(II) complex of 4-amino-1,4-dihydro-3-(2-pyridyl)-5-thioxo 1,2,4-triazole). Its chelating capability involves the thioxo and amino groups, as documented by the X-ray crystal structure (18). A0 and cisplatin showed a comparable cytotoxic activity in the human fibrosarcoma HT1080 cell line, where the concentrations of the two drugs needed to produce a 50% decrease in cell viability after 48 h, IC50, were 12 and 9 µM, respectively. The cytotoxicity showed by these complexes resulted significantly specific for tumor cells when compared with the normal counterparts (cultured human fibroblasts).

The primary characterization of the biological properties of A0 was the study of the cell death process induced by this compound. In contrast to the literature data, which attributed the cytotoxicity of copper complexes to apoptosis induction, the typical apoptotic-markers were not increased by A0. The difference in the morphology of cells treated with cisplatin or with copper complexes was dramatic. While cisplatin induced all the typical apoptotic features, A0-treated cells were well distinguishable for the appearance of a massive cytoplasmic vacuolization (19). The absence of an apoptotic morphology showed by A0-treated cells was consistent with cytofluorimetric analysis (lack of nuclear fragmentation), confocal microscopy (lack of phosphatidylserine exposure) and biochemical assays (no increase in caspase-3 activity), demonstrating that A0 did not trigger typical apoptosis (19). In contrast, cisplatin completely fulfilled its pro-apoptotic fame thus becoming an optimal term of comparison. Unexpectedly, A0 was able to inhibit completely the activation of caspase-3 stimulated by cisplatin. We think that the inhibition of caspase-3 activity could favor the switch of the cell death pathway triggered by A0 from apoptosis to an alternative process.

In parallel, the nature of A0-induced vacuoles was also investigated. Vacuoles were neither autophagic nor referable to a massive accumulation of proteins and lipids, and were independent from endocytosis. Electron microscopy yielded an accurate analysis of the progression of the vacuolization process, confirmed the scarcity of material inside the vacuoles and, more importantly, demonstrated their origin from the endoplasmic reticulum. As a whole, these results led us to conclude that A0 caused the induction of Type IIIB cell death (20), more recently named "paraptosis" (21). The first molecular approach for the elucidation of the processes involved in paraptosis appeared in 2000 in a paper by Sperandio et al. In that study, paraptosis was definitively distinguished from apoptosis, not only from a morphological point of view, but also through the identification of a few molecular paraptotic "players". This type of cell death could be induced following the deregulated expression of insulin-like growth factor I receptor (IGF-IR) in several mammalian cell lines, as well as in primary fibroblasts. In recent years, an increasing number of paraptotic death processes were identified in diverse fields, including development, cancer therapeutics and neurodegenerative disorders (22–24).

Our study was the first identification of an anticancer compound able to induce a paraptotic type of programmed cell death. For this reason, the comprehension of MOA and structure-activity relationship of A0 appeared to be of interest. The spontaneous desulfuration of the complex suggested that the reactivity of Cu-thioamido group was a determinant for the activity of A0. To test this hypothesis further, the thioxo group of A0 was methylated transforming the strong nucleophilic thione functionality into a less coordinative thioether form. In this way, previously unfavored nitrogen coordination sites become more accessible to metals. All the various groups attached to the sulphur atom lower both the coordination capability of the ligands and the potency of A0. On the other hand, all the newly synthesized complexes induced, at high concentrations, the same paraptotic morphology caused by A0 (25).

New synthetic procedures were applied to obtain ligands with an aminomethyl function attached to the heterocyclic ring in place of the pyridyl residue present in the ligands of A0 (26). The copper complexes obtained demonstrated a higher water solubility compared with their counterparts but, despite their good stability, they were scarcely effective in inhibiting proliferation of the cancer cells. The decrease in biological activity probably reflects the loss of hydrophobic segments important for the interaction with lipophilic sites of the cell, like plasma and intracellular membranes. Nevertheless, the dislocation of the nitrogen atom of the pyridil ring from *meta* to *para* position, rendered the complex completely ineffective, suggesting that this atom also participates in the coordination of copper (unpublished results). These results point to the triazole copper complex as a new class of compounds in which the N,S coordination enhance the cytotoxic activity.

As far as the mechanism of action of A0 is concerned, we obtained a clear cut evidence of the A0 ability to increase both the cell content of copper and the oxidized form of glutathione (25). The copper accumulation, and the consequent oxidative stress, demonstrated in HT1080 cells, provided a solid basis to link the chemical properties of the metal compound with some aspects of the cell response detailed below. We also demonstrated that the spectrum of activity of the A0 is determined by the different ability to accumulate copper upon incubation with the drug. This criterion of selectivity could be exploited to link specifically the toxicity of A0 to cancer cells with alterations in copper metabolism.

Our previous observation that in HT1080 cells the copper complex A0 induces paraptotic-like cell death and cisplatin induces apoptosis, (19) has been recently extended to the study of the sensitivity pattern of a panel of 25 human tumor cell lines to the two agents. The results obtained clearly indicate that the responses to the two drugs are independent, thus supporting the hypothesis of two distinct MOAs. Moreover, no cross resistance between A0 and cisplatin was found in two pairs of cisplatin-resistant/sensitive cell lines, C13*/2008 (ovarian carcinoma) and the newly established HT1080PTR/HT1080.

Various methods have been used to elucidate the intracellular effects of A0 and the consequent cell responses to the incubation in the presence of the complex. The genome-wide analysis of the transcriptional response induced by A0 allowed to find out some answers to these issues. The microarray results yielded a molecular fingerprint of the cell response to A0 and definitively demonstrated that A0 MOA was unrelated to that of cisplatin. Not only A0 elicited an integrated genetic program to face copper accumulation and oxidative stress, but it also turned on a strong response to endoplasmic reticulum (ER) stress. Indeed, A0 increased the expression of proteins involved in polypeptide folding, such as GRP78 and DNAJB9, known components of the unfolded protein response (UPR), and in the elimination of misfolded proteins by the ER-associated protein degradation (ERAD) system. Moreover A0 induced also ER stress-related pro-death genes like GADD34, CHOP and its target TRB-3, thus identifying new players of the paraptotic process.

In A0-treated cells the inhibition of translation that prevents further accumulation of unfolded proteins was associated to the phosphorylation of the translation initiation factor eIF2 subunit alpha (eIF2α), which controls the first regulated step of protein synthesis. The relevance of this event in the A0-induced cell death process was investigated comparing the response of Mouse Embryonic Fibroblasts (MEFs) homozygous for the mutation which eliminates the phosphorylation site of eIF2α (A/A), with the wild type counterpart (S/S). The results demonstrated that phospho-eIF2α enhanced the death of A0-treated cells, likely through the induction of its pro-death targets (i.e. GADD34 and CHOP).

A model that sketches the responses of a tumor cell population to conventional chemotherapeutic drugs is reported in Fig. 1. According to the model, cells can die

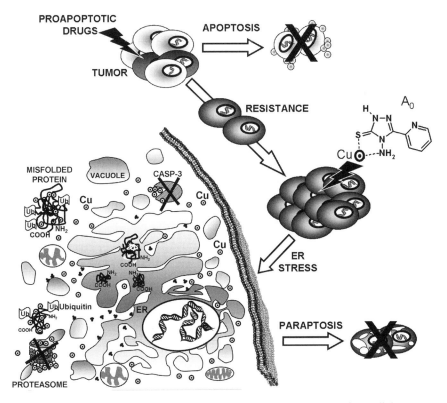

Fig. 1 A0, an alternative to classical pro-apoptotic drugs? A0 induces intracellular copper accumulation. Cu, represented free in the cytoplasm for simplicity, interacts with various cell components causing the loss of function of caspase-3 and proteasome as well as oxidative damage to other proteins. The consequent accumulation of damaged/misfolded unbiquitinylated proteins, determines ER stress and dilatation, massive vacuolization and, eventually, paraptosis

or, alternatively, can survive, if they are apoptosis-resistant. It is known, indeed, that impaired apoptosis contributes to a multidrug resistant phenotype and leads to chemotherapy failure. Under these conditions, the prosecution of treatment with pro apoptotic drugs is scarcely effective while compounds that trigger an alternative type of programmed cell death may still work. Since the copper complex A0 causes copper overload in cancer cells, ER stress and, eventually, paraptotic-like cell death it could be the starting point for the identification of innovative apoptosis-independent therapeutic strategies.

References

1. Rademaker-Lakhai JM, van den Bongard D, Pluim D, Beijnen JH, Schellens JH. A phase I and pharmacological study with imidazolium-trans-DMSO-imidazole-tetrachlororuthenate, a novel ruthenium anticancer agent. Clin Cancer Res 2004;10:3717–27.
2. Jakupec MA, Arion VB, Kapitza S, et al. KP1019 (FFC14A) from bench to bedside: preclinical and early clinical development–an overview. Int J Clin Pharmacol Ther 2005;43:595–6.
3. Meyers CA, Smith JA, Bezjak A, et al. Neurocognitive function and progression in patients with brain metastases treated with whole-brain radiation and motexafin gadolinium: results of a randomized phase III trial. J Clin Oncol 2004;22:157–65.
4. Hofheinz RD, Dittrich C, Jakupec MA, et al. Early results from a phase I study on orally administered tris(8-quinolinolato)gallium(III) (FFC11, KP46) in patients with solid tumors–a CESAR study (Central European Society for Anticancer Drug Research–EWIV). Int J Clin Pharmacol Ther 2005;43:590–1.
5. Wang T, Guo Z. Copper in medicine: homeostasis, chelation therapy and antitumor drug design. Curr Med Chem 2006;13:525–37.
6. Sorenson JR, Wangila GW. Co-treatment with copper compounds dramatically decreases toxicities observed with cisplatin cancer therapy and the anticancer efficacy of some copper chelates which supports the conclusion that copper chelate therapy may be markedly more effective and less toxic than cisplatin therapy. Curr Med Chem 2007;14:1499–503.
7. Prohaska JR, Gybina AA. Intracellular copper transport in mammals. J Nutr 2004;134:1003–6.
8. Rae TD, Schmidt PJ, Pufahl RA, Culotta VC, O'Halloran TV. Undetectable intracellular free copper: the requirement of a copper chaperone for superoxide dismutase. Science 1999;284:805–8.
9. Lutsenko S, Barnes NL, Bartee MY, Dmitriev OY. Function and regulation of human copper-transporting ATPases. Physiol Rev 2007;87:1011–46.
10. Cappuccino JG, Banks S, Brown G, George M, Tarnowski GS. The effect of copper and other metal ions on the antitumor activity of pyruvaldehyde bis(thiosemicarbazone). Cancer Res 1967;27:968–73.
11. Crim JA, Petering HG. The antitumor activity of Cu(II)KTS, the copper (II) chelate of 3-ethoxy-2-oxobutyraldehyde bis(thiosemicarbazone). Cancer Res 1967;27:1278–85.
12. Filomeni G, Cerchiaro G, Da Costa Ferreira AM, et al. Pro-apoptotic activity of novel Isatin-Schiff base copper(II) complexes depends on oxidative stress induction and organelle-selective damage. J Biol Chem 2007;282:12010–21.
13. Thati B, Noble A, Creaven BS, Walsh M, Kavanagh K, Egan DA. Apoptotic cell death: a possible key event in mediating the in vitro anti-proliferative effect of a novel copper(II) complex, [Cu(4-Mecdoa)(phen)(2)] (phen = phenanthroline, 4-Mecdoa = 4-methylcoumarin-6,7-dioxactetate), in human malignant cancer cells. Eur J Pharmacol 2007;569:16–28.

14. Ahmed F, Adsule S, Ali AS, et al. A novel copper complex of 3-benzoyl-alpha methyl benzene acetic acid with antitumor activity mediated via cyclooxygenase pathway. Int J Cancer 2007;120: 734–42.
15. Mookerjee A, Mookerjee Basu J, Dutta P, et al. Overcoming drug-resistant cancer by a newly developed copper chelate through host-protective cytokine-mediated apoptosis. Clin Cancer Res 2006;12:4339–49.
16. Chen D, Cui QC, Yang H, et al. Clioquinol, a therapeutic agent for Alzheimer's disease, has proteasome-inhibitory, androgen receptor-suppressing, apoptosis-inducing, and antitumor activities in human prostate cancer cells and xenografts. Cancer Res 2007;67:1636–44.
17. Chen D, Cui QC, Yang H, Dou QP. Disulfiram, a clinically used anti-alcoholism drug and copper-binding agent, induces apoptotic cell death in breast cancer cultures and xenografts via inhibition of the proteasome activity. Cancer Res 2006;66:10425–33.
18. Dallavalle F, Gaccioli F, Franchi-Gazzola R, et al. Synthesis, molecular structure, solution equilibrium, and antiproliferative activity of thioxotriazoline and thioxotriazole complexes of copper II and palladium II. J Inorg Biochem 2002;92:95–104.
19. Tardito S, Bussolati O, Gaccioli F, et al. Non-apoptotic programmed cell death induced by a copper(II) complex in human fibrosarcoma cells. Histochem Cell Biol 2006;126:473–82.
20. Clarke PG. Developmental cell death: morphological diversity and multiple mechanisms. Anat Embryol (Berl) 1990;181:195–213.
21. Sperandio S, de Belle I, Bredesen DE. An alternative, nonapoptotic form of programmed cell death. Proc Natl Acad Sci USA 2000;97:14376–81.
22. Jadus MR, Chen Y, Boldaji MT, et al. Human U251MG glioma cells expressing the membrane form of macrophage colony-stimulating factor (mM-CSF) are killed by huma monocytes in vitro and are rejected within immunodeficient mice via paraptosis that is associated with increased expression of three different heat shock proteins. Cancer Gene Ther 2003;10:411–20.
23. Abraham MC, Lu Y, Shaham S. A morphologically conserved nonapoptotic program promotes linker cell death in *Caenorhabditis elegans*. Dev Cell 2007;12:73–86.
24. Rao RV, Poksay KS, Castro-Obregon S, et al. Molecular components of a cell death pathway activated by endoplasmic reticulum stress. J Biol Chem 2004;279:177–87.
25. Tardito S, Bussolati O, Maffini M, et al. Thioamido coordination in a thioxo-1,2,4-triazole copper(II) complex enhances nonapoptotic programmed cell death associated with copper accumulation and oxidative stress in human cancer cells. J Med Chem 2007;50:1916–24.
26. Gaccioli F, Franchi-Gazzola R, Lanfranchi M, et al. Synthesis, solution equilibria and anti-proliferative activity of copper(II) aminomethyltriazole and aminomethylthioxotriazoline complexes. J Inorg Biochem 2005;99:1573–84.

Section D
Clinical Applications

Platinum Compounds and Radiation

Lea Baer, Franco M. Muggia, and Silvia C. Formenti

Abstract Combining concurrent radiation with platinum compounds has been the subject of both preclinical and clinical cancer research for over two decades. The property of platinum to enhance the effect of radiation on a variety of tumors has been successfully translated to the treatment of head and neck, non-small cell lung (NSCLC), and cervical cancer.

Several molecular pathways accounting for the mechanisms of radiation potentiation and sensitization have been described. Platinums create DNA adducts causing cross links which eventually lead to double strand DNA breaks. Such damage to the DNA triggers the cellular mismatch repair (MMR) apparatus, leading to cell cycle arrest and apoptosis. This pathway can be harnessed to enhance radiotherapy by targeting the subset of hypoxic tumor cells, resistant to the traditional effects of radiation.

Noticeably, in tumors with either a genetic defect or a gene rendered nonfunctional due to promoter hyper-methylation in the MMR pathway, resistance to both chemotherapies and ionizing radiation occurs. Concurrent administration of both modalities though, has shown to overcome this form of resistance. The mechanism underlying the combined effects includes platinum interference with repair mechanisms of sub lethal radiation damage to DNA and radiation potentiation of the effects of platinum by enhancing uptake and binding to DNA.

Experience from the clinic suggests that many variables govern the success of the combination. Specifically, the kind of platinum compound chosen and its dosing and scheduling during radiotherapy varies among tumor sites. The more manageable toxicity profile of carboplatin makes it a particularly attractive candidate for combined modality treatments. In a phase III CALBG and ECOG study, 283 patients with unresectable stage III NSCLC received radiosensitization with carboplatin. Complete Response (CR) rate was 18% in the chemo-radiation arm vs. 10% in the radiation-only arm, without significant difference detected in the 4-year survival rates (13% vs. 10%). Conversely, in cervical cancer the combination of

L. Baer, F.M. Muggia, and S.C. Formenti (✉)
Department of Radiation Oncology, New York University School of Medicine,
New York, NY, USA
e-mail: silvia.formenti@med.nyu.edu

A. Bonetti et al. (eds.), *Platinum and Other Heavy Metal Compounds
in Cancer Chemotherapy*, DOI: 10.1007/978-1-60327-459-3_26,
© Humana Press, a part of Springer Science + Business Media, LLC 2009

211

carboplatin and radiotherapy resulted in a survival improvement compared to other chemoradiation regimes.

A better insight of the genomics and biology of cancer will soon provide clinicians with the necessary rationale to devise multimodality protocols that target individual tumor pathways of resistance. Combinations of platinum agents with ionizing radiation could then be selectively offered to carriers of cancers with genetic and phenotypic characteristics that make them more likely to be vulnerable to this approach.

Keywords Radiotherapy; Platinum Compounds

Introduction

This review highlights some of the mechanisms mediating damage shared by platinum compounds and radiation, as well as some of the areas of demonstrated synergy when the two modalities are combined. While there is not an exhaustive report on the subject, this chapter offers an opportunity to reflect on the advantages of a multidisciplinary approach, which is also likely to reflect on improved local control in locally advanced and unresectable tumors. Moreover, while DNA repair pathways are rapidly being elucidated and their relevance to human tumors is more understood, interest in harnessing both platinum compounds and ionizing radiation is revived.

Platinum compounds create DNA adducts forming covalent bonds with specific purine bases, resulting in DNA intra- and inter-strand cross links and changes in DNA conformation. Such damage to the DNA not only inhibits DNA synthesis and causes delay in the S phase, but also triggers the cellular mismatch repair (MMR) apparatus leading to cell cycle arrest and apoptosis.

Resistance to platinum compounds may be an inherent trait of the particular tumor type or cells (possibly related to progenitor or "stem cells"), or may be acquired by some cells following exposure to a platinum. Such resistance has been attributed to mutations in various genes resulting in either limited uptake of the drug (1–3), increased intracellular levels of glutathione (GSH) (4), absence of damage induced apoptosis (5, 6) or by enhanced repair of the DNA damage (7, 8).

Noticeably, the same pathways governing response to platinum are relevant to radio response. Perego et al. tested platinum compounds against a panel of yeast mutants based on hypersensitivity to ionizing radiation due to mutations in genes involved in DNA repair and cell cycle control (9). This testing enabled the researchers to characterize a corresponding hypersensitivity to specific platinum compounds.

Combining Platinum with Radiation: Rationale and Preclinical Data

The concomitant use of radiation and the systemic delivery of chemotherapy have the potential to enhance local tumor control, decrease risk of distant relapse and consequently improve survival. Ideally this is to be achieved without increased toxicity to normal tissue. The enhancement of cell kill can be achieved with the combination of chemotherapy agents targeting the same sites as radiation, e.g. the DNA, or a different site altogether, thus resulting in a cumulative damage-triggering cell death.

Platinum analogues given concurrently with ionizing radiation enhance cell kill by several mechanisms. These mechanisms include enhanced formation of toxic platinum intermediates in the presence of radiation-induced free radicals, inhibition of DNA repair, radiation induced increase in cellular platinum uptake, and cell cycle arrest (10–13).

Radiosensitization is defined as an enhancement of radiation effect obtainable when the sensitizing drug is completely non-toxic at the dose level at which it is used (14). Such enhancement is particularly important in the treatment of the hypoxic cell fraction found in solid tumors. Such cells are undertreated by ionizing radiation due to lack or limited formation of free radicals, leading to sub lethal and potentially lethal DNA damage. The combined modality treatment inhibits the recovery of the hypoxic cells from the sub lethal damage, therefore causing sensitization and enhancing cell kill. The potential formation of toxic platinum compounds in the presence of radiation further targeting intra and extracellular sites in the field of radiation, accounts for the radiopotentiating effect.

The radiosensitizing and potentiating effects have been demonstrated in solid tumors not necessarily sensitive to platinum by itself (15). The administration of platinum to a platinum-sensitive tumor on the other hand, has the added benefit of addressing systemic disease as well, in the presence of adequate dose delivery.

The combination of platinum analogues and radiation has been investigated since the early seventies with work done on animal models and in vitro. The documented synergy in these early studies was later, further investigated in an effort to elucidate the underlying radiobiologic mechanisms. The seminal work by Wodinsky et al., published in 1974, has shown improved survival in mice bearing P388 lymphocytic leukemia when treated with combination cisplatin and radiation (16). Soon after studies by Richmond et al. (17, 18) have demonstrated enhanced DNA damage and lethality induction by the same combination in bacterial spores and *E. coli*.

The underlying mechanisms of this apparent synergy are yet to be fully understood but the inhibition of repair of potentially lethal damage (19) and the radiosensitization of hypoxic tumor cells (20) emerged as the most likely explanations. The sensitization of hypoxic cells by cisplatin was found to operate through reactive free radicals, in part through the interactions of radiation-induced reactive Pt(I) intermediates, and in part through the involvement of thermodynamic and kinetic aspects of Pt(II)-DNA binding during irradiation (10). The putative mechanism of PLD was further supported by preclinical studies showing greater benefit in combining chemotherapy and fractionated radiation (21). While the combined approach yielded the most benefit at the G1 phase of mammalian cell cycle, the difference when compared to other cell cycle phases was small and probably not clinically significant (22). The optimal sequencing of the two modalities was explored by Douple and Richmond in their work with the mouse mammary tumor MTG-B model (23). Tumor regression was maximized when cisplatin was given an hour before radiation when compared to post irradiation injection of cisplatin.

Combining Platinum and Radiation: Clinical Examples

At present concomitant chemoradiation is used in treatment of a variety of solid tumors warranting radiation for loco-regional control. These tumors include head and neck, small and non-small cell lung cancer, esophageal, rectal and anal cancers, gastric and pancreatic cancers, cervical and bladder cancers, glioblastoma and locally advanced breast cancer. The treatment of these tumors may be pre-operative, adjuvant or definitive with different scheduling and dosing schemes utilized accordingly.

Head and Neck Cancer

Platinum compounds were first introduced to the treatment of patients with advanced head and neck squamous cell carcinoma (HNSCC) with response rates (RR) of 30% (24) and with subsequent higher RR achieved in induction therapy (25).

Single agent carboplatin was also explored with similar, although somewhat inferior, results (26).

In 2000, Pignon et al., published a meta-analysis of 63 trials comparing chemora-diation to radiation alone, with a total of 10,741 patients enrolled in these trials (27). The addition of chemotherapy has resulted in a pooled hazard ratio of death of 0.90 ($p < 0.0001$), corresponding to an absolute survival benefit of 4% at 2 and 5 years in favor of chemotherapy. A meta-analysis of the six trials comparing concomitant or alternating chemoradiation versus the sequential treatment with chemotherapy and radiation, demonstrated the superiority of the former. A hazard ratio of 0.91 in favor of the concomitant or alternating approach was observed. The publication of two phase two trials combining 5-fluorouracil (5FU) and cisplatin with radiation and reporting RR of 67 and 70% and complete response rates (CR) of 19 and 27%, made this combination a common practice (28, 29). Two large trials comparing multi-drug chemoradiation to radiation alone, with either standard fractionation or twice daily radiation, have demonstrated improved loco-regional control and improved survival (30, 31). Wendt et al. reported on 298 patients randomized to 5FU and cisplatin with concurrent radiation twice daily or radiation alone (30). The 3-year loco regional was improved from 17 to 36% with the combined treatment and overall survival was improved from 24 to 48%, both results statistically sig-nificant. The GORTEC trial reported on 222 patients with oropharyngeal cancers treated with carboplatin and 5FU and radiation compared to radiation alone (31). Similar improvements were reported in 3-year loco regional control (66% vs. 42%, in favor of chemoradiation) and an overall survival (51% vs. 31%, respectively). When combination chemotherapy was compared to chemoradiation with a single agent, the combinations achieved higher response rates, but with added toxicity and no statistically significant survival benefit (32, 33).

The taxanes were introduced to the treatment of HNSCC during the previous decade. Both paclitaxel and docetaxel demonstrated significant activity as a single agent (34) and were incorporated into chemoradiation regimens. Taxanes were combined with either cisplatin or carboplatin, with acceptable toxicity profile and an encouraging RR showed organ preservation rates in advanced disease stages (35–38).

Non-Small Cell Lung Cancer (NSCLC)

As platinum based chemoradiation was studied in a multitude of clinical trials with a variety of dosing schemes and scheduling, the optimal treatment approach is yet to be defined. In a recent systematic review, El-Sharouni et al., compared the clinical results of radiotherapy alone versus concurrent or sequential chemoradiation, for inoperable NSCLC stage III (39). The mean median survival duration for radiotherapy only was 10.4 months. For sequential chemo- and radiotherapy it was increased to 13.0 months. When radiotherapy in the sequential regimen was accompanied by chemotherapy, the mean median duration was 15.8. For concurrent radiochemotherapy it was further increased to 16.4 months. The mean 2- and 3-year overall survivals for radiotherapy alone, sequential and concurrent radiochemotherapy were 17.1 and 10, 23.8 and 18.5, and 32.5 and 25.7%, respectively. Concurrent chemoradiotherapy is superior to the sequential treatment with both, and should be the treatment of choice.

Cancer of the Cervix

In 1998, the National Cancer Institute published a clinical alert, regarding the role of concurrent cisplatin based chemotherapy and radiation treatment of cervical cancer patients. The clinical alert was prompted by the maturation of data from five randomized trials conducted in the US in the 1990s (40–44). Collectively, these five trials, the GOG 85, RTOG-9001, GOG 120, SWOG-8797/GOG-109 and GOG-123, enrolled a total of 1,894 women in various disease stages. The superiority of concurrent chemoradiation to radiation alone was evident in all of the trials. The concurrent administration of cisplatin-based chemotherapy led to improvement in both local and distant control, therefore improving survival.

Following the clinical alert a sixth randomized trial was reported by the NCI of Canada (45). This multi institutional trial failed to demonstrate an added benefit of a similar concurrent cisplatin based chemotherapy regimen when compared to radiation alone in the treatment of locally advanced cervical cancer. It is important to note the small trial size and the higher prevalence of untreated severe anemia in the chemoradiation arm.

A pooled analysis of all six trials maintained the survival and local control advantage of the concurrent approach.

While carboplatin seems to be an attractive radiosensitizing agent due to its milder toxicity profile, several phase II trials evaluating its performance in advanced cervical cancer have reported lower response rates than seen with cisplatin (46, 47). The feasibility of concurrent carboplatin and radiation given continuously (48), weekly (49, 50), twice weekly (51) or once every three weeks (52) has been reported.

At present the platinum compound of choice remains cisplatin but a clearer definition of scheduling and dosing is still pending.

Oxaliplatin – Radiation: Potential Therapeutic Gains

While cisplatin and carboplatin have been both studied extensively in a variety of solid tumors, there is paucity of information regarding the incorporation of the newer compound, oxaliplatin, in chemoradiation regimens. The established role for oxaliplatin in the treatment of colorectal cancer (53, 54), made it an attractive candidate for radiosensitization studies in the treatment of locally advanced rectal cancer. The efficacy and feasibility of such an approach was demonstrated in pre-clinical (55, 56) and phase I-II trials (57–61). NSABP R-04, a randomized phase III trial of >1,600 patients, has begun to accrue patients and will compare neoadjuvant radiation with either infusion 5-FU with or without oxaliplatin versus capecitabine with or without oxaliplatin (62).

A pioneer phase III study from China published in 2005, compared standard radiotherapy with or without weekly oxaliplatin in the treatment of locally advanced nasopharyngeal carcinoma (NPC) (63): 115 patients were randomly assigned to either radiotherapy (RT) alone or concurrent chemoradiotherapy (CCRT). CCRT with oxaliplatin $70 \, mg/m^2$ weekly was administered for six doses from the first day of RT. 97% of the patients completed all planned doses of oxaliplatin, and no grade 3–4 toxicities were observed. After a median follow-up time of 24 months, significant differences in overall survival (100% vs. 77%, $p = 0.01$), relapse-free survival (96% vs. 83%, $p = 0.02$), and metastasis-free survival (92% vs. 80%, $p = 0.02$) were observed, all in favor of the CCRT arm.

Novel Compounds and Targeted Therapy

The incorporation of novel platinum compounds in chemoradiation studies may possibly offer improved toxicity profile with an equal or superior clinical benefit. Satraplatin (BMS-182751, JM-216), a novel oral cisplatin analog, has demonstrated a synergistic effect when combined with radiation in preclinical studies of various tumor models (64–66) and with a single agent phase I study reporting myelotoxicity as the dose limiting toxicity (67). A seminal phase I study evaluated the feasibility and toxicity of escalating doses of Satraplatin and concomitant radiation in the treatment of patients with advanced malignancies of the chest (68). Myelotoxicity was again the dose limiting toxicity, with 30 mg/m2/day for five days, the recommended dose for future chemoradiation studies. Phase II studies are needed to evaluate the possible clinical value of this combination.

The altered pharmacokinetics and toxicity profiles described, with the advent of liposomal encapsulated dosage forms of cisplatin (69, 70) may have important implications on the synergy targeted by the combined approach. Seminal work done with such slow-release vehicles combined with radiation have shown superior responses and improved survival in canines bearing nasal cavity tumor (71).

The combination of a platinum compound with targeted therapy is currently investigated in the treatment of various solid tumors. Cetuximab is a chimeric human- mouse monoclonal antibody that targets the epidermal growth factor receptor (EGFR), which is frequently overexpressed in non-small cell lung cancer (NSCLC). A phase II trial testing cetuximab in combination with a carboplatin and paclitaxel doublet as first-line chemotherapy in NSCLC, showed a 1 year survival rate of 45% and median survival of 11 months, with another phase II trial exploring cetuximab in combination with carboplatin and gemcitabine, reporting similar results (72). A phase II randomized trial tested cisplatin/vinorelbine with or without cetuximab as first-line therapy in 86 patients with advanced non-small cell lung cancer. The overall efficacy was slightly superior in the cetuximab arm and a phase III trial is currently ongoing to definitively determine the role of cetuximab in this setting.

In a phase III trial, Bonner et al. reported a significant survival benefit in patients with locally advanced HNSCC treated with a high-dose radiotherapy and weekly cetuximab when compared with radiotherapy alone (73). As chemoradiation with platinum is currently the standard of care for these patients, the combination of cis-platin (given every 3 weeks) and cetuximab with concurrent radiation was explored in a Phase II study as a definitive treatment of locally advanced HNSCC (74). The encouraging 3 year loco-regional control rate of 71%, progression-free survival rate of 56% and overall survival of 76%, will hopefully be validated in an ongoing phase III trial – RTOG 2303 – comparing cetuximab and concurrent radiation with and without cisplatin (q3w) (75).

Bevacizumab (Avastin) is a humanized monoclonal antibody directed against vascular endothelial growth factor (VEGF). In preclinical models, the administration of anti-angiogenesis therapies improves tumor oxygenation by normalizing tumor vasculature and interstitial pressure (76–78) and improves response to radiation (79–81). A phase I trial evaluated the combination of bevacizumab, capecit-abine, oxaliplatin, and radiation therapy in patients with rectal cancer. Eleven patients were enrolled with six documented clinical responses: two patients had a pathologic complete response, and 3 had microscopic disease only. One patient experienced a postoperative abscess, another a syncope episode, and one a subclini-cal myocardial infarction during adjuvant chemotherapy (82).

Pharmaco and Radiation Genomics: The DNA
Repair Crossroad

Pharmacogenomics and radiation genomics are emerging fields that may predict individual response to treatment (83). Germline mutations of the DNA repair path-way, relevant to both platinum and radiation sensitivity, result in impaired response

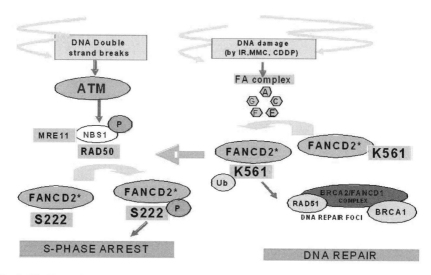

Fig. 1 The Fanconi anemia/BRCA pathway and inactivation of BRCA1 in breast/ovarian cancer. Modified from Olopade and Wei (84)

to DNA damage and increased cancer susceptibility. Alternatively the promoter of these genes can be methylated. In either case, sensitivity to these treatments can be exploited. Figure 1 summarizes the complex interaction between DNA repair signal transduction pathways (84). The Fanconi anemia/BRCA pathway plays a major role in these signaling and $FANCD_2$ protein functions at the intersection of two signaling pathways. In response to ionizing radiation mediated double-strand (DBS), ATM phosphorylates the NBS_1 protein. Phosphorylation of the NSB_1 is required for $FANCD_2$ phosphorylation at serine 222 (S222), leading to activation of an S phase checkpoint, and the FA complex mediates the UB of $FANCD_2$ at lysine 561. Activated $FANCD_2$ is translocated to chromatin and DNA repair foci, which contain the $BRCA_1$ protein and $BRCA_2/FANCD_1$ protein complex. $BRCA_2/FANCD_1$ binds to RAD_{51} and to DNA, promoting a DNA repair response. The Ub-$FANCD_2$ also co-localizes with NSB-MRE_{11}-RAD_{50} complex in DNA damage nuclear foci.

Thus inactivation of $BRCA_1$ or $BRCA_2$ leads to hypersensitivity to DNA damaging agents utilized in the treatment of breast/ovarian cancers arising in mutation carriers.

The co-localization of poly-ADP-ribose-polymerase-1 ($PARP_1$) has been noted in platinum-damaged DNA pointing to the importance of base-excision repair (BER) during platinum treatment. Cancers arising in a BRCA1 or BRCA2 deficient background are deficient in homology-directed DNA repair (or homologous recombination, HR) that is required for error-free repair of the duplex breaks caused by excision of platinum-DNA adducts. Conditional mouse models with breast tissue-specific mutation of BRCA1 are reminiscent of human basal-like (triple-negative) breast cancer (85). These cancers respond well to cisplatin and do not become resistant, highlighting the importance of irreversible inactivation of HR in platinum sensitivity (86). In fact, a newly described mechanism of resistance in these tumors appears to be the emergence of additional mutations that restore a functional BRCA protein (87, 88). Cells defective in HR are hypersensitive to PARP inhibitors that have recently undergone clinical development (89, 90). Trials with the PARP-1 inhibitors in ovarian, breast and lung cancers arising in mutation carriers are currently accruing (91). In addition, PARP inhibition is associated with increased cytotoxicity to DNA methylating drugs, topoisomerase 1 inhibitors (90) and ionizing radiation, thus logically leading to a search for enhanced anti-tumor activity through combining of the modalities.

In conclusion, the partnership between ionizing radiation and platinum compounds is sustained by the rapidly emerging scientific evidence. A more rational use of the combination requires acceptance of its superiority when in concurrence as well as in integration with the targeted therapy.

References

1. Sharp SY, Rogers PM, Kelland LR. Transport of cisplatin and bis-acetato-amminedichlorocyclohexylamine Platinum(IV) (JM216) in human ovarian carcinoma cell lines: identification of a plasma membrane protein associated with cisplatin resistance. Clin Cancer Res 1995;1:981–9.
2. Shen DW, Goldenberg S, Pastan I, Gottesman MM. Decreased accumulation of [14C]carboplatin in human cisplatin-resistant cells results from reduced energy-dependent uptake. J Cell Physiol 2000;183:108–16.
3. Gately, DP, SB Howell. Cellular accumulation of the anticancer agent cisplatin: a review. Br J Cancer 1993;67:1171–6.
4. Kondo Y, Kuo SM, Watkins SC, Lazo JS. Metallothionein localization and cisplatin resistance in human hormone-independent prostatic tumor cell lines. Cancer Res 1995;55:474–7.
5. Perego P, Righetti SC, Supino R et al. Role of apoptosis and apoptosis-related proteins in the cisplatin-resistant phenotype of human tumor cell lines. Apoptosis 1997;2:540–8.
6. Pestell KE, Medlow CJ, Titley JC, Kelland LR, Walton MI. Effect of p53 status on sensitivity to platinum complexes in a human ovarian cancer cell line. Mol Pharmacol 2000;57:503–11.
7. Fink D, Nebel S, Aebi S, et al. The role of DNA mismatch repair in platinum drug resistance. Cancer Res 1996;56:4881–6.
8. Lage H, Dietel M. Involvement of the DNA mismatch repair system in antineoplastic drug resistance. J Cancer Res Clin Oncol 1999;125:156–65.
9. Perego P, Zunino F, Carenini N, et al. Sensitivity to cisplatin and platinum-containing compounds of Schizosaccharomyces pombe rad mutants. Mol Pharmacol 1998;54:213–9.
10. Richmond RC, Khokhar AR, Teicher BA, Double EB. Toxic variability and radiation sensitization by Pt(II) analogs in *Salmonella typhimurium* cells. Radiat Res 1984;99:609–26.
11. Yang LX, Double EB, Wang HJ. Irradiation enhances cellular uptake of carboplatin. Int J Radiat Oncol Biol Phys 1995;33:641–6.
12. Servidei T, Ferlini C, Riccardi A, et al. The novel trinuclear platinum complex BBR3464 induces a cellular response different from cisplatin. Eur J Cancer 2001;37:930–8.
13. Moreland NJ, Illand M, Kim YT, Paul J, Brown R. Modulation of drug resistance mediated by loss of mismatch repair by the DNA polymerase inhibitor aphidicolin. Cancer Res 1999;59:2102–6.

14. Steel GG, Peckham MJ. Exploitable mechanisms in combined radiotherapy-chemotherapy: the concept of additivity. Int J Radiat Oncol Biol Phys 1979;5:85–91.
15. Overgaard J, Khan AR. Selective enhancement of radiation response in a C3H mammary carcinoma by cisplatin. Cancer Treat Rep 1981;65:501–3.
16. Wodinsky I, Swiniarski J, Kensler CJ, Venditti JM.Combination radiotherapy and chemotherapy for P388 lymphocytic leukemia in vivo. Cancer Chemother Rep 2 1974;4:73–97.
17. Richmond RC, Zimbrick JD, Hykes DL. Radiation-induced DNA damage and lethality in E. coli as modified by the antitumor agent cis-dichlorodiammineplatinum (II). Radiat Res 1977;71:447–60.
18. Richmond RC, Powers EL. Radiation sensitization of bacterial spores by cis-dichlorodiammineplatinum(II). Radiat Res 1976;68:251–7.
19. Dritschilo A, Piro AJ, Kelman AD. The effect of cis-platinum on the repair of radiation damage in plateau phase Chinese hamster (V-79) cells. Int J Radiat Oncol Biol Phys 1979;5:1345–9.
20. Stratford IJ, Williamson C, Adams GE. Combination studies with misonidazole and a cis-platinum complex: cytotoxicity and radiosensitization in vitro. Br J Cancer 1980;41:517–22.
21. Dewit L. Combined treatment of radiation and cisdiamminedichloroplatinum (II): a review of experimental and clinical data. Int J Radiat Oncol Biol Phys 1987;13:403–26.
22. Szumiel I, Nias AH. The effect of combined treatment with a platinum complex and ionizing radiation on chinese hamster ovary cells in vitro. Br J Cancer 1976; 33:450–8.
23. Douple EB, Richmond RC. Enhancement of the potentiation of radiotherapy by platinum drugs in a mouse tumor. Int J Radiat Oncol Biol Phys 1982;8:501–3.
24. Muggia FM, Rozencweig M, Louie AE. Role of chemotherapy in head and neck cancer: systemic use of single agents and combinations in advanced disease. Head Neck Surg 1980;2: 196–205.
25. Wittes R, Heller K, Randolph V, et al. Cis-Dichlorodiammineplatinum(II)-based chemotherapy as initial treatment of advanced head and neck cancer. Cancer Treat Rep 1979;63:1533–8.
26. Eisenberger M, Hornedo J, Silva H, Donehower R, Spaulding M, Van Echo D. Carboplatin (NSC-241–240): an active platinum analog for the treatment of squamous-cell carcinoma of the head and neck. J Clin Oncol 1986;4:1506–9.
27. Pignon JP, Bourhis J, Domenge C, Designé L. Chemotherapy added to locoregional treatment for head and neck squamous-cell carcinoma: three meta-analyses of updated individual data. MACH-NC Collaborative Group. Meta-Analysis of Chemotherapy on Head and Neck Cancer. Lancet 2000;355:949–55.
28. Amrein PC, Weitzman SA. Treatment of squamous-cell carcinoma of the head and neck with cisplatin and 5-fluorouracil. J Clin Oncol 1985;3:1632–9.
29. Kish JA, Weaver A, Jacobs J, Cummings G, Al-Sarraf M. Cisplatin and 5-fluorouracil infusion in patients with recurrent and disseminated epidermoid cancer of the head and neck. Cancer 1984;53:1819–24.
30. Wendt TG, Hartenstein RC, Wustrow TP, Lissner J. Cisplatin, fluorouracil with leucovorin calcium enhancement, and synchronous accelerated radiotherapy in the management of locally advanced head and neck cancer: a phase II study. J Clin Oncol 1989;7:471–6.
31. Calais G, Alfonsi M, Bardet E, et al. Randomized trial of radiation therapy versus concomitant chemotherapy and radiation therapy for advanced-stage oropharynx carcinoma. J Natl Cancer Inst 1999;91:2081–6.
32. Forastiere AA, Metch B, Schuller DE, et al. Randomized comparison of cisplatin plus fluorouracil and carboplatin plus fluorouracil versus methotrexate in advanced squamous-cell carcinoma of the head and neck: a Southwest oncology group study. J Clin Oncol 1992;10: 1245–51.
33. Jacobs C, Lyman G, Velez-García E, et al. A phase III randomized study comparing cisplatin and fluorouracil as single agents and in combination for advanced squamous cell carcinoma of the head and neck. J Clin Oncol 1992;10:257–63.
34. Schrijvers D, Vermorken JB. Taxanes in the treatment of head and neck cancer. Curr Opin Oncol 2005;17:218–24.

35. Clark JI, Hofmeister C, Choudhury A, et al. Phase II evaluation of paclitaxel in combination with carboplatin in advanced head and neck carcinoma. Cancer 2001;92:2334–40.

36. Basaran M, Bavbek SE, Güllü I, et al. A phase II study of paclitaxel and cisplatin combination chemotherapy in recurrent or metastatic head and neck cancer. J Chemother 2002;14:207–13.

37. Cmelak AJ, Murphy BA, Burkey B, Douglas S, Shyr Y, Netterville J. Taxane-based chemoirradiation for organ preservation with locally advanced head and neck cancer: results of a phase II multi-institutional trial. Head Neck 2007;29:315–24.

38. Chougule PB, Akhtar MS, Rathore R, et al. Concurrent chemoradiotherapy with weekly paclitaxel and carboplatin for locally advanced head and neck cancer: long-term follow-up of a brown university oncology group phase II study (HN-53). Head Neck 2008;30:289–96.

39. El-Sharouni SY, Kal HB, Battermann JJ, Schramel FM. Sequential versus concurrent chemo-radiotherapy in inoperable stage III non-small cell lung cancer. Anticancer Res 2006;26:495–505.

40. Whitney CW, Sause W, Bundy BN, et al. Randomized comparison of fluorouracil plus cisplatin versus hydroxyurea as an adjunct to radiation therapy in stage IIB-IVA carcinoma of the cervix with negative para-aortic lymph nodes: a gynecologic oncology group and Southwest oncology group study. J Clin Oncol 1999;17:1339–48.

41. Morris M, Eifel PJ, Lu J, et al. Pelvic radiation with concurrent chemotherapy compared with pelvic and para-aortic radiation for high-risk cervical cancer. N Engl J Med 1999;340:1137–43.

42. Rose PG, Bundy BN, Watkins EB, et al. Concurrent cisplatin-based radiotherapy and chemotherapy for locally advanced cervical cancer. N Engl J Med 1999;340:1144–53.

43. Keys HM, Bundy BN, Stehman FB, et al. Cisplatin, radiation, and adjuvant hysterectomy compared with radiation and adjuvant hysterectomy for bulky stage IB cervical carcinoma. N Engl J Med 1999;340:1154–61.

44. Peters WA III, Liu PY, Barrett RJ II, et al. Concurrent chemotherapy and pelvic radiation therapy compared with pelvic radiation therapy alone as adjuvant therapy after radical surgery in high-risk early-stage cancer of the cervix. J Clin Oncol 2000;18:1606–13.

45. Pearcey R, Brundage M, Drouin P, et al. Phase III trial comparing radical radiotherapy with and without cisplatin chemotherapy in patients with advanced squamous cell cancer of the cervix. J Clin Oncol 2002;20:966–72.

46. McGuire WP III, Arseneau J, Blessing JA, et al. A randomized comparative trial of carboplatin and iproplatin in advanced squamous carcinoma of the uterine cervix: a gynecologic oncology group study. J Clin Oncol 1989;7:1462–8.

47. Weiss GR, Green S, Hannigan EV, et al. A phase II trial of carboplatin for recurrent or metastatic squamous carcinoma of the uterine cervix: a Southwest oncology group study. Gynecol Oncol 1990;39:332–6.

48. Micheletti E, La Face B, Bianchi E, et al. Continuous infusion of carboplatin during conventional radiotherapy treatment in advanced squamous carcinoma of the cervix uteri IIB-IIIB (UICC). A phase I/II and pharmacokinetic study. Am J Clin Oncol 1997;20:613–20.

49. Corn BW, Hernandez E, Anderson L, Fein DA, Dunton CJ, Heller P. Phase I/II study of concomitant irradiation and carboplatin for locally advanced carcinoma of the uterine cervix: an interim report. Am J Clin Oncol 1996;19:317–21.

50. Higgins RV, Naumann WR, Hall JB, Haake M. Concurrent carboplatin with pelvic radiation therapy in the primary treatment of cervix cancer. Gynecol Oncol 2003;89:499–503.

51. Muderspach LI, Curtin JP, Roman LD, et al. Carboplatin as a radiation sensitizer in locally advanced cervical cancer: a pilot study. Gynecol Oncol 1997;65:336–42.

52. Dubay RA, Rose PG, O'Malley DM, Shalodi AD, Ludin A, Selim MA. Evaluation of concurrent and adjuvant carboplatin with radiation therapy for locally advanced cervical cancer. Gynecol Oncol 2004;94:121–4.

53. de Gramont A, Figer A, Seymour M, et al. Leucovorin and fluorouracil with or without oxaliplatin as first-line treatment in advanced colorectal cancer. J Clin Oncol 2000;18:2938–47.

54. André T, Boni C, Mounedji-Boudiaf L, et al. Oxaliplatin, fluorouracil, and leucovorin as adjuvant treatment for colon cancer. N Engl J Med 2004;350:2343–51.
55. Magné N, Fischel JL, Formento P, et al. Oxaliplatin-5-fluorouracil and ionizing radiation. Importance of the sequence and influence of p53 status. Oncology 2003;64:280–7.
56. Folkvord S, Flatmark K, Seierstad T, Røe K, Rasmussen H, Ree AH. Inhibitory effects of oxaliplatin in experimental radiation treatment of colorectal carcinoma: does oxaliplatin improve 5-fluorouracil-dependent radiosensitivity? Radiother Oncol 2008;86:428–34.
57. Turitto G, Panelli G, Frattolillo A, et al. Phase II study of neoadjuvant concurrent chemio-radiotherapy with oxaliplatin-containing regimen in locally advanced rectal cancer. Front Biosci 2006;11:1275–9.
58. Valentini V, Coco C, Minsky BD, et al. Randomized, Multicenter, Phase IIB study of preoperative chemoradiotherapy in T3 mid-distal rectal cancer: raltitrexed + oxaliplatin + radiotherapy Versus cisplatin + 5-Fluorouracil + radiotherapy. Int J Radiat Oncol Biol Phys 2008;70:403–12.
59. Hospers GA, Punt CJ, Tesselaar ME, et al. Preoperative chemoradiotherapy with capecitabine and oxaliplatin in locally advanced rectal cancer. A phase I-II multicenter study of the Dutch colorectal cancer group. Ann Surg Oncol 2007;14:2773–9.
60. Gambacorta MA, Valentini V, Coco C, et al. Chemoradiation with raltitrexed and oxaliplatin in preoperative treatment of stage II-III resectable rectal cancer: phase I and II studies. Int J Radiat Oncol Biol Phys 2004;60:139–48.
61. Rödel C, Grabenbauer GG, Papadopoulos T, Hohenberger W, Schmoll HJ, Sauer R. Phase I/II trial of capecitabine, oxaliplatin, and radiation for rectal cancer. J Clin Oncol 2003;21:3098–104.
62. Benson AB III. New approaches to assessing and treating early-stage colon and rectal cancers: cooperative group strategies for assessing optimal approaches in early-stage disease. Clin Cancer Res 2007;13:6913s–20s.
63. Zhang L, Zhao C, Peng PJ, et al. Phase III study comparing standard radiotherapy with or without weekly oxaliplatin in treatment of locoregionally advanced nasopharyngeal carcinoma: preliminary results. J Clin Oncol 2005;23:8461–8.
64. Amorino GP, Mohr PJ, Hercules SK, Pyo H, Choy H. Combined effects of the orally active cisplatin analog, JM216, and radiation in antitumor therapy. Cancer Chemother Pharmacol 2000;46:423–6.
65. van de Vaart PJ, Klaren HM, Hofland I, Begg AC. Oral platinum analogue JM216, a radio-sensitizer in oxic murine cells. Int J Radiat Biol 1997;72:675–83.
66. Wosikowski K, Lamphere L, Unteregger G, et al. Preclinical antitumor activity of the oral platinum analog satraplatin. Cancer Chemother Pharmacol 2007;60:589–600.
67. McKeage MJ, Raynaud F, Ward J, et al., Phase I and pharmacokinetic study of an oral platinum complex given daily for 5 days in patients with cancer. J Clin Oncol 1997;15:2691–700.
68. George CM, Haraf DJ, Mauer AM, et al. A phase I trial of the oral platinum analogue JM216 with concomitant radiotherapy in advanced malignancies of the chest. Invest New Drugs 2001;19:303–10.
69. Sugiyama T, Kumagai S, Nishida T, et al. Experimental and clinical evaluation of cisplatin-containing microspheres as intraperitoneal chemotherapy for ovarian cancer. Anticancer Res 1998;18:2837–42.
70. Meerum Terwogt JM, Groenewegen G, Pluim D, et al. Phase I and pharmacokinetic study of SPI-77, a liposomal encapsulated dosage form of cisplatin. Cancer Chemother Pharmacol 2002;49:201–10.
71. Lana SE, Dernell WS, Lafferty MH, Withrow SJ, LaRue SM. Use of radiation and a slow-release cisplatin formulation for treatment of canine nasal tumors. Vet Radiol Ultrasound 2004;45:577–81.
72. Lilenbaum RC. The evolving role of cetuximab in non-small cell lung cancer. Clin Cancer Res 2006;12:4432s–5s.
73. Bonner JA, Harari PM, Giralt J, et al. Radiotherapy plus cetuximab for squamous-cell carcinoma of the head and neck. N Engl J Med 2006;354:567–78.

74. Pfister DG, Su YB, Kraus DH, et al. Concurrent cetuximab, cisplatin, and concomitant boost radiotherapy for locoregionally advanced, squamous cell head and neck cancer: a pilot phase II study of a new combined-modality paradigm. J Clin Oncol 2006;24:1072–8.
75. Shirai K, O'Brien PE. Molecular targets in squamous cell carcinoma of the head and neck. Curr Treat Opt Oncol 2007;8:239–51.
76. Teicher BA, Holden SA, Ara G, et al. Influence of an anti-angiogenic treatment on 9L gliosarcoma: oxygenation and response to cytotoxic therapy. Int J Cancer 1995;61:732–7.
77. Lee CG, Heijn M, di Tomaso E, et al. Anti-Vascular endothelial growth factor treatment augments tumor radiation response under normoxic or hypoxic conditions. Cancer Res 2000;60:5565–70.
78. Griffin RJ, Williams BW, Wild R, Cherrington JM, Park H, Song CW. Simultaneous inhibition of the receptor kinase activity of vascular endothelial, fibroblast, and platelet-derived growth factors suppresses tumor growth and enhances tumor radiation response. Cancer Res 2002;62:1702–6.
79. Tong RT, Boucher Y, Kozin SV, Winkler F, Hicklin DJ, Jain RK. Vascular normalization by vascular endothelial growth factor receptor 2 blockade induces a pressure gradient across the vasculature and improves drug penetration in tumors. Cancer Res 2004;64:3731–6.
80. Yuan F, Chen Y, Dellian M, Safabakhsh N, Ferrara N, Jain RK. Time-dependent vascular regression and permeability changes in established human tumor xenografts induced by an anti-vascular endothelial growth factor/vascular permeability factor antibody. Proc Natl Acad Sci USA 1996;93:14765–70.
81. Dings RP, Loren M, Heun H, et al. Scheduling of radiation with angiogenesis inhibitors anginex and Avastin improves therapeutic outcome via vessel normalization. Clin Cancer Res 2007;13:3395–402.
82. Citrin D, Menard C, Camphausen K. Combining radiotherapy and angiogenesis inhibitors: clinical trial design. Int J Radiat Oncol Biol Phys 2006;64:15–25.
83. Lymberis SC, Parhar PK, Katsoulakis E, Formenti SC. Pharmacogenomics and breast cancer. Pharmacogenomics 2004;5:31–55.
84. Olopade OI, Wei M. FANCF methylation contributes to chemoselectivity in ovarian cancer. Cancer Cell 2003;3:417–20.
85. Rottenberg S, Nygren AO, Pajic M, et al. Selective induction of chemotherapy resistance of mammary tumors in a conditional mouse model for hereditary breast cancer. Proc Natl Acad Sci USA 2007;104:12117–22.
86. Liu X, Holstege H, van der Gulden H, et al. Somatic loss of BRCA1 and p53 in mice induces mammary tumors with features of human BRCA1-mutated basal-like breast cancer. Proc Natl Acad Sci USA 2007;104:12111–6.
87. Swisher EM, Sakai W, Karlan BY, Wurz K, Urban N, Taniguchi T. Secondary BRCA1 mutations in BRCA1-mutated ovarian carcinomas with platinum resistance. Cancer Res 2008;68:2581–6.
88. Sakai W, Swisher EM, Karlan BY, et al., Secondary mutations as a mechanism of cisplatin resistance in BRCA2-mutated cancers. Nature 2008;451:1116–20.
89. Bryant HE, Schultz N, Thomas HD, et al. Specific killing of BRCA2-deficient tumours with inhibitors of poly(ADP-ribose) polymerase. Nature 2005;434:913–7.
90. Smith LM, Willmore E, Austin CA, Curtin NJ. The novel poly(ADP-Ribose) polymerase inhibitor, AG14361, sensitizes cells to topoisomerase I poisons by increasing the persistence of DNA strand breaks. Clin Cancer Res 2005;11:8449–57.
91. Lewis C, Low JA. Clinical poly(ADP-ribose) polymerase inhibitors for the treatment of cancer. Curr Opin Investig Drugs 2007;8:1051–6.

Treating Cisplatin-Resistant Cancer: A Systematic Analysis of Oxaliplatin or Paclitaxel Salvage Chemotherapy

Britta Stordal, Nick Pavlakis, and Ross Davey

Abstract The objective of this study was to examine the preclinical and clinical evidence for the use of oxaliplatin or paclitaxel salvage chemotherapy in patients with cisplatin-resistant cancer.

Medline was searched for (a) cell models of acquired resistance, reporting cisplatin, oxaliplatin, and paclitaxel sensitivities; and (b) clinical trials of single-agent oxaliplatin or paclitaxel salvage therapy for cisplatin/carboplatin-resistant ovarian cancer. Oxaliplatin is widely regarded as being active in cisplatin-resistant cancer. In contrast, data in cell models suggests that there is cross-resistance between cisplatin and oxaliplatin in cellular models with resistance levels that reflect clinical resistance (less than tenfold). Oxaliplatin, as a single agent, had a poor response rate in patients with cisplatin-resistant ovarian cancer (8%, $n = 91$). In the treatment of platinum-resistant cancer, oxaliplatin performed better in combination with other agents, suggesting that the benefit of oxaliplatin may lie in its more favorable toxicity and its ability to be combined with other drugs, rather than an underlying activity in cisplatin resistance. Oxaliplatin, therefore, should not be considered broadly active in cisplatin-resistant cancer.

Cellular data suggest that paclitaxel is active in cisplatin-resistant cancer. 68.1% of cisplatin-resistant cells were sensitive to paclitaxel. As a single agent, paclitaxel had a response rate of 22% in patients with platinum-resistant ovarian cancer ($n = 1,918$), a significant increase from the response of oxaliplatin ($p < 0.01$). Paclitaxel-resistant cells were also sensitive to cisplatin, suggesting that alternating between agents may be beneficial. Studies of single-agent paclitaxel in platinum-resistant ovarian cancers where patients had previously received paclitaxel had an improved response rate of 35.3% $n = 232$ ($p < 0.01$), suggesting that pretreatment with paclitaxel improves the response of salvage paclitaxel therapy.

Cellular models reflect the resistance observed in the clinical treatment of ovarian cancer, as the cross-resistant agent oxaliplatin has a lower response rate compared to

B. Stordal (✉), N. Pavlakis, and R. Davey
Bill Walsh Cancer Research Laboratories, Department of Medical Oncology,
Royal North Shore Hospital, and the University of Sydney, Australia
e-mail: bstordal@med.usyd.edu.au or britta.stordal@dcu.ie

A. Bonetti et al. (eds.), *Platinum and Other Heavy Metal Compounds in Cancer Chemotherapy*, DOI: 10.1007/978-1-60327-459-3_27,
© Humana Press, a part of Springer Science + Business Media, LLC 2009

the non-cross-resistant agent paclitaxel. Alternating therapy with cisplatin and paclitaxel may therefore lead to an improved response rate in ovarian cancer.

Keywords Cisplatin; Oxaliplatin; Paclitaxel; Resistance; Ovarian cancer; Salvage chemotherapy

Oxaliplatin has been widely regarded as potentially useful for the treatment of cisplatin-resistant cancer. The evidence cited for oxaliplatin activity in cisplatin-resistant cancer comes, in general, from studies of highly cisplatin-resistant cell lines with low-level oxaliplatin resistance, or from review articles summarizing these findings and oxaliplatin in general. While highly resistant models are useful to understand the possible mechanisms of resistance, drug resistance in the clinical setting typically occurs at lower levels of resistance (1, 2), and may therefore involve different mechanisms of resistance.

Cisplatin and oxaliplatin target the DNA, whereas paclitaxel, a taxane, causes toxicity by stabilizing polymerized microtubules. Due to their differing mechanisms of action, platinums and taxanes are often combined in cancer therapy. Our laboratory has found that when cells become resistant to platinum, they often become sensitive to taxanes (3, 4). Preliminary reading of the literature suggested that the reverse is also true, i.e., that taxane-resistant cell lines can be sensitive to platinum. We undertook this systematic review to identify, describe, and critique the clinical and cellular evidence for the use of oxaliplatin or paclitaxel in patients with cisplatin-resistant cancer.

Resistant cell models are developed in the laboratory by repeatedly exposing cancer cells in culture to chemotherapy. The surviving resistant cells are then compared to the parental sensitive cells using a cell viability assay such as the MTT assay or the clonogenic assay. The IC_{50} (drug concentration causing 50% growth inhibition) for these paired cell lines can be used to determine the increase in resistance (known as fold resistance) by the following equation:

$$\text{Fold resistance} = IC_{50} \text{ of platinum resistant cell line}/IC_{50} \text{ of parental cell line}$$

The literature search for models of acquired platinum resistance that report cross-resistance data for both cisplatin and oxaliplatin identified 27 cell lines (5). For each cell line, the fold oxaliplatin resistance was plotted against the fold cisplatin resistance, allowing an analysis of the pattern of cross-resistance (Fig. 1a). The definition of cross-resistance is a matter of debate in the literature. Some studies consider two drugs cross-resistant only if a similar level of resistance is observed. For the purposes of this review, we have defined cross-resistance between cisplatin and oxaliplatin as greater than or equal to twofold resistance to both drugs. This definition is therefore based on what would be clinically observed as cross-resistance.

Figure 1a shows that the majority of models of acquired platinum resistance are cross-resistant to both cisplatin and oxaliplatin, having at least twofold resistance

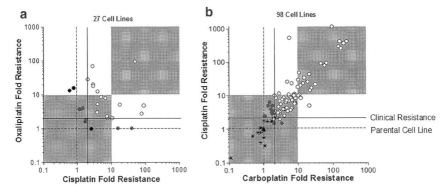

Fig. 1 Cross-resistance between (**a**) cisplatin and oxaliplatin, and (**b**) cisplatin and carboplatin, in cell models of acquired platinum resistance. The *dotted line* at 1 indicates the fold resistance of the parental cell lines. The *solid line* at 2 indicates the level of clinical platinum resistance. Cross-resistant models are indicated with open circles, non-cross-resistant with grey cirles, hypersensitive with black circles, non-resistance is indicated with black stars

to both drugs. The lower-level resistant models, below tenfold, tend to be cross-resistant at a similar level to both drugs. However, the higher-level resistant models, above tenfold, are highly resistant to their selecting drug, and then exhibit a lower level of resistance to the other drug. This suggests that a common mechanism of low-level resistance to both cisplatin and oxaliplatin develops at clinical levels of drug treatment, whereas the resistance mechanisms that develop at higher drug concentrations are likely to be more specific for the selecting drug. This is in contrast to the cross-resistance relationship between cisplatin and carboplatin, which shows cross-resistance at low- and high-level resistance, indicated by grey shading (6) (Fig. 1b).

The literature search for models of acquired resistance that report cross-resistance data for both cisplatin and paclitaxel identified 137 cell lines (6). For each cell line, the fold paclitaxel resistance was plotted against the fold cisplatin resistance, allowing an analysis of the pattern of cross-resistance between the two compounds (Fig. 2a). 13.9% of cell lines found in the literature review were below twofold resistance to both compounds, and therefore classed as non-resistant, indicated with black stars in Fig. 2a. It is the minority of cell models of acquired resistance that are cross-resistant (open circles) to both cisplatin and paclitaxel (16.8%). The majority of cells are either non-cross-resistant (grey circles; 40.9%), with no gain of resistance to the other compound, or hypersensitive (black circles; 28.5%), becoming more sensitive than the parental cancer cell line they were derived from. 71 cell lines were resistant to cisplatin; 48 of these were non-cross-resistant or hypersensitive to paclitaxel (67.6%). 69 cell lines were resistant to paclitaxel; 46 of these were non-cross-resistant or hypersensitive to cisplatin (66.6%). This suggests an inverse relationship between cisplatin and paclitaxel resistance in resistant cell models where resistance to one leads to sensitivity to the other. A similar inverse relationship was observed between cisplatin and docetaxel, carboplatin and paclitaxel, and

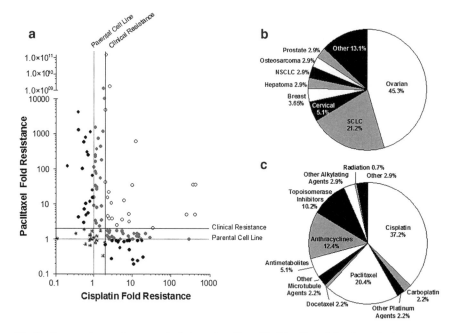

Fig. 2 Cross-resistance between cisplatin and paclitaxel in (**a**) cell models of acquired resistance. The *dotted line* at 1 indicates the fold resistance of the parental cell lines. The *solid line* at 2 indicates the level of clinical platinum resistance. Cross-Resistant modles are indicated with open circles, Non-Cross Resistant with grey cirles, Hypersensitive with black circles, Non-Resistance is indicated with black stars. Characteristics of the resistant models in the cisplatin/paclitaxel systematic review: (**b**) types of carcinoma and (**c**) chemotherapeutics used to develop the resistant models (6)

carboplatin and docetaxel, suggesting that an inverse resistance relationship exists between platinum and taxane chemotherapy (6).

The resistant cell lines found in the cisplatin/paclitaxel systematic review were diverse in the type of carcinoma (Fig. 2b). Ovarian (45.3%) and SCLC (21.2%) were the most common carcinomas used to develop cell lines. However, the other 16 types of carcinoma suggest that the inverse relationship between cisplatin and paclitaxel resistance is not cell-type-specific, and could apply to all cancers. The chemotherapeutics used to develop the resistant models were also diverse; the most common were cisplatin (37.2%) and paclitaxel (20.4%) (Fig. 2c). The other 31 agents are diverse mechanistically, suggesting that when cells become resistant to any agent, there are two distinct paths available: one that leads to cross-resistance to cisplatin, and the other that leads to cross-resistance to paclitaxel.

Cisplatin combination chemotherapy is the cornerstone of treatment of ovarian carcinomas. Initial platinum responsiveness in ovarian cancer is high, but up to 80% of patients will eventually relapse and become platinum resistant (7). Clinical platinum resistance is variably defined in the clinic and, as such, it is difficult to make comparisons of treatment activity between trials. However, many second-line ovarian carcinoma studies use Markman's criteria (8), where disease progression with a platinum-free interval of less than 6 months is considered platinum-resistant. Our search of the literature for single-agent oxaliplatin salvage therapy in platinum-resistant ovarian carcinoma identified four studies. The response rate (RR) of the platinum-resistant cohort was a very low RR of 8%, $n = 91$, compared to the platinum-sensitive cohort RR of 42%, $n = 50$ ($p < 0.05$, χ^2 test) (5). This suggests that there is no special activity of oxaliplatin in cisplatin-resistant cancer, and correlates with the *in vitro* data suggesting that there is cross-resistance between cisplatin and oxaliplatin at clinically relevant levels of resistance. Oxaliplatin performed better in combination with other agents for the treatment of cisplatin-resistant cancer, suggesting that the benefit of oxaliplatin may lie in its more favorable toxicity and its ability to be combined with other drugs, rather than an underlying activity in cisplatin resistance (5). Oxaliplatin, therefore, should not be considered broadly active in cisplatin-resistant cancer.

Our search of the literature for single-agent paclitaxel salvage therapy in platinum-resistant ovarian carcinoma identified 56 studies. In order to analyze whether the inverse relationship between cisplatin and paclitaxel resistance observed in resistant cell models is apparent in clinical trials, the studies were divided into two groups: paclitaxel naïve ovarian cancer or paclitaxel pretreated ovarian cancer. The paclitaxel naïve cisplatin-resistant patients had a higher response rate of 22%, $n = 1,918$, compared to the 8% response rate to oxaliplatin ($p < 0.01$). This again correlates with the *in vitro* data, there is a better response to the non-cross-resistant agent paclitaxel than to the cross-resistant agent oxaliplatin (Fig. 3). What was unexpected was that platinum-resistant patients who had previously received

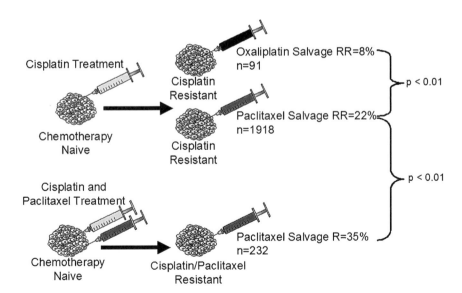

Fig. 3 Summary of response rates to oxaliplatin and paclitaxel salvage chemotherapy in cisplatin-resistant ovarian cancer. Significant differences were determined by the χ^2 test

paclitaxel therapy responded better to single-agent paclitaxel (RR 35.3%, $n = 232$) than the paclitaxel naïve patients (RR 22.7%, $n = 1,918$) ($p < 0.01$, χ^2 test) (Fig. 3) (6). Both cohorts of patients presented very similar age status, performance status, FIGO stage, and number of cycles of prior chemotherapy, and although there was a difference in histology, this did not account for this difference in response rates (6). Usually, if patients have received a drug and experienced disease progression, they are less likely to respond to therapy with a subsequent exposure to the same drug. Although one must be cautious in interpreting these summary findings due to the potential for biases in pooling of patients across studies, if the findings do reflect the true clinical response to these agents, they suggest that initial co-treatment with platinum and paclitaxel may improve the outcome of paclitaxel salvage therapy.

Conclusions

Oxaliplatin is not highly active in cisplatin-resistant cancer, and this appears to be due to cross-resistance between cisplatin and oxaliplatin at clinically relevant levels of resistance. This provides some insight into the mechanisms of resistance to these agents; low-level resistance provides cross-resistance to both, but, at higher levels of resistance, the mechanisms diverge. Paclitaxel has higher activity in cisplatin-resistant ovarian cancer, supporting the inverse resistance phenotype observed in cell models. Paclitaxel salvage chemotherapy has higher activity in ovarian cancer patients who have received prior paclitaxel therapy, suggesting that alternating between agents could improve response rates.

References

1. Kawai H, Kiura K, Tabata M, et al. Characterization of non-small-cell lung cancer cell lines established before and after chemotherapy. Lung Cancer 2002;35:305–14.
2. Kuroda H, Sugimoto T, Ueda K, et al. Different drug sensitivity in two neuroblastoma cell lines established from the same patient before and after chemotherapy. Int J Cancer 1991; 47:732–7.
3. Stordal BK, Davey MW, Davey RA. Oxaliplatin induces drug resistance more rapidly than cisplatin in H69 small cell lung cancer cells. Cancer Chemother Pharmacol 2006;58:256–65.
4. Henness S, Davey MW, Harvie RM, Davey RA. Fractionated irradiation of H69 small-cell lung cancer cells causes stable radiation and drug resistance with increased MRP1, MRP2, and topoisomerase IIα expression. Int J Radiat Oncol Biol Phys 2002;54:895–902.
5. Stordal B, Pavlakis N, Davey R. Oxaliplatin for the treatment of cisplatin-resistant cancer: A systematic review. Cancer Treat Rev 2007;33:347–57.
6. Stordal B, Pavlakis N, Davey R. A systematic review of platinum and taxane resistance from bench to clinic: an inverse relationship. Cancer Treat Rev 2007;33:688–703.
7. Dieras V, Bougnoux P, Petit T, et al. Multicentre phase II study of oxaliplatin as a single-agent in cisplatin/carboplatin ± taxane-pretreated ovarian cancer patients. Ann Oncol 2002;13:258–66.
8. Markman M, Hoskins W. Responses to salvage chemotherapy in ovarian cancer: a critical need for precise definitions of the treated population. J Clin Oncol 1992;10:513–4.

Platinum Compounds in Lung Cancer: Current Status

Kevin Tay, Martin Gutierrez, and Giuseppe Giaccone

Abstract Randomized clinical studies and meta-analyses of the literature have confirmed the improved survival of platinum-based chemotherapy doublets, that are considered standard therapy in patients with advanced non–small cell lung cancer (NSCLC) with a good performance status. The use of platinum compounds have also demonstrated a slight survival advantage over nonplatinum-based chemotherapy. Cisplatin remains the platinum agent of choice in the management of patients with NSCLC in both the advanced and adjuvant setting based on the results from recent meta-analyses. However, carboplatin may be offered to patients in advanced stages of the disease due to its more favorable toxicity profile. To date, four targeted agents (bevacizumab, cetuximab, erlotinib and gefitinib) have been studied in combination with platinum-based chemotherapy in the treatment of advanced NSCLC. Only bevacizumab has been shown to significantly prolong survival when added to carboplatin/paclitaxel as demonstrated in a large phase III study. However, issues of toxicity limit this treatment regimen to selected patients. The combination of bevacizumab with cisplatin and gemcitabine appears promising but is still awaiting the final results of the unpublished survival data. Preliminary studies indicate that molecular tumor markers may be able to identify tumors that are more likely to respond to chemotherapy. Excision repair cross-complementation group 1 (ERCC1) and Ribonucleotide Reductase M1 (RRM1) are two such genes critical to DNA synthesis and DNA damage repair pathways that have been studied. The results from the first prospective phase III randomized trial suggest that customizing chemotherapy based on ERCC1 expression in patients with advanced NSCLC is a feasible approach. In the future, selection of patients based on pharmacogenetics may help identify patients who will optimally benefit from specific therapies.

Keywords Platinum compounds; Bevacizumab; Cetuximab; Excision repair cross-complementation group 1 (ERCC1); Ribonucleotide reductace MI (RRMI)

K. Tay (✉), M. Gutierrez, and G. Giaccone
Medical Oncology Branch, National Cancer Institute, National Institutes of Health, Bethesda, MD, USA
e-mail: giacconeg@mail.nih.gov

A. Bonetti et al. (eds.), *Platinum and Other Heavy Metal Compounds in Cancer Chemotherapy*, DOI: 10.1007/978-1-60327-459-3_28,
© Humana Press, a part of Springer Science + Business Media, LLC 2009

Introduction

Lung cancer remains the leading cause of cancer death in the United States. An estimated 21,300 new diagnoses of lung cancer and 160,000 deaths are expected to occur in 2007 (1). Although surgery may be curative in the early-stage of the disease, an excess of 70% of patients with non–small cell lung cancer (NSCLC) are at an advanced stage of the disease at diagnosis and are not candidates for surgery. For many years, the treatment options for this group of patients were limited to the best supportive care. However, over the last two decades, several randomized trials and meta-analyses provided evidence that patients with NSCLC who receive chemotherapy demonstrated a moderate survival advantage, improvement in symptom control and quality of life when compared to the best supportive care alone (2, 3). The meta-analysis of 52 Randomized Controlled Trials (RCTs) in 1995 by the Non–Small Cell Lung Cancer Collaborative Group, when comparing cisplatin-based chemotherapy with the best supportive care alone showed that chemotherapy was associated with a 27% reduction in risk of death and a 10% absolute improvement in the 1 year survival (4).

Platinum compounds constitute the mainstay of therapy for a wide range of malignancies including NSCLC. Platinum compounds exert their cytotoxic effects by covalently binding to purine DNA bases at the N^7 positions of guanine and adenine. The main DNA lesions produced by both cisplatin and its analogs, accounting for over 90% of platinum-DNA adducts, are at the G–G, A–G and G–X–G intrastrand cross-links. These adducts disrupt the normal functions of cellular DNA via nucleotide substitution, deletions, chromosomal rearrangements or activation of cell-signalling pathways that result in apoptosis (5). A number of randomized trials have demonstrated that platinum-based combinations resulted in an improved outcome when compared with a single-agent in patients with advanced NSCLC. Further support from a 2004 meta-analysis that included 13,601 patients in 65 trials showed that the two-drug regimens were associated with a significant increase in both response rate and survival (26 vs. 13% objective response rate with a single agent therapy, and 35 vs. 30% 1-year survival) (6).

During the 1990s, the introduction of third-generation (3G) drugs such as gemcitabine, taxanes and vinorelbine emerged as active agents as monotherapy. That quickly led to the use of 3G agents in combination with platinum compounds. Since then, several trials with 3G platinum-based regimens have shown superior response and survival rates over second-generation (2G) platinum-based combinations (7, 8). The issue of whether three drug combinations are superior to two drugs have also been evaluated in several trials. A 2004 meta-analysis that identified 28 trials comparing the three-drug with two-drug combinations concluded that by adding a third drug, the response rate did significantly increase but no difference in the overall survival was shown and three-drug regimens were associated with more toxicities (6). Two multicenter trials using 3G platinum-based regimens published after this meta-analysis also showed similar findings (9, 10).

The use of platinum compounds, particularly cisplatin, in the elderly have always been of concern with respect to the tolerability of therapy. Despite these concerns, no studies to date have shown that patients who are older/elderly patients are associated with a significantly worse outcome compared to younger patients on chemotherapy. The recently published Multicenter Italian Lung Cancer in the Elderly Study-2P (MILES-2P) trial further validates that cisplatin-based combination therapy are feasible and active in the treatment of elderly patients with advanced NSCLC (11).

Performance status (PS) is an important prognostic factor and experiences from earlier trials have shown that patients with advanced NSCLC with poor performance status fared poorly, with more adverse results and worse survival outcomes. However with the advent of improved supportive therapy, a recent Phase II PS-2 specific study was able to show that platinum-based combination chemotherapy may be a feasible treatment option with acceptable toxicity, even though survival in these patients remains inferior to that of PS-0 to PS-1 patients (12). On the basis of these data, current international guidelines recommend the use of platinum-based third-generation chemotherapy doublets as standard of care for first-line treatment for patients with good performance status.

Nonplatinum Regimens

Third-generation (3G) agents are, in general, better tolerated than their predecessors, and some of them have been reported to produce a significant survival advantage as a single-agent over best supportive care alone in patients with advanced NSCLC (13–16). In the meta-analysis by Hotta et al. (17) comparing these 3G agents alone vs. a combination with platinum compounds demonstrated a higher objective response rate and a 13% improvement in survival in favor of the combination regimens, which reaffirms the evidence that single drug therapy is not recommended as the standard treatment. However, this survival benefit comes at the expense of higher toxicities in the combination regimens. Consequently, the activity and tolerability of these 3G agents led many investigators to evaluate the efficacy of doublet combination of third generation agents so as to avoid the use of platinum compounds in the treatment of advanced NSCLC.

Several randomized trials have been carried out to address the question whether nonplatinum combinations are as effective and can be used as an alternative therapy to the classical platinum-based combinations. The results were conflicting with at least two phase III trials yielding inferior overall survival rates in the nonplatinum regimens (18, 19). A large literature-based meta-analysis by D'Addario et al. (20) of 37 randomized phase II and III trials that included a total of 7,633 patients demonstrated that the use of platinum-based doublet regimens were associated with a 62% increase in the odds ratio (OR) for response (OR 1.62, 95% confidence interval (CI), 1.46–1.8; $p < 0.0001$). The 1-year survival rate was increased by 5% with platinum-based regimens (34 vs. 29%; OR 1.21; $p = 0.0003$). However when single-agent trials were excluded, the survival benefit disappeared when platinum-based combinations were compared with nonplatinum-based combinations only

(OR = 1.11; p = 0.17). Furthermore, the platinum-based regimens were associated with higher toxicities, particularly hematological toxicity, nephrotoxicity and nausea/vomiting but no difference in febrile neutropenia rate or in toxic death rate.

Another recent meta-analysis assessed 11/eleven phase III trials comprising a total of 4,602 patients, and randomizing platinum-based doublets vs. nonplatinum combinations. The results were similar with the earlier meta-analysis,the platinum-based regimens were associated with a decreased risk of death at 1 year (OR 0.88, 95% CI, 0.78–0.99; p = 0.044). There was a non statistically significant increase in toxic-related death in the platinum-based regimens. Again, the nonplatinum-based combinations showed a more favorable toxicity profile than platinum-based ones (21).

Both these two meta-analysis showed a small survival advantage with platinum-based chemotherapy without a significant increase in risk of toxic related death. This benefit was however counterbalanced, by an increase in nonfatal toxicity in the platinum-based regimens. From current data, platinum-based doublet chemotherapy should still remain the standard of care in patients with advanced NSCLC, but nonplatinum-based doublet may be an acceptable option in some patients, particularly in those who have concerns about toxic effects.

Cisplatin vs. Carboplatin

Carboplatin has often been substituted for cisplatin in combination regimens due to its more favorable toxicity profile. However, cisplatin is superior to carboplatin in several solid tumors, such as germ cell tumors, bladder cancer, head and neck cancer and potentially others. Schiller et al. (2002) compared cisplatin plus paclitaxel with three other combination regimens of cisplatin plus gemcitabine, cisplatin plus docetaxel and paclitaxel plus carboplatin in advanced NSCLC. No major differences were observed in objective response rate, survival and toxicity (22). Similar findings were reported in a trial comparing paclitaxel plus carboplatin with vinorelbine plus cisplatin (23).

The therapeutic equivalence of these two drugs have come into question in recent years. The first meta-analysis that looked at this issue, included eight trials with a total of 2,948 patients comparing carboplatin-based regimens with cisplatin-based regimens. It did reveal a higher rate of objective response but no statistically significant survival advantage was found in the cisplatin-based regimens when all trials were included in the analysis. However, a subgroup analysis revealed that combinations of cisplatin plus a new agent yielded an 11% longer survival than carboplatin plus the same new agent (Hazard ratio (HR) = 1.106; 95% CI, 1.005–1.218; p = 0.039) (24). The validity of the results from this meta-analysis was called into question because of the use of abstracted data instead of individual patient's data.

The cisplatin vs. carboplatin (CISCA) meta-analysis by Ardizzoni et al. (25) based on individual patient data from 2,968 patients in nine trials that compared a cisplatin with a carboplatin-based regimen in advanced NSCLC essentially revealed similar findings as the earlier meta-analysis. Carboplatin-based regimens appeared slightly less effective in prolonging survival with a median survival of 8.4 months and 1-year survival probability of 34%, compared with a median survival of 9.1 months and a 1-year survival probability of 37% in the cisplatin-treated patients. Although the risk of death was higher with carboplatin-treated patients, the difference was not statistically significant. (HR of mortality = 1.07, 95% CI, 0.99–1.15; $p = 0.10$). Similarly, when the analysis was restricted to more recent trials with third-generation platinum-based regimens, a statistically significant improvement was observed in the cisplatin-based regimens (HR of mortality 1.11, 95% CI, 1.01–1.21).

Further theory supports that the cisplatin-based third generation regimen should remain the standard therapy came from another recent meta-analysis which included only trials with platinum-based combinations with a newer agent vs. nonplatinum-based combinations. In line with the result from the two previous meta-analysis, the use of cisplatin-based doublet regimens is associated with a slightly higher 1-year survival rate (Relative risk (RR) = 1.16, 95% CI, 1.06–1.27; $p = 0.001$), while carboplatin-based doublet regimens have little or no effect on 1-year survival when compared to nonplatinum-based combinations (RR = 0.95, 95% CI, 0.85–1.07; $p = 0.43$) (26).

The equivalence of carboplatin and cisplatin in the adjuvant setting is even less certain. All of the phase III studies performed (27–29), which affirmed the benefit of adjuvant chemotherapy after resection of NSCLC incorporated cisplatin-based combinations except for one. The Lung Adjuvant Cisplatin Evaluation meta-analysis was conducted on the five largest, cisplatin-based studies (ALPI, BLT, IALT, JBR.10 and ANITA). It found a 5.3% absolute survival advantage at 5 years (HR 0.89, 95% CI, 0.82–0.96; $p = 0.004$) for overall adjuvant cisplatin therapy. (30). CALGB 9633 was the only adjuvant trial to use carboplatin and was also the only trial to evaluate patients with stage 1B disease, which did not demonstrate a survival benefit from chemotherapy in this subset of patients (31). The ongoing E1505 trial which is being performed to investigate the role of bevacizumab in addition to adjuvant chemotherapy also excluded carboplatin from its treatment arms. Therefore the use of carboplatin in the adjuvant setting cannot be recommended. Overall, the evidence to date indicates that cisplatin may be the platinum agent of choice for patients with advanced NSCLC although, due to a lower toxicity and the poor life expectancy of the advanced disease, carboplatin can also be offered (32). However, in the adjuvant setting cisplatin should still be used instead.

Targeted Therapy with Platinum Compounds

Advances in the knowledge of tumor biology have led to the development of several targeted therapies in the management of NSCLC. Based on promising results from phase II trials both as monotherapy and in combination with platinum agents in patients with advanced NSCLC, several randomized phase III trials have been published in the last few years addressing this issue. Bevacizumab in combination with carboplatin-paclitaxel as first-line therapy, is the only targeted agent to have demonstrated improved survival outcomes compared with chemotherapy alone in patients with advanced NSCLC.

The Eastern Cooperative Oncology Group (ECOG) conducted a randomized study (E4599) in which 878 patients with locally advanced, metastatic or recurrent nonsquamous NSCLC were assigned to receive paclitaxel plus carboplatin with or without bevacizumab (15 mg/kg). The addition of bevacizumab to chemotherapy reduced the risk of death by 21% (HR 0.79, 95% CI, 0.67–0.92; p = 0.003) with a median survival time of 12.3 months in the bevacizumab arm and 10.3 months in the control arm. An improvement in the median progression-free survival was also seen in the bevacizumab arm, 6.2 months vs. 4.5 months in the control arm (HR 0.66, p < 0.001). A major concern in this study was the significantly increased toxicities in the bevacizumab arm, in particular, the rates of clinically significant bleeding were 4.4 and 0.7% in the bevacizumab and chemotherapy only arms, respectively (p < 0.001). Furthermore, there were two treatment-related deaths in the chemotherapy group and 15 treatment-related deaths in the bevacizumab group, of which five deaths were attributed to pulmonary hemorrhage (33). The results of this study suggest that addition of bevacizumab can improve survival in patients with advanced NSCLC with the risk of increased adverse results and treatment-related deaths. A subset analysis of ECOG 4599 to evaluate the outcomes for elderly patients was recently published. The addition of bevacizumab did not demonstrate any survival advantage compared with chemotherapy alone and was associated with a higher degree of toxicity and treatment-related deaths (34).

Another randomized phase III study (the Avastin in Lung [AVAiL] trial) involving over 1,000 patients was done with the same objectives in mind but with bevacizumab added in combination with cisplatin and gemcitabine instead. Two doses of bevacizumab were being investigated: 7.5 and 15 mg/kg. Progression-free survival and response rates were significantly increased in the bevacizumab arm. The median progression-free survival times were 6.1, 6.7 and 6.5 months, respectively, for chemotherapy alone, chemotherapy plus bevacizumab 7.5 mg/kg (HR 0.75, 95% CI, 0.62–0.90; p = 0.002) and chemotherapy plus bevacizumab 15 mg/kg (HR 0.82, 95% CI, 0.68–0.98; p = 0.03). The survival data have so far not been disclosed (35).

The results of both ECOG 4599 and AVAiL trials suggest that the addition of bevacizumab to platinum agents have better efficacy outcomes than chemotherapy alone. However, there were disparities in the progression-free survival time between the two control chemotherapy arms in the trials. The progression-free survival time was 4.5 months in patients with carboplatin-based control arm in the ECOG 4599 study compared with 6.1 months in patients with cisplatin-based control arm in the AVAiL trial. This raises the question if the addition of bevacizumab in the ECOG 4599 trial conferred a survival advantage simply because carboplatin is inferior to cisplatin.

To date, there have been four other randomized phase III trials conducted with two epidermal growth factor receptor (EGFR) tyrosine kinase inhibitors – Gefitinib and Erlotinib, as first-line therapy in combination with platinum-based regimens in patients with advanced NSCLC. Two of the randomized phase III trials using erlotinib, each including over 1,000 patients, did not demonstrate a benefit in response rate, time to progression, or survival with the addition of erlotinib to either carboplatin and paclitaxel (TRIBUTE) (36) or cisplatin and gemcitabine (TALENT) (37) compared to the same platinum-based regimens alone. Similar results were reported from both INTACT 1 and 2 trials (38, 39), when gefitinib was added to either cisplatin and gemcitabine or carboplatin and paclitaxel respectively. Both trials failed to show any improvement in survival compared with chemotherapy alone.

The benefit of adding cetuximab to chemotherapy as first-line therapy for patients with advanced NSCLC has been investigated in two randomized phase II study. Rosell et al. (LUCAS) (40) compared 86 patients with EGFR-expressing advanced NSCLC using cisplatin and vinorelbine with or without cetuximab. The addition of cetuximab increased the response rate from 28 to 35%, prolonged median progression-free survival time (4.6 vs. 5.0 months) and improved the median survival time (7.3 vs. 8.3 months). A recently published randomized phase II trial confirms the feasibility of adding cetuximab to platinum-based chemo-therapy as first-line treatment of advanced NSCLC (41). In this study, 65 patients were randomized to receive either cisplatin or carboplatin and gemcitabine with or without cetuximab. Patients receiving cetuximab had a higher response rate (27.7 vs. 18.2%; 95% CI 17.3–40.2 vs. 9.8–29.6%), median progression-free survival (5.09 vs. 4.21 months; 95% CI 3.81 5.49 vs. 4.17–5.98) and median overall sur-vival (11.99 vs. 9.26 months; 95% CI 8.8–15.18 vs. 7.43–11.79).

However, it is unclear whether this level of benefit would be seen in a phase III study despite these encouraging results. To validate these results, two large randomized phase III trials that evaluate the role of cetuximab in combination with chemotherapy as first-line treatment in advanced NSCLC have recently closed to accrual (BMS 099 and EMR 62202-046 FLEX). A press release indicated that sur-vival was increased by the addition of cetuximab to cisplatin-vinorelbine. However, the final data have as yet not been disclosed.

Future Strategies to Guide Therapy

Several gene markers that are linked to drug resistance have been discovered in recent years. The excision repair cross-complementation group 1 (ERCC1) is one such critical gene in the nucleotide excision repair pathway. It is the primary DNA repair mechanism that recognizes and removes platinum-induced DNA adducts. In-vitro studies have shown that high levels of ERCC1 messenger RNA (mRNA) in cell lines of ovarian, cervical, testicular, bladder, and non–small cell lung can-cers is associated with cisplatin resistance (42). These data have been corroborated by small, retrospective clinical studies in several solid tumors including advanced NSCLC. One study examined the expression of ERCC1 mRNA from paraffin-embedded tumor specimens in stage IV. NSCLC patients treated with cisplatin and gemcitabine. Patients with low levels of ERCC1 mRNA were reported to have better survival and response rate than those with high levels, although the only difference between survival and response was statistically significant (43). On the other hand, a high expression of ERCC1 as determined by quantitative, real-time RT-PCR, has been associated with improved survival in patients with NSCLC (44).

Olaussen et al. analyzed ERCC1 expression in operative samples obtained from patients that had been enrolled in the International Adjuvant Cancer Trial (IALT). Patients with ERCC1-negative tumors, as determined by immunohistochemical analysis, appeared to have a survival benefit from adjuvant cisplatin-based chemotherapy (adjusted HR for death, 0.65; 95% CI, 0.50–0.86; $p = 0.002$), whereas patients with ERCC1-positive tumors did not. However, among patients who did not receive adjuvant chemotherapy, the presence of ERCC1 protein in tumors was associated with a survival advantage (adjusted HR for death, 0.66; 95% CI, 0.49–0.90; $p = 0.009$) (45).

On the basis of these encouraging results, Cobo et al. conducted the first prospective phase III randomized trial testing the concept of customized chemotherapy based on ERCC1 expression in patients with advanced NSCLC. Patients were randomized in a 1:2 ratio to either the control arm (cisplatin/docetaxel) or to the genotypic arm where chemotherapy was tailored according to the levels of ERCC1. Patients with low ERCC1 levels received the same platinum-based combination as the control arm, whereas those with high ERCC1 levels were treated with a nonplatinum-based combination (docetaxel/gemcitabine). Patients in the genotypic arm achieved a higher response rate than those in the control arm (51.2 vs. 39.3%; $p = 0.02$). The improved response remained statistically significant when the two sub-groups were compared to the control arm. However, there were no differences in progression-free survival and overall survival between the two arms. This study underscores the feasibility of utilizing such an approach in selecting the appropriate chemotherapy regimen in patients with advanced NSCLC (46).

Another gene critical to DNA synthesis and DNA damage repair pathways is the ribonucleotide reductase M1 (RRM1). The RRM1 gene encodes the regulatory subunit of ribonucleotide reductase, the rate limiting enzyme involved in DNA synthesis (47–49). RRM1 plays a role in tumor invasion and metastasis. Its effects are thought to be mediated by the actions of a bifunctional phosphatase, phosphatase and tensin homologue (PTEN). PTEN is an inhibitor of cell proliferation and decreases cell migration and invasiveness via the reduction of phosphorylation of focal adhesion kinases (50). RRM1 is also the molecular target of gemcitabine (2',2'-difluorodeoxycytidine) (51–53).

Earlier work from smaller studies had suggested that NSCLC patients with high levels of RRM1 expression as compared with low levels demonstrated improved disease-free and overall survival (54). A larger study done by Zheng et al. further validated RRM1 as a marker of clinical outcome in patients with NSCLC. In that study of 187 patients with completely resected stage I NSCLC, the group of patients with tumors that had high expression of RRM1 as compared with low expression correlated with an improved median disease-free survival (>120 vs. 54.5 months, HR 0.46; $p = 0.004$) and overall survival (120 vs. 60.2 months, HR 0.61; $p = 0.02$). The study also demonstrated that high levels of expression of both RRM1 and ERCC1 were associated with an excellent outcome as seen in the subgroup of patients, comprising 30% of the study cohort (55).

On the contrary, high levels of expression of these genes have been linked to poorer survival outcomes in NSCLC patients treated with gemcitabine and platinum-based regimens in retrospective analyses (43, 56). A prospective phase II clinical trial in patients with advanced NSCLC treated with two cycles of gemcitabine and carboplatin demonstrated that high levels of both ERCC1 and RRM1 were inversely correlated with tumor response (53). On the basis of these results from earlier studies, Simon et al. conducted a prospective phase II clinical trial to assess the efficacy of selecting chemotherapy based on RRM1 and ERCC1 expression in patients with advanced NSCLC. Patients with high expression of RRM1 were treated without gemcitabine and those with high expression of ERCC1 were treated without carboplatin. The results of the study compared favorably to other studies in similar patient population, with a response rate of 44%, a 1-year survival of 59% and median overall survival of 13.3 months (57).

The development of genomic-derived signatures to predict sensitivity to cisplatin is another approach that has the potential to customize chemotherapy to individual patients with NSCLC and perhaps in other cancers where cisplatin-based therapy is considered the standard of care (58). These preliminary results are promising and have demonstrated the feasibility of utilizing a biomarker-based therapeutic strategy in the management of patients with NSCLC. This has paved the way for future research in this area of individualizing therapy by identifying patients who will respond to treatment, thereby increasing the overall effectiveness of chemotherapy.

Conclusion

Advanced NSCLC remains a fatal disease with low response rates and short survival outcomes. Despite the introduction of newer and less toxic chemotherapeutic agents, platinum compounds remain the backbone of systemic treatment of NSCLC. Nonetheless, therapeutic choices should be tailored to individual patients, taking into account age, performance status, co-morbidities and toxicity profile of therapy. Platinum combinations with bevacizumab have shown to be of benefit over chemotherapy alone and targeted therapies will potentially be introduced. Selection of patients based on genomic approaches may well come into play in the near future and help identify patients who will optimally benefit from specific therapies.

References

1. Jemal A, Siegal R, Ward E, et al. Cancer statistics, 2007. CA Cancer J Clin 2007;57:43–66.
2. Cullen MH, Billingham LJ, Woodroffe, et al. Mitomycin, ifosfamide and cisplatin in unresectable non-small cell lung cancer: effects on survival and quality of life. J Clin Oncol 1999;17:3188–94.
3. Spiro SG, Rudd RM, Souhami RL, et al. Chemotherapy vs. supportive care in advanced non-small cell lung cancer: improved survival without detriment to quality of life. Thorax 2004;59:828–36.

4. Non-Small Cell Lung Cancer Collaborative Group. Chemotherapy in non-small cell lung cancer: a meta-analysis using updated data on individual patients from 52 randomized clinical trials. BMJ 1995;311:899–909.
5. Freidberg EC. How nucleotide excision repair protects against cancer. Nat Rev Cancer 2001;1:22–33.
6. Delbaldo C, Michiels S, Syz N, Soria JC, Le Chevalier T, Pignon JP. Benefits of adding a drug to a single-agent or a 2-agent chemotherapy regimen in advanced non-small-cell lung cancer: a meta-analysis. JAMA 2004;292:470–84.
7. Le Chevalier T, Scagliotti G, Natale R, et al. Efficacy of gemcitabine plus platinum chemotherapy compared with other platinum containing regimens in advanced non-small cell lung cancer: a meta-analysis of survivcal outcomes. Lung Cancer 2005;47:69–80.
8. Baggstrom M, Stinchombe T, Socinski M, et al. Third-Generation chemotherapy agents in the treatment of advanced non-small cell lung cancer: a meta-analysis. J Thorac Oncol 2007;2:845–53.
9. Paccagnella A, Oniga F, Bearz A, et al. Adding gemcitabine to paclitaxel/carboplatin combination increases survival in advanced non-small-cell lung cancer: results of a phase II-III study. J Clin Oncol 2006;24:681–7.
10. Comella P, Filippelli G, De Cataldis G, et al. Efficacy of the combination of cisplatin with either gemcitabine and vinorelbine or gemcitabine and paclitaxel in the treatment of locally advanced or metastatic non-small-cell lung cancer: a phase III randomised trial of the Southern Italy Cooperative Oncology Group (SICOG 0101). Ann Oncol 2007;18:324–30.
11. Gridelli C, Maione P, Illiano A, et al. Cisplatin plus gemcitabine or vinorelbine for elderly patients with advanced non-small cell lung cancer: the MILES-2P studies, J Clin Oncol 2007;25:4663–9.
12. Langer C, Li S, Schiller J, et al. Randomized phase II trial of paclitaxel plus carboplatin or gemcitabine plus cisplatin in Eastern Cooperative Oncology Group Performace Status 2 non-small cell lung cancer patients: ECOG 1599. J Clin Oncol 2007;25:418–23.
13. Effects of vinorelbine on quality of life and survival of elderly patients with advanced non-small cell lung cancer. The Elderly Lung Cancer Vinorelbine Italian Study Group. J Natl Cancer Inst 1999;91:66–72.
14. Anderson H, Hopwood R, Stephens R. Gemcitabine plus best supportive care (BSC) vs BSC in inoperable non-small lung cancer – a randomized trial with quality of life as the primary outcome. Br J Cancer 2000;83:447–53.
15. Ranson M, Davidson N, Nicolson M, et al. Randomized trial of paclitaxel plus supportive care versus supportive care for patients with advanced non-small cell lung cancer. J Natl Cancer Inst 2000;92:1074–80.
16. Roszkowski K, Pluzanska A, Krzakowski M, et al. A multicenter, randomized, phase III study of docetaxel plus best supportive care versus best supportive care in chemotherapy-naïve patients with metastatic or non-resectable localized non-small cell lung cancer. Lung Cancer 2000;27:145–57.
17. Hotta K, Matsuo K, Ueoka H, et al. Addition of platinum compounds to a new agent in patients with advanced non-small cell lung cancer: a literature based meta-analysis of randomized trials. Ann Oncol 2004;15:1782–9.
18. Gridelli C, Gallo C, Shepherd FA, et al. Gemcitabine plus vinorelbine compared with cisplatin plus vinorelbine or cisplatin plus gemcitabine for advanced non-small cell lung cancer: a phase III trial of the Italian GEMVIN Investigators an the National Cancer Institute of Canada Clinical Trials Group. J Clin Oncol 2003;21:3025–34.
19. Smit EF, van Meerbeeck JP, Lianes P, et al. Three-arm randomized study of two cisplatin based regimens and paclitaxel plus gemcitabine in advanced non small cell lung cancer: a phase III trial of the European organization for research and treatment of cancer. Lung Cancer Group EORTC 08975. J Clin Oncol 2003;21:3909–17.
20. D'Addario G, Pintilie M, Leighl NB, et al. Platinum-based versus non-platinum based chemotherapy in advanced non-small cell lung cancer: a meta-analysis of the published literature. J Clin Oncol 2005;49:2926–36.

21. Pujol JL, Barlesi F, Daures JP. Should chemotherapy combinations for advanced non-small cell lung cancer be platinum-based? A meta-analysis of phase III randomized trials. Lung Cancer 2006;51:335–45.
22. Schiller JH, Harrington D, Johnson DH, et al. Comparison of four chemotherapy regimens for advanced non-small cell lung cancer. N Engl J Med 2002;346:92–8.
23. Kelly K, Crowley J, Bunn PA, et al. Randomized phase III trial of paclitaxel plus carboplatin versus vinorelbine plus cisplatin in the treatment of patients with advanced non-small cell lung cancer: a Southwest oncology group trial. J Clin Oncol 2001;19:3210–8.
24. Hotta K, Matsuo K, Hiroshi U, et al. Meta-analysis of randomized clinical trials comparing cisplatin to carboplatin in patients with advanced non-small cell lung cancer. J Clin Oncol 2004;22:3852–9.
25. Ardizzoni A, Boni L, Tiseo M, et al. Cisplatin versus carboplatin-based chemotherapy in first-line treatment of advanced non-small cell lung cancer: an individual patient data meta-analysis. J Natl Cancer Inst 2007;99:847–57.
26. Rajeswaran A, Trojan A, Burnand B, Giannelli M. Efficacy and side effects of cisplatin and carboplatin-based doublet chemotherapeutic regimens versus non-platinum-based doublet chemotherapeutic regimens as first line treatment of metastatic non-small cell lung carcinoma: a systemic review of randomized controlled trials. Lung Cancer 2008;59(1):1–11.
27. Arriagada R, Bergman B, Dunant A, et al. Cisplatin-based adjuvant chemotherapy in patients with completely resected non-small cell lung cancer. N Engl J Med 2004;350:351–60.
28. Winston T, Livingston R, Johnson D, et al. Vinorelbine plus cisplatin vs observation in resected non-small cell lung cancer. N Engl J Med 2005;352:2589–97.
29. Douillard JY, Rosell R, Delena M, et al. Adjuvant vinorelbine plus cisplatin versus observation in patients with completely resected stage IB-IIIA non-small-cell lung cancer (Adjuvant Navelbine International Trialist Association [ANITA]): a randomised controlled trial Lancet Oncol 2006;7:719–27.
30. Pignon JP, Tribodet GV, Scagliotti G, et al. Lung adjuvant cisplatin evaluation (LACE): a pooled analysis of five randomized clinical trials including 4,584 patients. Prog Proc Am Soc Clin Oncol 2006;24:366 (abstract).
31. Strauss GM, Herndon JE, Maddaus MA, et al. Adjuvant chemotherapy in stage IB non-small cell lung cancer: update on cancer and leukemia group B (CALGB) protocol 9633. Prog Proc Am Soc Clin Oncol 2006;24:365 (abstract).
32. Jiang J, Liang X, Zhou X, Huang R, Chu Z. A meta-analysis of randomized controlled trials comparing carboplatin-based to cisplatin-based chemotherapy in advanced non-small cell lung cancer. Lung Cancer 2007;57:348–58.
33. Sandler A, Gray R, Perry MC, et al. Paclitaxel-carboplatin alone or with bevacizumab for non-small cell lung cancer. N Engl J Med 2006;355:2542–50.
34. Ramalingam SS, Dahlberg SE, Langer CJ, et al. Outcomes for elderly, advanced-stage non-small cell lung cancer patients treated with bevacizumab in combination with carboplatin and paclitaxel: analysis of Eastern Cooperative Oncology Group Trial 4599. J Clin Oncol 2008;26:60–5.
35. Manegold C, von Pawel J, Zatloukal P, et al. Randomized, double-blind multicenter phase III study of bevacizumab in combination with cisplatin and gemcitabine in chemotherapy-naïve patients with advanced or recurrent non-squamous non-small cell lung cancer: B017704. Prog Proc Am Soc Clin Oncol 2007;25:7514 (abstract).
36. Herbst RS, Prager D, Hermann R, et al. TRIBUTE: a phase III trial of erlotinib hydrochloride (OSI-774) combined with carboplatin and paclitaxel cehmotherapy in advanced non-small cell lung cancer. J Clin Oncol 2005;23:5892–99.
37. Gatzemeier U, Pluzanska A, Szczesna A, et al. Phase III study of erlotinib in combination with cisplatin and gemcitabine in advanced non-small cell lung cancer: The Tarceva Lung Cancer Investigation Trial. J Clin Oncol 2007;25:1545–52.
38. Giaccone G, Herbst RS, Manegold C, et al. Gefitinib in combination with gemcitabine and cisplatin in advanced non-small cell lung cancer: a phase III trial – INTACT 1. J Clin Oncol 2004;22:777–84.

39. Herbst RS, Giaccone G, Schiller J, et al. Gefitinib in combination with paclitaxel and carboplatin in advanced non-small cell lung cancer: a phase III trial – INTACT 2. J Clin Oncol 2004;22:785–94.

40. Rosell R, Robinet G, Szczesna A, et al. Randomized phase II study of cetuximab plus cisplatin/vinorelbine compared with cisplatin/vinorelbine alone as first-line therapy in EGFR-expressing advanced non-small cell lung cancer. Ann Oncol 2008;19:362–9.

41. Butts CA, Bodkin D, Middleman EL, et al. Randomized phase II study of gemcitabine plus cisplatin, with or without cetuximab, as first-line therapy for patients with advanced or metastatic non-small cell lung cancer. J Clin Oncol 2007;25:5777–84.

42. Altaha R, Liang X, Yu JJ, et al. Excision repair cross complementing-group 1: gene expression and platinum resistance. Int J Mol Med 2004;14:959–70.

43. Lord RV, Brabender J, Gandara D, et al. Low ERCC1 expression correlates with prolonged survival after cisplatin plus gemcitabine chemotherapy in non-small cell lung cancer. Clin Cancer Res 2002;8:2286–91.

44. Simon GR, Sharma S, Cantor A, et al. ERCC1 expression is a predictor of survival in resected patients with non-small cell lung caner. Chest 2005;127:978–83.

45. Olaussen KA, Dunant A, Fouret P, et al. DNA repair by ERCC1 in non-small cell lung cancer and cisplatin-based adjuvant chemotherapy. N Engl J Med 2006;355:983–91.

46. Cobo M, Dolores I, Massuri B, et al. Customizing cisplatin based on quantitative excision repair cross-complementing 1 mRNA expression: a phase III trial in non-small cell lung cancer. J Clin Oncol 2007;25:2747–54.

47. Filatov D, Ingemarson R, Johansson E, et al. Mouse ribonucleotide reductase: from genes to proteins. Biochem Soc Trans 1995;23:903–5.

48. Stubbe J. Ribonucleotide reductases in the twenty-first century. Proc Natl Acad Sci USA 1998;95:2723–4.

49. Pitterle DM, Kim YC, Jolicoeur EMC, et al. Lung cancer and the human gene for ribonucleotide reductase subunit M1 (RRM1). Mamm Genome 1999;10:916–22.

50. Gautam A, Li ZR, Bepler G. RRM1-induced metastasis suppression through PTEN-regulated pathways. Oncogene 2003;22:2135–42.

51. Davidson JD, Ma L, Flagella M, et al. An increase in the expression of ribonucleotide reductase large subunit 1 is associated with gemcitabine resistance in non-small cell lung cancer cell lines. Cancer Res 2004;64:3761–6.

52. Bergman AM, Eijk PP, van Haperen VW, et al. In vivo induction of resistance to gemcitabine results in increased expression of ribonucleotide reductase subunit M1 as a major determinant. Cancer Res 2005;65:9510–6.

53. Bepler G, Kusmartseva I, Sharma S, et al. RRM1-modulated in vitro and in vivo efficacy of gemcitabine and platinum in non-small cell lung cancer. J Clin Oncol 2006;24:4731–7.

54. Bepler G, Sharma S, Cantor A, et al. RRM1 and PTEN as prognostic parameters for overall and disease-free survival in patients with non-small cell lung cancer. J Clin Oncol 2004;22:1878–85.

55. Zheng Z, Chen T, Li X, et al. DNA synthesis and repair genes RRM1 and ERCC1 in lung cancer. N Engl J Med 2007;356:800–8.

56. Rosell R, Danenberg K, Alberola V, et al. Ribonucleotide reductase subunit 1 mRNA expression and survival in gemcitabine/cisplatin-treated advanced non-small cell lung cancer patients. Clin Cancer Res 2004;64:3761–6.

57. Simon G, Sharma A, Li X, et al. Feasibility and efficacy of molecular analysis-directed individualized therapy in advanced non-small cell lung cancer. J Clin Oncol 2007;25:2741–6.

58. Hsu DS, Balakumaran BS, Acharya CR, et al. Pharmacogenomic strategies provide a rational approach to the treatment of cisplatin-resistant patients with advanced cancer. J Clin Oncol 2007;25:4350–7.

Is Lipoplatinum Monotherapy an Active Alternative in Second Line Treatment of Metastatic Non–Small Cell Lung Cancer? A Phase II Trial

Alberto Ravaioli, Manuela Fantini, Fabrizio Drudi, Maximilian Papi, Enzo Pasquini, Maurizio Marangolo, Wainer Zoli, Ilaria Panzini, Britt Rudnas, Stefania VL Nicoletti, Cinzia Possenti, Emiliano Tamburini, Lorenzo Gianni, and Manuela Imola

Abstract Lipoplatin is a liposome encapsulated form of cisplatin. Phase I studies on Lipoplatin showed an excellent toxicity profile of the compound. Therefore we performed a phase II trial in heavily pre-treated patients with advanced non–small cell lung cancer (NSCLC).

This was an open label single-arm trial in patients with NSCLC with stage IV disease already pre-treated with first line chemotherapy. 63% of these patients were pre-treated with platinum containing regimens. Statistical analysis was performed with the SPSS statistical program (version 11.0). Survival curves were estimated by the Kaplan Meyer method. We administered Lipoplatin at the dose of $100\,mg/m^2$ every 14 days as second line chemotherapy. The primary endpoint was the response rate. The secondary endpoints were safety, time to progression and overall survival.

Nineteen patients with stage IV NSCLC, the median age being 64 were treated. Fifteen patients completed at least six cycles and were evaluated for response and toxicity. Four patients completed one cycle of therapy and were evaluated only for toxicity. We obtained one partial response (5.2%) and three stable diseases (15.9%). Median time to progression was 4 months and median survival time was 7.2 months.

In this study lipoplatin as second line treatment showed a lower activity in comparison to other drugs, but the same overall survival. New phase II studies with escalation of the dosage should be considered.

Keywords Lipoplatin; Non–small cell lung cancer; Phase II trial

A. Ravaioli (✉), M. Fantini, F. Drudi, M. Papi, E. Pasquini, M. Marangolo, W. Zoli, I. Panzini, B. Rudnas, S.VL. Nicoletti, C. Possenti, E. Tamburini, L. Gianni, and M. Imola
Department of Oncology and Oncoematology, Infermi Hospital, Rimini, Italy
e-mail: aravaiol@auslrn.net

A. Bonetti et al. (eds.), *Platinum and Other Heavy Metal Compounds in Cancer Chemotherapy*, DOI: 10.1007/978-1-60327-459-3_29,
© Humana Press, a part of Springer Science + Business Media, LLC 2009

243

Introduction

Non–small cell lung cancer (NSCLC) currently represents almost 85% of all lung cancers with many patients presenting an advanced stage of the disease at the time of diagnosis. Chemotherapeutic agents are important in the therapy of this aggressive disease, and there are data supporting the advantage of regimens containing platinum drugs in terms of clinical benefit, palliation and increase in overall survival.

Cisplatin plays a central role in lung cancer chemotherapy in spite of its toxicity (1, 2). The response rate ranges between 25 and 30% for chemonaive patients treated with cisplatin in combination with gemcitabine or taxanes. The efficacy of cisplatin is dose dependent, but the dose is limited by the significant risk of renal and gastrointestinal toxicity, ototoxicity and toxic neuropathy (3–6). Therefore one of the major aims for medical oncologists is to find new more effective therapeutic agents with lower toxicity (7).

Some new interesting platinum compounds, administered either orally or by i.v. infusion, are under clinical evaluation: satraplatin (JM216; bis-acetatoamminedichlorocyclohexylamine platinum) is a platinum complex developed in an attempt to circumvent tumour resistance which can be administered by the oral route; ZD-0473 (formerly JM-473 and AMD-473) is a sterically hindered platinum complex designed and synthesized by Johnson Matthey Technology and the Cancer Research Campaign (CRC) and under development as a potential treatment for cisplatin-resistant cancers; and, the antitumor polynuclear platinum drug BBR3464 which forms stronger intra- and interstrand cross-links (CLs) on DNA, the typical target of platinum drugs. Extensive scientific efforts are directed towards finding new and improved platinum anticancer agents. A promising approach is the encapsulation of cisplatin in sterically stabilized, long circulating PEGylated 100 nm liposomes. A liposomal cisplatin formulation known as SPI-77 showed excellent stability in plasma and had a longer circulation time, greater efficacy and lower toxicity than cisplatin (8) but failed in clinical trials due to inadequate release of the drug in the tumour.

In this paper we describe our experience with Lipoplatin™, another liposomal platinum drug recently developed by Regulon (California), in a phase II trial of patients with advanced NSCLC.

This liposome measures 110 nm in diameter and is composed by a lipid shell made of dipalmitoyl phosphatidyl glycerol, soy phosphatidyl-choline, cholesterol, and methoxy-polyethylene glycol-distearoyl phosphatidylethanolamine lipid conjugate, containing a central core of cisplatin, with a ratio of cisplatin to lipids of 8.9% cisplatin and 91.1% total lipids (Regulon, 715 North Shoreline Boulevard Mountain View, California 94043, Regulon, AE, 7 Grigoriou Afxentiou, Alimos 17455, Greece) (8). It does not appear to be readily detected by the macrophages and immune cells, it remains in circulation for a longer period and it accumulates preferentially in the tumour sites and metastases through their hyperpermeable tumour vasculature. It was developed in order to reduce the systemic toxicity of cisplatin and enhance targeting tumour (8–13).

Lipoplatin showed low toxicity and good anti-tumour activity in mouse xenografts (12). In a Phase I study Lipoplatin™ demonstrated very few adverse effects and a very low toxicity. Peak levels were reached in the blood in 8h at a concentration up to 50 times higher in malignant tissue compared to normal tissue (10, 11). Within the first 24h 23–40% of cisplatin is excreted in urine (14, 15); in contrast, the half life of Lipoplatin™ was 117.46h in plasma with a 40.7% of the drug excreted in the urine in about 3 days (9, 14, 15). Clinical trials were performed in advanced stages of head and neck, pancreatic and lung cancers (8, 16, 17). These studies demonstrated a favourable toxicity profile for the drug, some partial remissions and cases of stable disease (PR 8.3%, SD 33.3% in pancreatic cancer patients), with higher targeting properties and longer half-life compared to cisplatin. Currently, various clinical phase II and III trials are ongoing in lung cancer patients and preliminary results suggest that the drug is relatively safe and capable of producing some partial responses. The results from these trials have yet to be published. As there was insufficient data available, our group undertook additional preclinical and clinical studies of Lipoplatin™.

Methods

We tested the in vitro activity of Lipoplatin™ in four established NSCLC cell lines, including three sensitive lines (ChaGo-K1 broncogenic cell line, CAEP and RAL derived from epidermoid human carcinoma) and one cisplatin-resistant line (ChaGo-CPL, isolated in IRST[WZ] laboratory). We also tested the toxicity on peripheral blood stem cells obtained by leukaphereses from four lymphoma patients treated with chemotherapy. Cells were used in the exponential growth phase in all the experiments. The drugs used, cisplatin and Lipoplatin™, were solubilized in dimethylsulfoxide (DMSO, Sigma Aldrich) with the final DMSO concentration not exceeding 0.5%. In vitro chemosensivity assays were performed; the dose response curves were created with Excel software, Inhibition Growth 50 (IG_{50}), Lethal Growth 50 (LG_{50}) and Inhibitory Concentration 50 (IC_{50}) values were determined graphically from the plots. The toxicity to hematopoietic precursors was studied in liquid cultures incubated with different concentrations (cisplatin 2.2 µM for 6h and Lipoplatin 20 µM for 72h) with flow cytometric analysis (FACS Vantage flow cytometric, Becton Dickinson, San Diego California).

In the clinical setting we undertook a phase II study of second line treatment in advanced NSCLC to study the drug's efficacy in a subset of heavily pre-treated patients with stage IV NSCLC. The dose used for Lipoplatin™ was 100 mg/m² i.v. every 2 weeks, diluted in 500 ml of 5% dextrose and infused over 8h. No pre or post-hydratation was used. The toxicity was graded using modified NCI Common Toxicity Criteria (version 5/12/95). Toxicity was evaluated on a 1–4 grade scale. According to the grade of toxicity (grade 3 and 4) the investigator could reduce or interrupt the treatment. Disease progression was a cause for discontinuation of treatment in this study.

Day 1 of each cycle could be delayed up to 14 day in case of toxicity. The patient could receive a maximum of 12 cycles; treatment was stopped earlier if there was evidence of progressive disease, unacceptable toxicity or due to the patient's wish. No other treatments other than contraceptives, replacement steroids and radiation therapy to single lesions were allowed during the study.

This was an open label single-arm trial. Statistical analysis was performed with the SPSS (version 11.0) statistical program. Survival curves were estimated by the Kaplan-Meier method. The Simon two-stage phase II design was used, providing 80% power and a 0.05 level of overall significance to distinguish between the null and alternative hypotheses. Planned maximum sample size was 33 subjects. The sample size in the first stage was of 19 subjects and in the second stage it was of 15. A stopping rule was established at the first step if two or less of the first 19 subjects responded. This provided 95% confidence that the response rate was less that 10% for the regimen. Our primary end point objective was objective disease response. Subjects who experienced CR or PR were classified as responders. Secondary endpoints were the evaluation of time to progression and overall survival. The international index for dose adjustment was used. Evaluation of the response was performed by two reviewers independently. The discordant evaluations were reviewed by the authors with an attending radiologist.

Results

From in vitro experiments we proved that cisplatin has the same cytotoxic activity as Lipolatin™. Cisplatin has a stronger activity in one cell line (ChaGo-K1). On the contrary the bone marrow toxicity of Lipoplatin™ was milder than that of cisplatin the liposomal compound never reaching an IC_{50} (<0.02 µM) (Fig. 1).

In our phase II protocol we enrolled 19 patients from December 2003 to 2004. The base-line characteristics of patients are presented in Table 1. Fourteen males

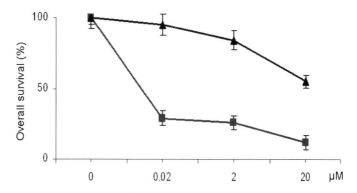

Fig. 1 Cytotoxic activity of Lipoplatin and cisplatin on bone marrow stem cells. *Filled triangle* lipoplatin; *filled square* cisplatin

Table 1 Patient characteristics

		Number	Percent	Range	Median
Age				42–78	64
Sex	Males	14	73.7	–	–
	Females	5	26.3		
Histology subtype	Adenocarcinoma	12	63.3		
	Squamous cell	4	21	–	–
	Mixed adenosquamosus	2	10.5		
	Anaplastic	1	5.2		
	Prior surgery	3	15.8	–	–
	Prior radiotherapy	9	47.3	–	–
First line chemotherapy	Gemcitabine–taxotere	6	31.5	–	–
	Gemcitabine–cisplatin	6	31.5	–	–
	Gemcitabine–carboplatin	6	31	–	–
	Gemcitabine	1	5.5	–	–

Table 2 Response rate, time to progression and survival

	CR	PR	SD	PD
Response rate	–	1 (5.2%)	3 (15.9)	15 (78.9)
	Median (months)	Range (months)	–	–
Time to progression	4	1–21	–	–
Survival time	7.2	1–12	–	–

and five females with stage IV NSCLC were enrolled. The average age was 64 years (range 42–78 years). The ECOG performance status was 0–2 in all patients. The histology of the disease was adenocarcinoma in 12 patients, squamous cell in 4 patients, mixed adeno-squamous in 2 patients and anaplastic in 1 patient. Three patients underwent surgery before relapse and sixteen did not. Nine patients had received prior radiation therapy. The first line of medical treatment was gemcitabine and taxotere in 6 patients, cisplatin and gemcitabine in 6, carboplatin and gemcitabine in 6 and gemcitabine alone in 1 patient.

Fifteen patients completed at least six cycles and were evaluated for response and toxicity. Four patients completed one cycle of therapy and were evaluated only for toxicity. Among the 15 patients with at least six cycles of therapy we observed one partial response (5.2%) and three cases of stable disease (15.9%). Median time to progression was 4 months (range 1–21) and median survival time was 7.2 months (219 days, 31.2 weeks) (Table 2). The 1 year survival rate was 16.6%. Very little toxicity was observed. The most frequent adverse events included: anaemia G1–2 (4 patients; 21%); mucositis G1–2 (2 patients; 10.5%); nausea and vomiting G1–2 (4 patients; 21%); and, asthenia G1–2 (3 patients; 15.7%). No grade 3–4 adverse events were observed.

Discussion

In the management of NSCLC patients treated with second line therapy clinicians must evaluate the benefit relative to the toxicities of an agent. Docetaxel (18–20), pemetrexed (21) and erlotinib (22, 23) have been reported to produce response rates between 7.1 and 9.1% with a survival time of nearly 7 months and an acceptable safety profile. These results leave a great deal of room for improvement. On the one hand they are only marginally effective and on the other hand the economic costs of these treatments is very high. For these two reasons (scientific and economic) many researchers and pharmaceutical companies are trying to find new compounds with more clinical efficacy. Many of these drugs are under evaluation in phase II and III clinical trials.

Lipoplatin™ is one of these drugs. This molecule at the dosage used has a very low toxicity and a clinical efficacy not so different from the more established agents. On the basis of our experience, however, we think that Lipoplatin™, at the dosage used in this trial, has unsatisfactory activity although it has a very low toxicity. Furthermore, we think that the drug is inadequately studied at the dosage chosen in phase II trials ($100 \, mg/m^2$ every 2 weeks). In our opinion this formulation should be further evaluated to identify the optimal dose in single agent phase II trials and would propose a dose of $125 \, mg/m^2$ every 2 weeks.

Acknowledgment This work was supported by Istituto Oncologico Romagnolo; project number IOR RN 2003.

References

1. Rosenberg B, VanCamp L, Trosko JE, Mansour VH. Platinum compounds: a new class of potent antitumor agents. Nature 1969;222:385–6.
2. McKeage MJ. Comparative adverse effect profiles of platinum drugs. Drug Saf 1995;13:228–44.
3. Arany I, Safirstein RL. Cisplatin nephrotoxicity. Semin Nephrol 2003;23:460–4.
4. Townsend DM, Deng M, Zhang L, Lapus MG, Hanigan MH. Metabolism of cisplatin to a nephrotoxin in proximal tubule cells. J Am Soc Nephrol 2003;14:1–10.
5. Humes HD. Insights into ototoxicity. Analogies to nephrotoxicity. Ann NY Acad Sci 1999;884:15–8.
6. Caraceni A, Martini C, Spatti G, Thomas A, Onofrj M. Recovering optic neuritis during systematic cisplatin and carboplatin chemotherapy. Acta Neurol Scand 1997;96:260–1.
7. Ali BH, Al Moundhri MS. Agents ameliorating or augmenting the nephrotoxicity of cisplatin and other platinum compounds: a review of some recent research. Food Chem Toxicol 2006;44:1173–83.
8. Boulikas T, Vougiouka M. Cisplatin and platinum drugs at the molecular level. Oncol Rep 2003;10:1663–82.
9. Stathopoulos GP, Boulikas T, Vougiouka M, et al. Pharmacokinetics and adverse reactions of new liposomal cisplatin (Lipoplatin): phase I study. Oncol Rep 2005;13:589–95.
10. Boulikas T. Low toxicity and activity of a novel liposomal cisplatin (lipoplatin) in mouse xenografts. Oncol Rep 2004;12:3–12.

11. Boulikas T, Stathopoulos GP, Volakakis N, Vougiouka M. Systemic Lipoplatin infusion results in preferential tumor uptake in human studies. Anticancer Res 2005;25:3031–9.
12. Bandak S, Goren D, Horowitz A, Tzemach D, Gabizon A. Pharmacological studies of cisplatin encapsulated in long-circulating liposomes in mouse tumor models. Anticancer Drugs 1990;10:911–20.
13. Devarajan P, Tarabishi R, Mishra J, et al. Low renal toxicity of lipoplatin compared to cisplatin in animals. Anticancer Res 2004;24:2193–200.
14. Gormley PE, Bull JM, LeRoy AF, Cysyk R. Kinetics of *cis*-dichlorodiammineplatinum. Clin Pharmacol Ther 1979;25:351–7.
15. Belt RJ, Himmelstein KJ, Patton TF, Bannister SJ, Sternson LA, Repta AJ. Pharmacokinetics of non-protein-bound platinum species following administration of *cis*-dichlorodiammineplatinum(II). Cancer Treat Rep 1979;63:1515–21.
16. Jehn CF, Boulikas T, Kourvetaris A, Possinger K, Lüftner D. Pharmacokinetics of liposomal cisplatin (lipoplatin) in combination with 5-FU in patients with advanced head and neck cancer: first results of a phase III study. Anticancer Res 2007;27:471–5.
17. Stathopoulos GP, Boulikas T, Vougiouka M, Rigatos SK, Stathopoulos JG. Liposomal cisplatin with gemcitabine in pretreated advanced pancreatic cancer patients: a phase I–II study. Oncol Rep 2006;15:1201–4.
18. Shepherd FA, Dancey J, Ramlau R, et al. Prospective randomized trial of docetaxel versus best supportive care in patients with non-small-cell lung cancer previously treated with platinum-based chemotherapy. J Clin Oncol 2000;18:2095–103.
19. Gandara DR, Vokes E, Green M, et al. Activity of docetaxel in platinum-treated non-small-cell lung cancer. Results of a phase II multicenter trial. J Clin Oncol 2000;18:131–5.
20. Fossella FV, Lee JS, Shin DM, et al. Phase II study of docetaxel for advanced or metastatic platinum refractory non-small-cell lung cancer. J Clin Oncol 1995;13:645–51.
21. Hanna N, Shepherd FA, Fossella FV, et al. Randomized phase III trial of pemetrexed versus docetaxel in patients with non-small cell lung cancer previously treated with chemotherapy. J Clin Oncol 2004;22:1589–97.
22. Smith J. Erlotinib: small-molecule targeted therapy in the treatment of non-small-cell lung cncer. Clin Ther 2005;27:1513–34.
23. Tsao MS, Sakurada A, Cutz JC, et al. Erlotinib in lung cancer: molecular and clinical predictors of outcome. N Engl J Med 2005;353:133–44.

Combining Platinums in Gastric Cancer

Florian Lordick and Dirk Jäger

Abstract The role for systemic treatment in gastric cancer has become more evident over the past years. Perioperative chemotherapy increases the cure rates in localized stages. At the same time, palliative chemotherapy has shown to prolong survival and maintain the patients' quality of life in advanced disease.

Cisplatin in combination with 5-fluorouracil with or without an anthracycline now has a definite role in the treatment of patients with advanced disease. Newer studies support the addition of docetaxel to cisplatin plus 5-fluorouracil-based chemotherapy. The DCF regimen (docetaxel, cisplatin and 5-fluorouracil) is now a new reference regimen for the treatment of advanced stomach cancer. Recent studies suggest that oxaliplatin is as effective as cisplatin. Oxaliplatin was shown to be associated with slightly less toxicity, except sensory neuropathy which is more common with oxaliplatin. Therefore, oxaliplatin can replace cisplatin in combination chemotherapy regimens given in advanced disease.

The role of cisplatin for the preoperative (neoadjuvant) treatment of gastric cancer in locally advanced stages has now been established. Two randomized trials have been published recently. Patients with stage II and stage III stomach cancer and carcinoma of the gastroesophageal junction who received 8–9 weeks of preoperative cisplatin-5-fluorouracil-based chemotherapy had a significantly better overall survival chances compared to surgery alone.

The effectiveness and feasibility of chemotherapy in the postoperative (adjuvant) phase is less clear. There is no proven role for the use of cisplatin-containing combination chemotherapy in the postoperative setting. Studies employing platinum combinations in the adjuvant setting failed to show an improvement in survival.

Keywords Gastric cancer; Systemic chemotherapy; Cisplatin; Docetaxel; 5-fluorouracil

F. Lordick (✉) and D. Jäger
National Center for Tumor Diseases, Department of Medical Oncology,
University of Heidelberg, Heidelberg, Germany
e-mail: florian.lordick@med.uni-heidelberg.de

A. Bonetti et al. (eds.), *Platinum and Other Heavy Metal Compounds in Cancer Chemotherapy*, DOI: 10.1007/978-1-60327-459-3_30,
© Humana Press, a part of Springer Science + Business Media, LLC 2009

Epidemiology of Stomach Cancer

In the early nineteenth century, adenocarcinoma of the stomach was the most common malignancy in the US and Europe, but its incidence declined throughout the twentieth century and has now reached a plateau. From a world wide perspective, stomach cancer incidence still ranks number three in men and number four in women. Across continents, incidence rates vary from 3.4 per 100,000 patients per year among females in North America to 26.9 per 100,000 patients per year among males in Asia (1). Overall 5-year relative survival rates of ~20% (2, 3) in most areas of the world, except in Japan where mass screening programs, and treatment may contribute to superior 5-year survival rates of ~60% (4). With nearly 700,000 deaths, stomach cancer follows lung cancer as the second most common cancer leading to death worldwide (1).

Stomach cancers are anatomically classified as non-cardia and cardia cancers. Because non-cardia cancers constitute the majority of stomach cancer cases worldwide, overall stomach cancer incidence rates are predominated by this disease entity. The decrease of non-cardia cancer in the Western world probably reflects a diminishing prevalence of Helicobacter pylori infection due to improved sanitation, increasing availability of fresh fruits and vegetables, and decreasing use of salt- and smoke-based food preservation methods (1). However, non-cardia stomach cancer remains common in many geographic regions, including China, Japan, Eastern Europe, and Central/South America.

In contrast to non-cardia cancers, incidence rates of gastric cardia cancers have either increased or remained constant in Western countries (5, 6). While Helicobacter pylori is a strong risk factor for non-cardia gastric cancer it is inversely associated with the risk of gastric cardia cancer. These findings bolster the hypothesis that the decreasing prevalence of Helicobater pylori during the past century may have contributed to lower rates of non-cardia cancer and higher rates of cardia cancer in Western countries (7).

Activity of Cisplatin and Other Cytotoxic Drugs in Stomach Cancer

Cisplatin was found to be among the drugs with the highest in vitro activity against stomach cancer in preclinical studies (8).

Due to methodological flaws in many studies the real activity of many cytotoxic drugs given as monotherapy for stomach cancer remains relatively unknown. 5-fluorouracil (5-FU), doxorubicin, epirubicin, cisplatin, etoposide, and mitomycin C have led to responses in 15–20% of chemo-naïve tumours and were therefore considered to be active drugs (Table 1).

Cisplatin is one of the most active drugs in the treatment of gastroesophageal cancer. Response rates up to 25% were reported in chemo-naïve patients (9). While it was not profoundly studied in gastric cancers, oxaliplatin has shown in several

Table 1 Different cytotoxic drug activities when given as monotherapy in advanced stomach cancer (literature excerpt)

Class/Compound	No. of patients	CR/PR [%]
Platinum compounds		
Cisplatin	139	19
Carboplatin	41	5
Anti-metabolites		
5-Fluorouracil	416	21
UFT	188	28
Capecitabine	44	28
S-1	106	31
Pemetrexed	38	21
Gemcitabine	26	4
Anthracyclines		
Doxorubicin	141	17
4-Epirubicin	80	19
Taxanes		
Paclitaxel	98	17
Docetaxel	123	21
Other classes		
Irinotecan	66	23
Mitomycin C	211	30
Vinorelbin	29	7
BCNU	55	18

CR complete response; *PR* partial response

phase II and two phase III combination chemotherapy studies that its activity is comparable to that of cisplatin.

5-FU is considered to be one cornerstone of chemotherapy for stomach cancer. It was given as an intravenous bolus on five consecutive days or once every week. 5-fluorouracil displays its anti-proliferative activity above all on cells in the S-phase of the cell cycle and it has a plasma half-life of only 10–20 min. Therefore, continuous infusion is potentially superior to bolus infusion. 5-FU was infused in considerably different schedules, e.g. at a dose of 1,000 mg/m^2/day on 5 consecutive days (usually in combination with cisplatin every 3–4 weeks), as weekly high-dose infusion (with up to 3 g/m^2/for 24 h) or as a low-dose protracted infusion (300 mg/m^2/day continuous infusion over a couple of weeks). Until now, the optimal dosing and scheduling of 5-FU is unknown. Moynihan et al. observed responses in 31% of patients treated with protracted infusional 5-fluorouracil (10).

Different 5-fluorouracil prodrugs that allow for oral administration were developed in the recent years. Despite augmented intratumoural 5-fluorouracil concentrations that can be reached with these drugs, no increased gastrointestinal toxicity was observed. The most extensive experience, particularly in East Asia, does exist with uracil-tegafur (UFT) and S-1. S-1 (tegafur plus gimeracil and oteracil) showed considerable activity given as a monotherapy with response rates up to 48% in phase II studies (11, 12). Capecitabine has also shown activity as a monotherapy in advanced stomach cancer (13).

Novel classes of cytotoxic drugs have been investigated in stomach cancer. Topoisomerase-I-inhibitors, particularly irinotecan (14), the taxanes paclitaxel (15, 16) and docetaxel (17) and the multi-target anti-folate pemetrexed (18) have proven activity. In contrast, gemcitabine and vinorelbine, were only marginally active in stomach cancer (19, 20).

In conclusion, a number of older and newer cytotoxic drugs are active in gastro-esophageal cancer. With the newer compounds a considerable expansion of treatment options has occurred. But complete remissions are rarely achieved with monotherapy alone and response durations are relatively short with a median between 2 and 6 months. While in Japan monotherapy has been considered to be a standard of care until recently (21), many oncologists in the Western hemisphere favour combination regimens against the background of a suggested correlation between tumour response to first-line chemotherapy and the prognosis in stomach cancer (22) and on the basis of randomized trials that have been published during the past decade.

The Clinical Rationale for Platinum Combinations in Stomach Cancer

A recently published meta-analysis of 7 randomized trials including a total of 508 patients (23) showed that the addition of cisplatin to an anthracycline-5-fluorouracil based combination regimen does lead to a significant improvement in the overall survival in patients with advanced stomach cancer (Hazard ratio [HR] = 0.83; 95% confidence interval [CI] = 0.76–0.91; $p < 0.001$). Although some of the randomized trials did not meet their primary endpoint and did not show a significant improvement in overall survival by the addition of cisplatin, the cisplatin-containing regimens showed a consistently 10–20% higher tumour response rate compared with the non-cisplatin containing regimens (24, 25). The lack of an improvement in overall survival was probably due to the small sample size of the trials that were statistically underpowered and could therefore not prove smaller increments in survival. The largest of these trials, that randomized 274 patients to receive ECF (epirubicin, cisplatin, 5-fluorouracil) or FAMTX (5-fluorouracil, adriamycin, methotrexate) showed a significant improvement in the tumour response rate (46% [95% CI, 37–55%] with ECF, and 21% [95% CI, 13–28%] with FAMTX; $P = 0.00003$). The median survival was 8.7 months with ECF and 6.1 months with FAMTX ($P = 0.0005$). The 2-year survival rates were 14% (95% CI, 8–20%) for the ECF arm, and 5% (95% CI, 2–10%) for the FAMTX arm ($P = 0.03$). Histopathologically complete surgical resection following chemotherapy was achieved in ten patients in the ECF arm (three pathological complete responses to chemotherapy) and three patients in the FAMTX arm (no pathological complete responses). The authors concluded that the ECF regimen resulted in a response and survival advantage compared with FAMTX chemotherapy. The probability of long-term survival following surgical resection of residual disease was increased by this treatment and the high response rates seen with ECF supported its use in the neoadjuvant setting (26, 27).

After publication of these randomized trials in the end-nineties, cisplatin-based combination chemotherapy became an empiric standard of care for the treatment of advanced gastric cancer in the Western hemisphere countries. Since then, the most widely used regimes were ECF (epirubicin, cisplatin, 5-fluorouracil) and CF (cisplatin, 5-fluorouracil).

Combining Cisplatin with 5-Fluorouracil or Oral Fluoropyrimidines

5-fluorouracil and cisplatin in combination have been shown to possess synergistic cytotoxicity against human neoplasms (28, 29). It is thought that cisplatin enhances the anti-tumour effect of 5-fluorouracil by increasing the availability of the reduced folate necessary for tight binding of fluorodeoxyuridylate, a 5-fluorouracil metabolite, to deoxythymidylic acid synthase (30, 31).

In the clinical setting, the synergy of cisplatin and 5-fluororacil given as continuous infusion either for 24 h (2,600 mg/m^2) weekly or for 120 h (800 mg/m^2/day) every 4 weeks was demonstrated in two randomized trials. Both studies showed a more than 20% increase of tumour responses with the combination of cisplatin and 5-fluorouracil compared with 5-fluorouracil as a single agent. Also, an increase in progression-free survival was seen (21, 32).

The promising tumour response rates of oral fluoropyrimidines (Table 1), their ease of application and their favourable toxicity profile prompted the design and conduct of randomized controlled trials.

S-1 is an orally active combination of tegafur (a prodrug that is converted to fluorouracil on a cytochrome CYP2A6-dependent mechanism), gimeracil (an inhibitor of dihydropyrimidine dehydrogenase, which degrades fluorouracil), and oteracil (which inhibits the phosphorylation of fluorouracil in the gastrointestinal tract, thereby reducing the gastrointestinal toxic effects of fluorouracil) in a molar ratio of 1:0.4:1 (33, 34). S-1 showed a considerable activity given as a monotherapy with response rates up to 48% in phase II studies (11, 12, 35). Experiences outside of Japan are limited. But as a combination partner with cisplatin, first experiences in the Western hemisphere are also encouraging (36). A recently presented Japanese trial randomized 298 patients with advanced and previously untreated stomach cancer to receive either S-1 alone (40–60 mg twice daily for 28 days of a 6-week cycle) or S-1 (40–60 mg twice daily for 21 days of a 5-week cycle) plus cisplatin (60 mg/m^2 on day 8) (37). The combination led to a > 20% increased tumour response rate (54% for cisplatin/S-1 vs. 31% for S-1; $p = 0.0018$) and a significant increase in progression-free survival (6.0 months vs. 4.0 months; HR = 0.567; $p < 0.001$) and in overall survival (13.0 months vs. 11.0 months; HR = 0.774; $p = 0.0366$). This study represents a mile stone in the treatment of advanced stomach cancer in Japan, as for the first time a better overall survival with a cisplatin-fluoropyridine combination treatment compared with single-agent fluoropyrimidine was demonstrated. The authors concluded that these results define a new standard of care for the treatment of advanced stomach cancer in Japan. However, the value of cisplatin plus S-1 remains to be determined in a non-Japanese population. For this reason, the first-line advanced gastric cancer study (FLAGS) was performed which recruited more than 1,000 patients from April 2005 to February 2007 in the United States and Europe to receive either cisplatin and 5-fluoruracil or cisplatin ($100 mg/m^2$ on day 1) and S-1 ($24 mg/m^2$ twice daily on days 1–21) repeated every four weeks. The primary endpoint of the FLAGS study is overall survival (superiority of cisplatin/S-1). The results are expected in 2009.

Capecitabine is an oral fluoropyrimidine that is activated in tumour tissue by a three-step enzymatic conversion culminating with thymidine phosphorylase (38). Capecitabine is an established oral alternative to fluorouracil for the treatment of localized and advanced colorectal cancer (39, 40) and it has been safely combined with oxaliplatin without loss of efficacy (41–43). Phase 1 evaluation in esophagogastric cancer supports the safety of capecitabine when administered twice daily (44) and in combination with epirubicin and cisplatin, with indications of efficacy (45). Cisplatin $80 mg/m^2$ on day 1 plus capecitabine $2,000 mg/m^2/day$ on days 1–14 every three weeks (XP) was compared with cisplatin $80 mg/m^2$ on day 1 plus 5-fluorouracil $1,000 mg/m^2/day$ on days 1–4 every three weeks (FP) in a recently presented randomized multicenter trial performed in Asia, Eastern Europe and South America (46). The primary endpoint of this study was to demonstrate non-inferiority in progression-free survival (PFS) of XP vs. FP. XP led to a significantly higher tumour response rate (41%, 95% CI 33–47%) compared with FP (29%, 95% CI 22–37%; $p = 0.030$). The primary endpoint of this study was met with the PFS being 5.6 months (median) with XP vs. 5.0 with FP (HR = 0.81, 95% CI = 0.63–1.04). Also overall survival was clearly not inferior being 10.5 months (median) with XP vs. 9.3 with FP (HR = 0.85, 95% CI = 0.64–1.13). Toxicities tended to be slightly less common and/or less severe with XP compared with FP except hand-foot-syndromes that occurred more frequently in patients randomized to receive XP. An even larger randomized trial that was recently published (47) confirmed the finding that capecitabine $1,250 mg/m^2/day$ orally can replace 5-fluorouracil $200 mg/m^2/day$ as a continuous infusion in a regimen containing epirubicine $50 mg/m^2$ on day 1 repeated every three weeks plus either cisplatin $60 mg/m^2$ or oxaliplatin $130 mg/m^2$ both given on day 1 and repeated every three weeks. Again, response rates were slightly higher with the platin-capecitabine combination regimens compared with the platin-5-fluorouracil combinations, without reaching statistical significance. Overall survival, which was the primary endpoint of this trial, was 10.9 months with platin-capecitabine-epirubicin vs. 9.6 months with platin-5-fluorouracil-epirubicin (HR = 0.86, 95% CI = 0.80–0.99) giving proof to the study hypothesis that combining platin-epirubicin with capecitabine is not inferior to combining platin-epirubicin with 5-fluorouracil. Based on these trials and on the known preference of patients in favour of the use of oral agents compared to intravenously administered chemotherapeutic drugs (48) oncologists should consider substituting capecitabine for 5-fluorouracil in platin-combination chemotherapy regimens given for the treatment of advanced stomach cancer (49). Currently used chemotherapy regimens combining platin compounds with capecitabine are included in Table 2.

Table 2 Currently used platinum-based chemotherapy combination regimens for the treatment of stomach cancer (investigated in randomized controlled phase III trials)

Drugs		Dose and route [mg/m^2]	
Three-drug combinations			
ECF (26)			
Epirubicine	50	i.v. (30 min)	day 1
Cisplatin	60	i.v (60 min)	day 1
5-Fluorouracil	200	i.v. (continous infusion)	days 1–21
Repeated			day 22
ECX (47)			
Epirubicin	50	i.v. (30 min)	day 1
Cisplatin	60	i.v (60 min)	day 1
Capecitabine	1,250	p.o.	days 1–21
Repeated			day 22
EOF (47)			
Epirubicin	50	i.v. (30 min)	day 1
Oxaliplatin	130	i.v (120 min)	day 1
5-Fluorouracil	200	i.v. (continous infusion)	days 1–21
Repeated			day 22
EOX (47)			
Epirubicin	50	i.v. (30 min)	day 1
Oxaliplatin	130	i.v (120 min)	day 1
Capecitabine	1,250	p.o.	days 1–21
Repeated			day 22
DCF (57)			
Docetaxel	75	i.v. (60 min)	day 1
Cisplatin	75	i.v. (60 min)	day 1
5-Fluorouracil	750	i.v. (24 h)	days 1–5
Prophylactic use of granulocyte-stimulating growth factors (G-CSF) recommended			
Repeated			day 22
Two-drug combinations			
Cisplatin-5-Fluorouracil (46)			
Cisplatin	80	i.v. (60 min)	day 1
5-Fluorouracil	1,000	i.v. (24 h)	days 1–4
repeated			day 22
Cisplatin–Capecitabine (46)			
Cisplatin	80	i.v. (60 min)	day 1
Capecitabine	2,000	p.o.	days 1–14
Repeated			day 22
Cisplatin-S1 (Japan) (37)			
Cisplatin	60	i.v. (60 min)	day 8
S-1	40–60 twice daily	p.o.	days 1–21
Repeated			day 22
FLO (74)			
Oxaliplatin	85	i.v. (120 min)	day 1
Folinic acid	200	i.v. (120 min)	day 1
5-Fluorouracil	2,600	i.v. (48 h)	day 1
Repeated			day 22

Combining Cisplatin with Taxanes

There are limited phase II data available for paclitaxel-platinum combinations in advanced gastric cancer. Paclitaxel $175 \, mg/m^2$ over 3 h on day 1 combined with 5-FU $750 \, mg/m^2$ over 24 h on days 1–5 and cisplatin $20 \, mg/m^2$ over 2 h on days 1–5, every 28 days, achieved an overall response rate of 51% and a median survival duration of 6 months in a study of 41 patients with metastatic, unresectable advanced, or relapsed stomach cancer (50). The main toxicity was myelosuppression, with grade 3–4 neutropenia reported in 34% of patients. Another study of 45 patients (51) with previously untreated unresectable, locally advanced or metastatic gastric cancer assessed 8-week cycles (6 weeks with therapy followed by 2-week rest) with paclitaxel $175 \, mg/m^2$ as a 3-h infusion on days 1 and 22, cisplatin $50 \, mg/m^2$ as a 1-h infusion on days 8 and 29, and 5-fluorouracil $2 \, g/m^2$ given over 24 h, weekly, preceded by folinic acid $500 \, mg/m^2$ for over 2 h. The overall response rate was 51%, median PFS 9 months and OS 14 months. Grade 3–4 neutropenia was reported in 7 patients (15%); other grade 3–4 toxicities included nausea/vomiting in 5 patients (11%), alopecia in 22 patients (49%), and diarrhoea in 1 patient (2%).

Multiple phase II studies have investigated the efficacy of docetaxel as a single agent in patients with advanced stomach cancer. Overall response rates ranged from 16 to 24% when docetaxel was used as front-line therapy and from 0 to 21% when given to pre-treated patients. In both settings, a significant proportion of patients (close to 30%) achieved disease stabilisation (52). A phase II study was undertaken by the Swiss Group for Clinical Cancer Research (SAKK) and European Institute for Oncology (EIO) to investigate the efficacy and tolerability of docetaxel ($85 \, mg/m^2$) in combination with cisplatin ($75 \, mg/m^2$) (DC) administered every 3 weeks for up to eight cycles in 48 patients with advanced stomach cancer (53). In terms of efficacy, DC was associated with a favourable overall response rate (ORR) of 56% (including two complete responses), a median time to progression (TTP) of 6.6 months and a median overall survival (OS) of 9 months. In addition, DC was well tolerated with a predictable and manageable toxicity profile. As expected, the vast majority of grade 3–4 toxicities were haematological (neutropenia 81%, anaemia 32%, thrombocytopenia 4%). While there were nine episodes of febrile neutropenia, none was fatal. A phase I–II dose-finding study (54) was subsequently conducted by the same study group to establish the feasibility of adding a protracted continuous infusion of 5-FU $300 \, mg/m^2/day$ for 2 weeks to first-line DC (DCF) in patients with measurable, unresectable and/or metastatic gastric carcinoma. A similar overall response rate (51%; $n = 41$), median overall survival (9.3 months) and safety profile were observed with this DCF regimen. Consequently, a randomized, three-arm phase II study (SAKK 42/99) (55) was conducted in first line treatment of advanced stomach cancer. Patients were randomized to receive up to eight cycles every 3 weeks of either DC (docetaxel $85 \, mg/m^2$, cisplatin $75 \, mg/m^2$), DCF (like DC + continuous infusion of 5-fluorouracil $300 \, mg/m^2/day$ for 14 days) or ECF (epirubicin $50 \, mg/m^2$, cisplatin $60 \, mg/m^2$, continuous infusion 5-fluorouracil CI $200 \, mg/m^2/day$ for 21 days). The primary endpoint was overall response rate. Due to febrile neutropenia (ten occurrences in the first 21 included patients), the dose of docetaxel was decreased from $85\,mg/m^2$ to $75\,mg/m^2$, resulting in lesser febrile neutropenia occurrence. In all, grade 3–4 non-haematological toxicity was infrequent (less than 10% of patients) except alopecia (ranging from 20 to 47% in the three arms), nausea (18% in DC and DCF arms) and diarrhoea (15% in DCF arm). Preliminary results on 119 patients (40 in ECF, 38 in DC and 41 in DCF) showed the highest overall response rate in the DCF arm (36.6%) then the ECF (25.0%) and the DC (18.5%) and median time to progression of 7.8 months, 5.4 months and 4.4 months, respectively. Overall survival was higher in docetaxel-based regimens (median survival: 10.4 months and 11.0 months in DCF and DC, respectively) than in ECF arm (8.2 months).

The TAX 325 Study Group had undertaken a multinational, randomized phase II/III study in order to determine the most efficient docetaxel-containing regimen (DC or DCF) to be tested in a phase III trial against CF (cisplatin $100\,mg/m^2$ on day 1, and 5-fluorouracil $1,000\,mg/m^2/day$ as a continuous infusion on days 1–5 every 4 weeks), chosen as reference arm before the onset of phase II trial. CF was chosen as it was an accepted standard reference therapy for regulatory purposes, used worldwide and studied in advanced gastric cancer as well as the reference arm in two ongoing large phase III trials (21, 24). In the phase II study (56) 158 previously untreated patients with metastatic (accounting for 95% of patients) or locally advanced/recurrent stomach or gastro-esophageal adenocarcinoma received either DCF (docetaxel $75\,mg/m^2$ on day 1, cisplatin $75\,mg/m^2$ on day 1, and 5-fluorouracil $750\,mg/m^2/day$ as a continuous infusion on days 1–5) or DC (docetaxel $85\,mg/m^2$ and cisplatin $75\,mg/m^2$ on day 1), administered every 3 weeks until disease progression, unacceptable toxicity or consent withdrawal. The aim of the study was overall response rate and safety comparisons between the regimens. DCF was superior to DC for confirmed responses (43% vs. 26%, respectively) and median time to tumour progression (5.9 vs. 5.0 months, respectively, equating to a 20% reduction in the risk of progression), while median overall survival was slightly longer in the DC group (10.5 months) than in the DCF group (9.6 months) with similar 1-year survival (41.7% vs. 35.4%, respectively). The most frequent grade 3–4 toxicities were neutropenia (86% vs. 87%) and gastrointestinal events (56% vs. 30%); they were considered as manageable. In the phase III stage of the TAX 325 study (57) DCF was selected for further investigation by an independent data monitoring committee. The primary endpoint of the TAX 325 study was time to tumour progression. Unlike most previous trials in this setting, almost all patients (97%) had metastatic disease (81% with at least two metastatic sites), indicating that patients had a high tumour burden. In all, 227 patients were randomized to the DCF arm and 230 to the CF arm. Patients received a median of six cycles of DCF and four cycles of CF. DCF ($n = 221$) were significantly superior to CF ($n = 224$) for time to tumour progression ($p = 0.0004$) with a risk reduction of 32% (HR 1.46; 95% CI 1.19–1.82; median: 5.6 months vs. 3.7 months), for overall survival ($p = 0.02$) with a risk reduction of 23% (median: 9.2 months vs. 8.6 months; 1-year survival: 40% vs. 32%; 2-year survival: 18% vs. 9%), confirmed response rate (37% vs. 25%, $p = 0.01$) and median time to treatment failure (4.0 months vs 3.4 months, $p = 0.03$). Even though DCF was the more intense regimen, the difference between treatments was statistically significantly in favour of the DCF regimen for quality of life assessments (time to 5% definitive deterioration of Global Health Status vs. baseline: 6.5 months vs. 4.2 months, $p = 0.0121$) and clinical benefit (time to definitive deterioration of Karnofsky Performance Status by one category vs. baseline: 6.1 months vs. 4.8 months, $p = 0.088$) endpoints. DCF was also statistically significantly superior to CF for nearly all secondary quality of life analyses (time to definitive deterioration in social functioning, nausea/vomiting, appetite loss, pain and EuroQoL EQ-5D thermometer), with a trend for time to definitive deterioration in physical functioning ($p = 0.1349$), time to definitive 5% weight loss ($p = 0.0776$) and time to definitive worsening of appetite ($p = 0.1143$). No difference between treatments was observed for pain-free survival and time to first cancer pain requiring opioids (57–59). DCF was associated with increased toxicity compared with CF especially grade 3–4 neutropenia (82.3% vs. 56.8%) and febrile neutropenia/neutropenic infection (30% vs. 13.5%), diarrhoea (20.4% vs. 8.0%) and neurosensory toxicity (7.7% vs. 3.1%). In contrast, grade 3–4 stomatitis (20.8% vs. 27.2%) and anaemia (18.2% vs. 25.6%) occurred less frequently than with CF. The main cause of toxic deaths in both arms was infection (7 of 8 in DCF and 8 of 12 in CF), and they mainly occurred during the first cycle of chemotherapy. In all, 19% of patients in the DCF arm received secondary prophylaxis with granulocyte colony-stimulating factor (G-CSF) and 9% in the CF arm: among them the incidence of febrile neutropenia/neutropenic infection was only 12% vs. 15%, respectively. In patients aged at least 65 years, grade 3–4 infection (related to treatment) was more frequent with DCF (20%) than with CF (9%) (57). Primary prophylaxis with G-CSF would dramatically reduce the rate of complicated neutropenia associated with DCF. This treatment strategy is consistent with new European and North American guidelines that recommend the routine use of primary G-CSF prophylaxis when using a chemotherapy regimen that is associated with a high (>20%) risk of febrile neutropenia, such as DCF (60, 61).

The TAX 325 study has demonstrated that the addition of docetaxel to CF resulted in improved efficacy suggesting that it should now be incorporated in front-line strategies used for the treatment of patients with advanced stomach or gastro-esophageal cancer. Although DCF is associated with a high risk of febrile neutropenia, this complication may be prevented by primary G-CSF prophylaxis, a treatment strategy advocated in current practice guidelines. Other haematological and non-haematological toxicities are predictable, acceptable and manageable. Moreover, overall toxicity management can be improved further through proper patient selection, early intervention, improved awareness of the treatment complications and better patient education involving close management by cancer nurses and general practitioners.

Following the results of TAX 325 and docetaxel approvals by the authorities in the USA and Europe, the docetaxel-cisplatin-5-fluorouracil (DCF) triplet has become a new reference regimen in advanced gastric cancer. Numerous studies are ongoing to try to optimize both the efficacy and safety of existing regimens and to investigate the potential of new drug combinations in gastric cancer. Potential modifications of the DCF regimen include variations in the

DCF schedule, the substitution of cisplatin with oxaliplatin, the substitution of 5-fluorouracil with oral fluoropyrimidines, and the addition of biological agents. The modified DCF regimen was tested in a randomized phase II study (62) conducted in 106 patients with previously untreated metastatic stomach or oesophageal carcinoma who received either modified(m) DCF (docetaxel 30 mg/m^2 on days 1 and 8, cisplatin 60 mg/m^2 on day 1, and 5-FU 200 mg/m^2/day continuous infusion) every 3 weeks or mDX (docetaxel 30 mg/m^2 on days 1 and 8 and capecitabine 1,600 mg/m^2/day on days 1–14) every 3 weeks. The study showed a confirmed overall response rate (primary endpoint) of 47% for mDCF and 26% for mDX, median progression-free-survival 5.8 months vs. 4.6 months for mDCF and mDX, respectively. Safety and tolerability were satisfactory in both treatment arms, with diarrhoea, hand foot syndrome and febrile neutropenia each reported in less than 10% of patients in each arm. To reduce the haematological toxicity while maintaining the efficacy of DCF, split doses of docetaxel, cisplatin, leucovorin, and 5-fluorouracil were investigated (63). Chemotherapy-naive patients with advanced stomach or gastroesophageal adenocarcinomas received docetaxel 50 mg/m^2 and cisplatin 50 mg/m^2 on days 1, 15 and 29 and folinic acid 500 mg/m^2 plus 5-FU 2,000 mg/m^2 on days 1, 8, 15, 22, 29 and 36, every 8 weeks. Because significant dose reductions to <80% became necessary in most of patients, the regimen was amended after the first 15 patients to docetaxel 40 mg/m^2, cisplatin 40 mg/m^2, folinic acid 200 mg/m^2, and 5-FU 2,000 mg/m^2. Sixty patients were enrolled: 24 had locally advanced tumours and 36 had metastatic disease. The overall response rate was 47%. Twenty-three patients with locally advanced disease underwent secondary surgical resection (96%); complete resection (R0) was achieved in 87%. Overall, median time to progression and overall survival were 9.4 and 17.9 months, respectively (8.1 and 15.1 months, respectively, for patients with metastatic disease).

DCF and modifications (Table 3) are increasingly used in clinical routine. Other modifications of the DCF are under investigation in order to maintain the activity and to improve the tolerance of the original DCF regimen: e.g. replacing cisplatin by oxaliplatin and 5-FU by capecitabine (64, 65).

Substituting Oxaliplatin for Cisplatin

Oxaliplatin is a platinum compound that is complexed to a diaminocyclohexane carrier ligand. Like other platinum compounds, oxaliplatin stimulates apoptosis and ultimately cell death by inhibition of DNA replication and repair by means of adducts between pair bases. Oxaliplatin has demonstrated activity in tumours with intrinsic or acquired resistance to cisplatin (66–68). Whereas cisplatin is associated with dose-limiting renal toxicity, peripheral neuropathy and cumulative ototoxicity (69) the principal dose-limiting toxicity of oxaliplatin is cumulative sensory peripheral neuropathy, which may resolve over time. Other oxaliplatin-associated toxicities include neutropenia, diarrhoea and vomiting, which can be managed with appropriate

Table 3 The original DCF (docetaxel, cisplatin, 5-FU) chemotherapy regimen and recently published modifications

Regimen	No. of patients	CR/PR [%]	Febrile neutropenia (%)
DCF (57), every three weeks Docetaxel 75 mg/m^2 on day 1 Cisplatin 75 mg/m^2 on day 1 5-Fluorouracil 1,000 mg/m^2 on days 1–5	221	37	29
GASTRO-TAX (63), every seven weeks Docetaxel 40 mg/m^2 on days1, 15, 29 Cisplatin 40 mh/m^2 on days 1, 15, 29 Folinic acid 200 mg/m^2 on days 1, 8, 15, 21, 29, 36 5-Fluorouracil 2,000 mg/m^2 on days 1, 8, 15, 21, 29, 36	60	47	5
ATTAX (62), every three weeks Docetaxel 30 mg/m^2 on days 1, 8 Cisplatin 60 mg/m^2 on day1 5-Fluorouracil 200 mg/m^2/day continously	50	49	4
D-FOX (64), every two weeks Docetaxel 50 mg/m^2 on day 1 Oxaliplatin 85 mg/m^2 on day 1 5-Fluorouracil 2,200 mg/m^{2}on day 1 (48 h)	36	43	0
FLOT (65), every two weeks Docetaxel 50 mg/m^2 on day 1 Oxaliplatin 85 mg/m^2 on day 1 Folinic acid 200 mg/m^2 on day 1 5-Fluorouracil 2,600 mh/m^2 on day 1 (24 h)	59	53	2

CR complete remission; *PR* partial remission

prophylaxis and treatment. Oxaliplatin has demonstrated in vitro anti-tumour activity in human gastric cancer cell lines (70).

Results of several phase II studies using the FOLFOX regimen as first-line treatment in advanced gastric cancer were previously published and recorded a 45% and 43% response rate, respectively, a median time to progression of 6.2 months and median overall survival of 8.6 months in a French study (71) and a median overall survival of 9.6 months in a German study (72). In another German phase II study conducted in 48 patients with previously untreated metastatic stomach cancer (73) weekly 5-fluorouracil-oxaliplatin (FUFOX) demonstrated a favourable toxicity profile and achieved an overall response rate of 54%, median time to progression of 6.5 months and a median overall survival duration of 11.4 months. All these phase 2 studies showed relatively high and consistent degrees of activity.

Using ECF as a reference regimen, the UK National Cancer Research Institute's phase III REAL-2 study (47) was conducted in 1002 patients with previously untreated metastatic adeno-, squamous or undifferentiated carcinoma of the oesophagus, gastro-oesophageal junction or stomach. The study used a 2×2 factorial study design, in which patients were randomised to one of four treatment arms: ECF (epirubicin, cisplatin, 5-fluorouracil), ECX (epirubicin, cisplatin, capecitabine); EOF (epirubicin, oxaliplatin, 5-fluorouracil), EOX (epirubicin, oxaliplatin, capecitabine) with epirubicin given at a dose of 50mg/m^2, cisplatin 60mg/m^2, oxaliplatin 130mg/m^2, protracted venous infusion of 5-fluorouracil at $200 \text{mg/m}^2/\text{day}$ and oral capecitabine 625mg/m^2 twice daily, for a total of eight 3-week cycles. Characteristics were well-balanced between treatment arms, 89% patients had Eastern Cooperative Oncology Group (ECOG) performance status 0–1 and 77% had metastatic disease. Primary endpoints were overall survival comparison for capecitabine vs. 5-fluorouracil and oxaliplatin vs. cisplatin (non-inferiority margin of 1.23) and between all four regimens (superiority) using stratification by centre, locally advanced/metastatic cancer, Performance Status (PS) 0–1/2. In the intent-to-treat population, median survival was 9.9 months for ECF, 9.3 months for EOF, 9.9 months for ECX and 11.2 months for EOX. The non-inferiority primary endpoint (overall survival) was met for both the fluoropyrimidine (HR = 0.92, 95% CI: 0.80–1.10) and platinum (HR = 0.86, 95% CI: 0.8–0.89) comparisons of the respective per-protocol populations. The survival benefit for EOX compared to ECF was statistically significant ($p = 0.020$), with a HR of 0.80 (95% CI = 0.66–0.97). The overall response (complete/partial response) rates were consistently high at 40.7%, 46.4%, 42.4% and 47.9% for the ECF, ECX, EOF and EOX regimens, respectively, with no significant difference between groups. Grade 3–4 neutropenia was more commonly associated with cisplatin (ECF, 41.7%; ECX, 51.1%) than with oxaliplatin (EOF, 29.9%; EOX, 27.6%). Grade 3–4 non-hematological toxicity was reported for 36%, 33%, 42% and 45% of patients in the ECF, ECX, EOF and EOX groups, respectively. The authors concluded that oxaliplatin may substitute for cisplatin and capecitabine for 5-FU without decreasing efficacy, with improved convenience and favourable safety; EOX seems to be associated with significantly improved efficacy compared to ECF.

In the German study FLO/FLP (5-fluorouracil, leucovorin, cisliplatin) (74), 112 patients were randomized to receive FLO (5-FU $2,600 \text{mg/m}^2$ 24-h infusion, folinic acid 200mg/m^2, and oxaliplatin 85mg/m^2, every 2 weeks) and 110 patients to FLP (5-FU $2,000 \text{mg/m}^2$ 24-h infusion, folinic acid 200mg/m^2 weekly, and cisplatin 50mg/m^2, every 2 weeks). The primary endpoint was time to tumour progression. In all, 162 patients (FLO, 80; FLP, 81) had disease progression with a median time to progression of 5.7 months for FLO and 3.8 months for FLP (p = 0.081). Response to FLO (34%) was superior to FLP (27%), with 15% and 30% of patients having disease progression as best response to FLO and FLP, respectively ($p = 0.012$). Median treatment duration was 4.3 months with FLO and 3 months with FLP.

FLO was associated with significantly less NCI-CTC grade 1–4 leucopenia, nausea, alopecia, fatigue, and renal toxicity and FLP was associated with significantly less peripheral neuropathy ($p < 0.05$). Severe adverse events related to treatment were less frequent with FLO (8.9%) as compared to FLP (18.6%) ($p = 0.046$).

In conclusion, oxaliplatin seems to be at least as active and less toxic compared to cisplatin in combination regimens in gastric cancer and can therefore replace cisplatin. Currently used regimens incorporating oxaliplatin are integrated into Table 2.

Platinum Combinations in the Multimodality Treatment of Stomach Cancer

The value of adjuvant chemotherapy has generated controversial debates for years. But recent results from two randomized European trials have demonstrated a consistent survival advantage for perioperative chemotherapy in patients presenting with locally advanced stomach cancer and cancer at the gastroesophageal junction deemed to be resectable (clinical stages II and III according to Union International Contre le Cancer [UICC]). Perioperative treatment consisted of 8–9 weeks of preoperative platinum-5-fluorouracil-based chemotherapy and another 9–12 weeks of the same chemotherapy for those who were able to tolerate postoperative treatment (75, 76). Results are shown in Table 4. As overall survival was shown to be increased with perioperative chemotherapy, cisplatin-5-fluorouracil-based regimens have become a standard of care for the treatment of stage II and III stomach cancer in many institutions in the Western hemisphere.

A couple of randomized trials have also been performed to investigate the value of postoperative adjuvant treatment. European studies mostly focused on

Table 4 Perioperative chemotherapy in stage II and stage III stomach cancer. Phase III studies

Author	No. of patients	Stages (UICC)	CTx	R0 (%)	HR PFS (95% CI)	HR OS (95% CI)	5-year survival (%)
Cunningham et al. (75)	250	II and III	ECF × 3 preop., ×3 postop., ×3	69%	0.66 (0.53–0.81)	0.75 (0.60–0.93)	36
	253		none	66%			23
Boige et al. (76)	113	II and III	CF × 2 preop., × 4 postop.	87%	0.65 (0.48–0.89)	0.69 (0.50–0.95)	38
	111		none	74%			24

CT computed tomography; *CTx* chemotherapy; *(E)CF* (epirubicin), cisplatin, 5-fluorouracil; *HR* hazard ratio; *OS* overall survival; *PFS* progression-free survival; *UICC* Union International Contre le Cancer

intensive combination chemotherapy regimens, usually associated with considerable toxicities. These trials have never demonstrated any significant improvement in survival by adjuvant chemotherapy. Meanwhile, several meta-analyses on the effect of adjuvant chemotherapy in gastric cancer have been published (77). In the largest meta-analysis from a Scandinavian group of investigators it was shown that smaller survival advantages were seen in those studies performed in Asia. The cause of this difference is not apparent, but interestingly platinum-based combination chemotherapies were not used in Asia in the postoperative (adjuvant) setting and toxicities were reported to be much less compared with the European trials. In a recently published trial, Japanese investigators have shown that S-1 (80mg/m^2 day 1–28, repeated day 43) given for one year after curative resection including a D2 lymphadenectomy did significantly improve the overall survival (78). 90% of the patients included had nodal positive disease. A similar survival advantage over surgery alone, investigated in a smaller and prematurely terminated study, has been published with the use of adjuvant uracil-tegafur (UFT) for 16 months (79). Postoperative S-1 is now a new standard of care for node positive R0 D2 resected patients in Japan. The oral 5-FU prodrugs, above all S-1, should clearly be studied in the adjuvant setting outside of Japan.

In the US, adjuvant chemoradiation has been adopted as a standard of care. This recommendation was based on the results of the Intergroup study 0116 that compared 5-fluorouracil-based chemoradiation with no adjuvant treatment after curative resection of locally advanced stomach cancer. Survival was significantly better with adjuvant chemoradiation. Again, platinum compounds were not applied in this trial (80). Italian investigators asked the question of the additional value of cisplatin in the adjuvant chemotherapy of gastric cancer. They recently published results of a study that showed no benefit at all when cisplatin and epirubicin were added to adjuvant 5-fluorouracil/folinic acid in patients with serosa negative but nodal positive disease (81). A point to note is that only 9% of the patients were able to finish adjuvant cisplatin-containing combination chemotherapy as planned. This clearly shows that tolerable and feasible regimens should be preferred when adjuvant chemotherapy in stomach cancer is used. At present, no data support the preferred use of more toxic (cisplatin-) based combination chemotherapy regimens compared to 5-fluorouracil alone in the adjuvant setting.

Platinum Compounds in Newer Combination Regimens with Biologically Targeted Agents

Currently, some promising data arise from studies investigating monoclonal antibodies directed against epidermal growth factor receptors EGFR (Her-1) and ErbB2/Her2 as well as against vascular endothelial growth factor (VEGF). In the majority of these phase II trials the antibodies are combined with platinum-based regimens (82–84).

References

1. Kamangar F, Dores GM, Anderson WF. Patterns of cancer incidence, mortality, and prevalence across five continents: defining priorities to reduce cancer disparities in different geographic regions of the world. J Clin Oncol 2006;24:2137–50.
2. Cunningham SC, Kamangar F, Kim MP, et al. Survival after gastric adenocarcinoma resection: eighteen-year experience at a single institution. J Gastrointest Surg 2005;9:718–25.
3. Faycal J, Bessaguet C, Nousbaum JB, et al. Epidemiology and long term survival of gastric carcinoma in the French district of Finistere between 1984 and 1995. Gastroenterol Clin Biol 2005;29:23–32.
4. Tsubono Y, Hisamichi S. Screening for gastric cancer in Japan. Gastric Cancer 2000;3:9–18.
5. Blot WJ, Devesa SS, Kneller RW, Fraumeni JF Jr. Rising incidence of adenocarcinoma of the esophagus and gastric cardia. JAMA 1991;265:1287–9.
6. Devesa SS, Fraumeni JF. The rising incidence of gastric cardia cancer. J Natl Cancer Inst 1999;91:747–9.
7. Kamangar F, Dawsey SM, Blaser MJ, et al. Opposing risks of gastric cardia and noncardia gastric adenocarcinomas associated with Helicobacter pylori seropositivity. J Natl Cancer Inst 2006;98:1445–52.
8. Park JG, Kramer BS, Lai SL, Goldstein LJ, Gazdar AF. Chemosensitivity patterns and expression of human multidrug resistance-associated MDR1 gene by human gastric and colorectal carcinoma cell lines. J Natl Cancer Inst 1990;82:193–8.
9. Leichman L, Berry BT. Experience with cisplatin in treatment regimens for esophageal cancer. Semin Oncol 1991;18:64–72.
10. Moynihan T, Hansen R, Anderson T, et al. Continuous 5-fluorouracil infusion in advanced gastric carcinoma. Am J Clin Oncol 1988;11:461–4.
11. Ohtsu Y, Sakata N, Horikoshi Y, et al. A phase II study of S-1 in patients with advanced gastric cancer. Proc Am Soc Clin Oncol 1998;17:262 (abstract).
12. Koizumi W, Kurihara M, Nakano S, Hasegawa K. Phase II study of S-1, a novel oral derivative of 5-fluorouracil, in advanced gastric cancer. For the S-1 cooperative gastric cancer study group. Oncology 2000;58:191–7.
13. Hong YS, Song SY, Lee SI, et al. A phase II trial of capecitabine in previously untreated patients with advanced and/or metastatic gastric cancer. Ann Oncol 2004;15:1344–7.
14. Futatsuki K, Wakui A, Nakao I, et al. Late phase II study of irinotecan hydrochloride (CPT-11) in advanced gastric cancer. CPT-11 gastrointestinal cancer study group. Gan To Kagaku Ryoho 1994;21:1033–8.
15. Ajani JA, Fairweather J, Dumas P, Patt YZ, Pazdur R, Mansfield PF. Phase II study of Taxol in patients with advanced gastric carcinoma. Cancer J Sci Am 1998;4:269–74.
16. Ohtsu A, Boku N, Tamura F, et al. An early phase II study of a 3-hour infusion of paclitaxel for advanced gastric cancer. Am J Clin Oncol 1998;21:416–9.
17. Sulkes A, Smyth J, Sessa C, et al. Docetaxel (Taxotere) in advanced gastric cancer: results of a phase II clinical trial. EORTC early clinical trials group. Br J Cancer 1994;70:380–3.
18. Bajetta E, Celio L, Buzzoni R, et al. Phase II study of pemetrexed disodium (Alimta) administered with oral folic acid in patients with advanced gastric cancer. Ann Oncol 2003;14:1543–8.
19. Sessa C, Aamdal S, Wolff I, et al. Gemcitabine in patients with advanced malignant melanoma or gastric cancer: phase II studies of the EORTC early clinical trials group. Ann Oncol 1994;5:471–2.
20. Kulke MH, Muzikansky A, Clark J, et al. A Phase II trial of vinorelbine in patients with advanced gastroesophageal adenocarcinoma. Cancer Invest 2006;24:346–50.
21. Ohtsu A, Shimada Y, Shirao K, et al. Randomized phase III trial of fluorouracil alone versus fluorouracil plus cisplatin versus uracil and tegafur plus mitomycin in patients with unresectable, advanced gastric cancer: the Japan clinical oncology group study (JCOG9205). J Clin Oncol 2003;21:54–9.

22. Ichikawa W, Sasaki Y. Correlation between tumor response to first-line chemotherapy and prognosis in advanced gastric cancer patients. Ann Oncol 2006;17:1665–72.
23. Wagner AD, Grothe W, Haerting J, Kleber G, Grothey A, Fleig WE. Chemotherapy in advanced gastric cancer: a systematic review and meta-analysis based on aggregate data. J Clin Oncol 2006;24:2903–9.
24. Vanhoefer U, Rougier P, Wilke H, et al. Final results of a randomized phase III trial of sequential high-dose methotrexate, fluorouracil, and doxorubicin versus etoposide, leucovorin, and fluorouracil versus infusional fluorouracil and cisplatin in advanced gastric cancer: a trial of the European organization for research and treatment of cancer gastrointestinal tract cancer cooperative group. J Clin Oncol 2000;18:2648–57.
25. Cocconi G, Carlini P, Gamboni A, et al. Cisplatin, epirubicin, leucovorin and 5-fluorouracil (PELF) is more active than 5-fluorouracil, doxorubicin and methotrexate (FAMTX) in advanced gastric carcinoma. Ann Oncol 2003;14:1258–63.
26. Webb A, Cunningham D, Scarffe JH, et al. Randomized trial comparing epirubicin, cisplatin, and fluorouracil versus fluorouracil, doxorubicin, and methotrexate in advanced esophagogastric cancer. J Clin Oncol 1997;15:261–7.
27. Waters JS, Norman A, Cunningham D, et al. Long-term survival after epirubicin, cisplatin and fluorouracil for gastric cancer: results of a randomized trial. Brit J Cancer 1999;80:269–72.
28. Schabel FM Jr, Trader MW, Laster WR Jr, Corbett TH, Griswold DP Jr. Cis-Dichlorodiammineplatinum (II): combination chemotherapy and cross-resistance studies with tumors of mice. Cancer Treat Rep 1979;63:1459–73.
29. Rooney M, Kish J, Jacobs J, et al. Improved complete response rate and survival in advanced head and neck cancer after three-course induction therapy with 120-hour 5-FU infusion and cisplatin. Cancer 1985;55:1123–8.
30. Scanlon KJ, Newman EM, Lu Y, Priest DG. Biochemical basis for cisplatin and 5-fluorouracil synergism in human ovarian carcinoma cells. Proc Natl Acad Sci USA 1986;83:8923–5.
31. Shirasaka T, Shimamoto Y, Ohshimo H, Saito H, Fukushima M. Metabolic basis of the synergistic antitumor models in vivo. Cancer Chemother Pharmacol 1993;32:167–72.
32. Lutz MP, Wilke H, Wagener DJ, et al. Weekly infusional high-dose fluorouracil (HD-FU), HD-FU plus folinic acid (HD-FU/FA), or HD-FU/FA plus biweekly cisplatin in advanced gastric cancer: randomized phase II trial 40953 of the European organisation for research and treatment of cancer gastrointestinal group and the Arbeitsgemeinschaft Internistische Onkologie. J Clin Oncol 2007;25:2580–5.
33. Shirasaka T, Shimamoto Y, Ohshimo H, et al. Development of a novel form of an oral 5-fluorouracil derivative (S-1) directed to the potentiation of the tumor selective cytotoxicity of 5-fluorouracil by two biochemical modulators. Anticancer Drugs 1996;7:548–57.
34. Diasio RB. Clinical implications of dihydropyrimidine dehydrogenase inhibition. Oncology (Williston Park) 1999;13:17–21.
35. Sakata Y, Ohtsu A, Horikoshi N, Sugimachi K, Mitachi Y, Taguchi T. Late phase II study of novel oral fluoropyrimidine anticancer drug S-1 (1 M tegafur-0.4 M gimestat-1 M otastat potassium) in advanced gastric cancer patients. Eur J Cancer 1998;34:1715–20.
36. Lenz HJ, Lee FC, Haller DG, et al. Extended safety and efficacy data on S-1 plus cisplatin in patients with untreated, advanced gastric carcinoma in a multicenter phase II study. Cancer 2007;109:33–40.
37. Koizumi W, Narahara H, Hara T, Takagane A, Akiya T, Takagi M, Miyashita K, Nishizaki T, Kobayashi O, Takiyama W, Toh Y, Nagaie T, Takagi S, Yamamura Y, Yanaoka K, Orita H, Takeuchi M. S-1 plus cisplatin versus S-1 alone for first-line treatment of advanced gastric cancer (SPIRITS trial): a phase III trial. Lancet Oncol. 2008 Mar;9(3):215–21.
38. Miwa M, Ura M, Nishida M, et al. Design of a novel oral fluoropyrimidine carbamate, capecitabine, which generates 5-fluorouracil selectively in tumours by enzymes concentrated in human liver and cancer tissue. Eur J Cancer 1998;34:1274–81.
39. Van Cutsem E, Twelves C, Cassidy J, et al. Oral capecitabine compared with intravenous fluorouracil plus leucovorin in patients with metastatic colorectal cancer: results of a large phase III study. J Clin Oncol 2001;19:4097–106.

40. Twelves C, Wong A, Nowacki MP, et al. Capecitabine as adjuvant treatment for stage III colon cancer. N Engl J Med 2005;352:2696–704.

41. Porschen R, Arkenau HT, Kubicka S, et al. Phase 3 study of capecitabine plus oxaliplatin compared with fluorouracil and leucovorin plus oxaliplatin in metastatic colorectal cancer: a final report of the AIO colorectal study group. J Clin Oncol 2007;25:4217–23.

42. Díaz-Rubio E, Tabernero J, Gómez-Espana A, et al. Phase III study of capecitabine plus oxaliplatin compared with continuous-infusion fluorouracil plus oxaliplatin as first-line therapy in metastatic colorectal cancer: final report of the Spanish cooperative group for the treatment of digestive tumors trial. J Clin Oncol 2007;25:4224–30.

43. Cassidy J, Clarke S, Díaz-Rubio E, Scheithauer W, Figer A, Wong R, Koski S, Lichinitser M, Yang TS, Rivera F, Couture F, Sirzén F, Saltz L. Randomized phase III study of capecitabine plus oxaliplatin compared with fluorouracil/folinic acid plus oxaliplatin as first-line therapy for metastatic colorectal cancer. J Clin Oncol. 2008;26(12):2006–12.

44. Evans TR, Pentheroudakis G, Paul J, et al. A phase I and pharmacokinetic study of capecitabine in combination with epirubicin and cisplatin in patients with inoperable oesophago-gastric adenocarcinoma. Ann Oncol 2002;13:1469–78.

45. Cho EK, Lee WK, Im SA, et al. A phase II study of epirubicin, cisplatin and capecitabine combination chemotherapy in patients with metastatic or advanced gastric cancer. Oncology 2005;68:333–40.

46. Kang Y, Kang WK, Shin DB, et al. Randomized phase III trial of capecitabine/cisplatin (XP) vs. continuous infusion of 5-FU/cisplatin (FP) as first-line therapy in patients (pts) with advanced gastric cancer (AGC): efficacy and safety results. Proc Am Soc Clin Oncol 2006;24:4018 (abstract).

47. Cunningham D, Starling N, Rao S. Capecitabine and oxaliplatin for advanced esophagogastric cancer. N Engl J Med 2008;358:36–46.

48. Liu G, Franssen E, Fitch MI, Warner E. Patient preferences for oral versus intravenous palliative chemotherapy. J Clin Oncol 1997;15:110–5.

49. Van Cutsem E, Van de Velde C, Roth A, et al. Expert opinion on management of gastric and gastro-oesophageal junction adenocarcinoma on behalf of the European Organisation for Research and Treatment of Cancer (EORTC) – gastrointestinal cancer group. Eur J Cancer 2008;44:182–94.

50. Kim YH, Shin SW, Kim BS, et al. Paclitaxel, 5-fluorouracil, and cisplatin combination chemotherapy for the treatment of advanced gastric carcinoma. Cancer 1999;85:295–301.

51. Kollmannsberger C, Quietzsch D, Haag C, et al. A phase II study of paclitaxel, weekly, 24-hour continous infusion 5-fluorouracil, folinic acid and cisplatin in patients with advanced gastric cancer. Br J Cancer 2000;83:458–62.

52. Abbrederis K, Lorenzen S, von Weikersthal LF. Weekly docetaxel monotherapy for advanced gastric or esophagogastric junction cancer. Results of a phase II study in pretreated patients or patients with impaired performance status. Crit Rev Oncol Hematol 2008;66:84–90.

53. Roth A, Maibach R, Martinelli G, et al. Docetaxel (Taxotere)-cisplatin (TC): an effective drug combination in gastric carcinoma. Swiss group for clinical cancer research (SAKK), and the European Institute of Oncology (EIO). Ann Oncol 2000;11:301–6.

54. Roth A, Maibach R, Fazio N, et al. 5-Fluorouracil as protracted continuous intravenous infusion can be added to full-dose docetaxel (Taxotere)-cisplatin in advanced gastric carcinoma: a phase I-II trial. Ann Oncol 2004;15:759–64.

55. Roth A, Maibach R, Falk S, et al. Docetaxel-cisplatin-5FU (TCF) versus docetaxel-cisplatin (TC) versus epirubicin-cisplatin-5FU (ECF) as systemic treatment for advanced gastric carcinoma (AGC): a randomized Phase II trial of the Swiss group for clinical cancer research (SAKK). J Clin Oncol 2007;25:3217–23.

56. Ajani J, Fodor M, Tjulandin S, et al. Phase II multiinstitutional randomized trial of docetaxel plus cisplatin with or without fluorouracil in patients with untreated, advanced gastric, or gastroesophageal adenocarcinoma. J Clin Oncol 2005;23:5660–7.

57. Van Cutsem E, Moiseyenko V, Tjulandin S, et al. V325 study group. Phase III study of docetaxel and cisplatin plus fluorouracil compared with cisplatin and fluorouracil as first-line therapy for advanced gastric cancer: a report of the V325 study group. J Clin Oncol 2006;24:4991–7.

58. Ajani J, Moiseneyenko V, Tjuladin S, et al. Quality of life with docetaxel plus cisplatin and fluorouracil compared with cisplatin and fluorouracil from a phase III trial for advanced gastric or gastroesophageal adenocarcinoma: the V-325 study group. J Clin Oncol 2007;25: 3210–6.

59. Ajani J, Moiseneyenko V, Tjuladin S, et al. Clinical benefit with docetaxel plus fluorouracil and cisplatin compared with cisplatin and fluorouracil in a phase III trial of advanced gastric or gastroesophageal cancer adenocarcinoma: the V-325 study group. J Clin Oncol 2007;25:3205–9.

60. Aapro M, Cameron D, Pettengell R, et al. European Organisation for Research and Treatment of Cancer (EORTC) Granulocyte Colony-Stimulating Factor (G-CSF) guidelines working party EORTC guidelines for the use of granulocytecolony stimulating factor to reduce the incidence of chemotherapy-induced febrile neutropenia in adult patients with lymphomas and solid tumours. Eur J Cancer 2006;42:2433–53.

61. Smith T, Khatcheressian J, Lyman G, et al. 2006 update of recommendations for the use of white blood cell growth factors: an evidence-based clinical practice guideline. J Clin Oncol 2006;24:3187–205.

62. Tebbutt N, Sournina T, Strickland A, et al. ATTAX: randomised phase II study evaluating weekly docetaxel based chemotherapy combinations in advanced oesophagogastric cancer: final results of an AGITG trial. Proc Am Soc Clin Oncol 2007;25:4528 (abstract).

63. Lorenzen S, Hentrich M, Haberl C, et al. Split-dose docetaxel, cisplatin, and leucovorin/fluorouracil as first-line therapy in advanced gastric cancer and adenocarcinoma of the gastroesophageal junction: results of a phase II trial. Ann Oncol 2007;18:1673–9.

64. Ajani JA, Phan H, Ho L, et al. Phase I/II trial of docetaxel plus oxaliplatin and 5-fluorouracil (D-FOX) in patients with untreated, advanced gastric or gastroesophageal cancer. Proc Am Soc Clin Oncol 2007;25:4612 (abstract).

65. Al-Batran SE, Hartmann JT, Hofheinz R, et al. Modified FOLFOX in combination with docetaxel for patients with metastatic adenocarcinoma of the stomach or gastroesophageal junction: a multicenter phase II study of the Arbeitsgemeinschaft Internistische Onkologie (AIO). Proc Am Soc Clin Oncol 2007;25:4545 (abstract).

66. Mathé G, Kidani Y, Segiguchi M, et al. Oxalo-platinum or 1-OHP, a third-generation platinum complex: an experimental and clinical appraisal and preliminary comparison with cisplatinum and carboplatinum. Biomed Pharmacother 1989;43:237–50.

67. Raymond E, Faivre S, Woynarowksi J, Chaney S. Oxaliplatin: mechanism of action and antineoplastic activity. Semin Oncol 1998;5:4–12.

68. Raymond E, Faivre S, Chaney S, Woynarowski J, Cvitkovic E. Cellular and molecular pharmacology of oxaliplatin. Mol Cancer Ther 2002;3:227–35.

69. Hartmann J, Lipp H. Toxicity of platinum compounds. Expert Opin Pharmacother 2003;4:889–901.

70. Eriguchi M, Nonaka Y, Yanagie H, Yoshizaki I, Takeda Y, Sekiguchi M. A molecular biological study of anti-tumour mechanisms of an anti-cancer agent oxaliplatin against established human gastric cancer cell lines. Biomed Pharmacother 2003;57:412–5.

71. Louvet C, Andre T, Tigaud J, et al. Phase II study of oxaliplatin, fluorouracil, and folinic acid in locally advanced or metastatic gastric cancer patients. J Clin Oncol 2002;20:4543–8.

72. Al-Batran S, Atmaca A, Hegewisch-Becker S, et al. Phase II trial of biweekly infusional fluorouracil, folinic acid, and oxaliplatin in patients with advanced gastric cancer. J Clin Oncol 2004;22:658–63.

73. Lordick F, Lorenzen S, Stollfuss J, et al. Phase II study of weekly oxaliplatin plus infusional fluorouracil and folinic acid (FUFOX regimen) as first-line treatment in metastatic gastric cancer. Br J Cancer 2005;93:190–4.

74. Al-Batran SE, Hartmann J, Probst S, et al. . A randomized phase III trial in patients with advanced adenocarcinoma of the stomach receiving first-line chemotherapy with fluorouracil, leucovorin and oxaliplatin (FLO) versus fluorouracil, leucovorin and cisplatin (FLP). Proc Am Soc Clin Oncol 2006;24:4016 (abstract).

75. Cunningham D, Allum WH, Stenning SP, et al. Perioperative chemotherapy versus surgery alone for resectable gastroesophageal cancer. N Engl J Med 2006;355:11–20.

76. Boige V, Pignon JP, Saint-Aubert B, et al. Final results of a randomized trial comparing preoperative 5-fluorouracil (F)/cisplatin (P) to surgery alone in adenocarcinoma of stomach and lower esophagus (ASLE): FNLCC ACCORD07-FFCD 9703 trial. Proc Am Soc Clin Oncol 2007;25:4510 (abstract).

77. Lordick F, Siewert JR. Multimodal treatment for gastric cancer. Gastric Cancer 2005;8: 78–85.

78. Sakuramoto S, Sasako M, Yamaguchi T, et al. Adjuvant chemotherapy for gastric cancer with S-1, an oral fluoropyrimidine. N Engl J Med 2007;357:1810–20.

79. Nakajima T, Kinoshita T, Nashimoto A, et al. Randomized controlled trial of adjuvant uracil-tegafur versus surgery alone for serosa-negative, locally advanced gastric cancer. Br J Surg 2007;94:1468–76.

80. Macdonald JS, Smalley SR, Benedetti J, et al. Chemoradiotherapy after surgery compared with surgery alone for adenocarcinoma of the stomach or gastroesophageal junction. N Engl J Med 2001;345:725–30.

81. Cascinu S, Labianca R, Barone C, et al. Adjuvant treatment of high-risk, radically resected gastric cancer patients with 5-fluorouracil, leucovorin, cisplatin, and epidoxorubicin in a randomized controlled trial. J Natl Cancer Inst 2007;99:601–7.

82. Shah MA, Ramanathan RK, Ilson DH, et al. Multicenter phase II study of irinotecan, cisplatin, and bevacizumab in patients with metastatic gastric or gastroesophageal junction adenocarcinoma. J Clin Oncol 2006;24:5201–6.

83. Cortés-Funes H, Rivera F, Alés I, et al. Phase II of trastuzumab and cisplatin in patients (pts) with advanced gastric cancer (AGC) with HER2/neu overexpression/amplification. Proc Am Soc Clin Oncol 2007;25:4613 (abstract).

84. Lordick F, Lorenzen S, Hegewisch-Becker S, et al. 2007. Cetuximab plus weekly oxaliplatin/5FU/FA (FUFOX) in 1st line metastatic gastric cancer. Final results from a multicenter phase II study of the AIO upper GI group. Proc Am Soc Clin Oncol 2007;25:4514 (abstract).

Oxaliplatin-Based Chemotherapy for Colon Cancer

Andrea Bonetti and Lara Furini

Abstract For more than 40 years the treatment of colorectal cancer was based upon the use of 5-fluoruracil (5-FU) administered according to a variety of schedules, either alone or with several modulators. The response rate ranged between 10% and 20% with progression-free survival (PFS) of 6 months and overall survival of around 1 year. The introduction into the clinic of oxaliplatin, a diaminocyclohexane platinum analogue, and the demonstrated synergistic activity when combined with 5-FU, led to the popular scheme FOLFOX 4 and its simplified forms, including more recent evolutions with capecitabine as a substitute for leucovorin-modulated 5-FU. We learned from several randomised phase III trials that in the advanced setting these combinations could produce a response rate ranging from 37 to 50% with a progression-free survival of around 8–9 months. Furthermore, a small percentage of unselected patients initially considered inoperable may become resectable following chemotherapy. Oxaliplatin-based regimens can be further strengthened by the addition of a third component, either a traditional drug such as CPT11 or a targeted agent such as the anti VEGF antibody bevacizumab and the anti-EGFR receptor cetuximab. The sequential administration of all these active agents significantly improved the outcome of advanced colorectal cancer patients with several studies reporting median survivals exceeding 20 months. Two large phase III studies (the MOSAIC trial and the NSABP C07) enrolling patients with stage II and III colon cancer have consistently demonstrated a 5% absolute improvement in a 3-year DFS favouring the oxaliplatin-containing arms. In the MOSAIC trial the improved 3-year DFS translates in a statistically significant better 6-year survival only for stage III patients (73% vs. 68.6%).

Keywords Oxaliplatin-based chemotherapy; Advanced colorectal cancer; Adjuvant setting

A. Bonetti (✉) and L. Furini
Department of Oncology, Mater Salutis Hospital, Legnago, Italy
e-mail: andrea.bonetti@aulsslegnago.it

A. Bonetti et al. (eds.), *Platinum and Other Heavy Metal Compounds in Cancer Chemotherapy*, DOI: 10.1007/978-1-60327-459-3_31,
© Humana Press, a part of Springer Science + Business Media, LLC 2009

Introduction

Since its introduction into the clinic fifty years ago and up to the mid-1990s, 5-fluorouracil (5-FU) was the only effective agent for the treatment of colorectal cancer (1). During this period of time an extensive knowledge regarding the mechanisms of actions of the drug was gained (2). In particular it was learned that when given by prolonged venous infusion (PVI) the drug was associated with improved thimidylate syntase (TS) inhibition and less interference with DNA and RNA synthesis, as compared with the bolus schedules. 5-FU toxicity was also schedule-dependent, skin toxicity and diarrhoea being prevalent with PVI 5-FU, while neutropenia was more often observed with the bolus schedules. These observations provided the theoretical basis for the combination of the two modalities of 5-FU administration (bolus and PVI), along with the modulator leucovorin (LV) into the same schema, known as LV5FU2, developed in France by Aimery de Gramont at the end of the 1980s (3). In a randomised study, the program combining 5-FU bolus and continuous infusion nearly doubled response rate compared with bolus administration but without meaningful improvement of survival (4). When the cisplatin analogue oxaliplatin was introduced into the clinic, LV5FU2 seemed a good partner to combine with, bringing about the regimen known as "FOLFOX 3" and its evolutions (5).

The main clinical achievements in the treatment of stage IV (advanced) colorectal cancer and of stage II and III (radically resected, node negative and node positive, respectively) colon cancer during the 5-FU era can be summarised as follows:

1. Stage IV colorectal cancer patients derive a sizable benefit from the treatment with 5-FU, as compared with patients left untreated: increased overall survival from 6 months to around 1 year, better quality of life (6, 7)
2. Compared to 5-FU alone, 5-FU modulated by LV or methotrexate is associated with the doubling of the response rate (from 10 to 20%), which translates into a marginal improvement of overall survival (8, 9)
3. Compared to observation, six months of LV modulated bolus 5-FU chemotherapy given according to different schedules (Mayo clinic, Roswell Park, Machover) following radical resection of stage III colon cancer improved patient's overall survival and disease-free survival (10–12).

In this paper we will briefly review the main results obtained following the addition of oxaliplatin to the armamentarium of drugs available for the treatment of advanced colorectal cancer and radically resected (Stage II and III) colon cancer. The role of oxaliplatin in the multimodality treatment of rectal cancer and to improve resectability with curative intent in metastatic colorectal cancer is discussed elsewhere in this book.

Advanced Colorectal Cancer

As a single agent, oxaliplatin displays only a marginal activity in the clinic (13). However, when administered with 5-FU, the combination is highly synergistic.

The best example of this synergism comes from the 3-arm phase III trial by Rothenberg et al. (14) in which advanced colorectal cancer patients progressing following treatment with irinotecan, 5-FU and LV were randomised to receive 5-FU alone, oxaliplatin alone or the "FOLFOX 4" combination of the two drugs. Overall Response Rate (ORR) and Time to Progression (TTP) were similarly low in patients allocated to receive either 5-FU alone (0% ORR; 2.7 months TTP) or oxaliplatin alone (1.3% ORR; 1.6 months TTP) while better results were observed in the combination arm (9.9% ORR; 4.6 months TTP). *In vitro* data implies the down-regulation of TS protein expression by oxaliplatin as a possible molecular mechanism for the observed synergy (15). As front line treatment the "FOLFOX 4" regimen was tested against LV5FU2 in a randomised study which involved 420 patients, published in the year 2000 (16). Although patients randomised to receive up front the combination including oxaliplatin showed a better ORR (50.7% vs. 22.3%) and a longer TTP (9.2 months vs. 6 months), OS was not significantly improved (16.2 vs. 14.7 months). However, median OS observed in the LV5FU2 arm is about 3 months longer than that reported in the pre-oxaliplatin era, probably as a result of the introduction of oxaliplatin (or irinotecan) as a second line treatment.

In that same year 2000 the results of two trials in which patients were randomised to receive a combination of irinotecan and 5-FU or 5-FU alone were published. 5-FU was given according to different schedules: the weekly bolus infusion according to Roswell Park in the USA (17), weekly PVI (the "German schedule") or biweekly combination of bolus and PVI as in the LV5FU2 in Europe (18). The irinotecan-containing arms performed statistically better regarding all the investigated parameters (ORR, TTP and OS). Overall, these data prompted the head to head comparison of oxaliplatin- or irinotecan-containing regimens in five trials (Table 1). Looking at the most important parameter, OS, in 3 studies the two drugs tied while in the remaining oxaliplatin arms were the winners. However, the bigger of these two trials (20) deserves two comments: (1) oxaliplatin was combined with 5-FU given as bolus and PVI while irinotecan was administered in combination with bolus 5-FU,

Table 1 Published trials comparing oxaliplatin- and irinotecan-containing regimens

Reference	No. of Patients	Treatment	OR/CR (%)	Resection rate (%)	TTP (months)	OS (months)	p value
Tournigand (19)	226	FOLFOX 6	54/4.6	22	8.5	20.6	n.s.
		FOLFIRI	45/2.8	9		21.5	
Goldberg (20)	795	FOLFOX 4	45/8.6	4.1	8.7	19.5	
		IFL[a]	31/3	0.7	6.9	15	0.0001
		IROX	35/4	4.2	6.5	17.4	0.04
Comella (21)	274	OXAFAFU	44/14	4.3	7[b]	18.9	0.032
		IRIFAFU	31/12	2.2	5.8[b]	15.6	
Kalofonos (22)	295	OXA/LV/FU	33/	n.r.	7.6	17.4	n.s.
		IRI/LV/FU	32/5		8.9	17.6	
Colucci (23)	360	FOLFOX 4	34/5.2	n.r.	7	15	n.s.
		FOLFIRI	31/4.8		7	14	

[a]Bolus 5-FU
[b]Time to Treatment failure
n.r. not reported; *n.s.* not significant

in a regimen, the IFL, which lately emerged as too toxic (24); (2) when this trial was conducted oxaliplatin was not marketed in the USA and therefore only a minority of patients randomised to IFL could receive oxaliplatin upon progression. Overall, the main conclusions that can be drawn from these comparisons are the equivalence of the two drugs in terms of efficacy and the importance of exposing the majority of patients to both. The last concept was later strengthened by Grothey et al. (25). They collected data from seven published phase 3 trials and were able to demonstrate a correlation between the percentage of patients exposed to all active drugs (5-FU, Oxaliplatin, CPT11) and OS. In particular, when the percentage of patients receiving both doublets (5-FU oxaliplatin, 5-FU irinotecan) is close to 60%, OS is around 20 months, and it is irrespective of the sequence.

Further developments upon the 5-FU/oxaliplatin cornerstone were the combinations initially with irinotecan and more recently with the biological drugs bevacizumab and cetuximab. Triplets including irinotecan (5-FU/oxaliplatin/irinotecan) have been investigated in eleven phase I-II studies (26–36). Table 2 summarises the main results of these studies. Although the different schedules make any comparison difficult, it is easy to see that, as expected, dose limiting toxicities observed in all the trials were diarrhoea and neutropenia. A response rate ranging from 50 to 72% was observed in advanced colorectal cancer patients when triplets were administered as first line treatment, and from 24 to 27% in the studies evaluating triplets in 5-FU-refractory patients (27, 36). The front-line administration of a triplet, compared to a doublet including 5-FU and irinotecan, has been investigated in two randomised phase 3 trials. In the trial by the Hellenic Cooperative Group which involved 283 patients, although all the investigated parameters of efficacy were in favour of the triplet arm (ORR 43% vs. 34%; TTP 9.4 vs. 6.9 months; OS 21.5 vs. 19.5 months), no one reached statistical significance (37). The second trial included 244 patients and was performed by the Italian GONO Cooperative Group (38). In this paper the administration of the triplet was associated with improved ORR (60% vs. 34%, $p < 0.001$) longer OS (22.6 vs.16.7 months, $p = 0.032$) and an increased resectability rate (15% vs. 6%, $p = 0.033$). While the 5-FU-irinotecan regimen is the same in both trials, the schedule and the doses of the drugs in the triplet arms are different. This fact, along with differences in the treated populations may account for the discrepant results observed.

Bevacizumab is a monoclonal antibody which blocks the Vascular Endothelial Growth Factor, a critical mediator of angiogenesis (39, 40). It has been shown in randomised studies in previously untreated patients that the addition of bevacizumab to 5-FU alone (41) or to the combination of 5-FU and irinotecan (42) improves the efficacy of chemotherapy. In patients previously treated with 5-FU and irinotecan, the inclusion of bevacizumab into the FOLFOX 4 regimen significantly improves ORR (22.7% vs. 8.6%), TTP (7.3 vs. 4.7 months) and OS (12.9 vs. 10.8 months), when compared to the FOLFOX only arm (43). The results obtained when bevacizumab is given as a front-line treatment along with an oxaliplatin-containing regimen were presented last year. This study (NO 16966) (44, 45) began as a front line study in which patients were randomised to receive either FOLFOX 4 or XELOX (oxaliplatin 130 mg/m² as an intravenous injection

Table 2 Main results of published papers combining 5-FU, l-OHP and CPT11

Reference	No. of patients	Tumour type	CT line	MTD (mg/m²)/days of administration						Cycle length	DLT	RR (%)
				FA	5-FU bolus	5-FU pi	L-OHP	CPT11				
Souglakos (25)	31	Advanced CRC	I-line	(d-l) 200, on days 2–3	400 on days 2, 3	600 on days 2, 3 over 22 h	65 on day 2	150 on day 1		2 weeks	Diarrhoea/ neutropenia	58
Comella (26)	46	Advanced CRC (42)	II-line	(l)250 on day 2	800 on day 2	–	110 on day 1	200 on day 1		2 weeks	Diarrhoea/ neutropenia	27
Calvo (27)	26	Advanced CRC	I–II	(dl) 500 on days 1, 15		2,600 on days 1, 15 over 24 h	120 on day 1	250 on day 1		4 weeks	Diarrhoea/ neutropenia	69.2
Calvo (28)	53	Advanced CRC	I–II	(dl)500 on days 1, 15		2,500–2,600 on days 1–4[a]	120 on day 1	250–300 on day 1		4 weeks	Diarrhoea/ neutropenia	
Falcone (29)	42	Advanced CRC	I line	(d-l) 200 on day 1		3,800 on day 1 over 48 h	100 on day 1	175 on day 1		2 weeks	Diarrhoea/ neutropenia	71.4
Ychou (30)	34	several	II line	(d-l) 200 on days 1, 2	400 on days 1, 2	2,400 on day 1 over 46 h	85 on day 1	180 on day 1		2 weeks	Diarrhoea/ neutropenia	–
Goetz (31)	13	Several	I–II	(l) 20 on days 1, 8, 15, 22	320 on days 1, 8, 15, 22	–	50 on days 8, 22	75 on days 1, 15		6 weeks	Diarrhoea/ neutropenia	
	22	Several	I–II	(l) 20 on days 2–5	–	240 on days 2–5 over 90 min	85 on day 1	175 on day 1		3 weeks	Diarrhoea/ neutropenia	

(continued)

Table 2 (continued)

Reference	No. of patients	Tumour type	CT line	MTD (mg/m²)/days of administration					Cycle length	DLT	RR (%)
				FA	5-FU bolus	5-FU pi	L-OHP	CPT11			
Cals (32)	34	Advanced CRC	I-II line	–	–	3,000 on days 1, 8, 15, 22 over 24h	80 on days 8, 22	100 on days 1, 15	5 weeks	Diarrhoea	50
Masi (33)	32	Advanced CRC	I line	(d-l) 200 on day 1	–	3,200 on day 1 over 48h	85 on day 1	165 on day 1	2 weeks	Diarrhoea/ neutropenia	72
Seium (34)	30	Advanced CRC	I line	(l) 30 on days 1, 8, 15, 22	–	2,300 on days 1, 8, 15, 22 over 24h	70 on days 1, 15	100 on days 8, 22	5 weeks	Diarrhoea/ neutropenia	78
Bonetti (35)	27	Advanced CRC	II line	(l) 100 on days 1, 2	300 on days 1, 2	500 on days 1, 2 over 44h	75 on day 1	150 on day 2	2 weeks	Diarrhoea/ mucositis	24

[a]5-FU was given as an intra-arterial infusion at the dose of 2,500 mg/m²/day on days 1–4 to 32 patients with dominant liver metastases; 5-FU was given as an intravenous infusion at the dose of 2,600 mg/m²/day on days 1–4, combined with leucovorin 500 mg/m² on days 1 and 15 to the remaining 21 patients

on day 1 and capecitabine 1,000 mg/m^2 orally b.i.d on days 1–14 every 3 weeks). In August 2003 after the phase III bevacizumab data became available the protocol was amended to a 2 × 2 partially blinded study by adding 7.5 mg/kg of bevacizumab i.v. or placebo on day 1 every 3 weeks to XELOX and bevacizumab 5 mg/kg i.v. or placebo every two weeks to FOLOFOX 4; overall 2,034 patients were included. Main objectives of the study were twofold: (1) non inferiority of XELOX vs. FOLFOX 4; (2) bevacizumab plus chemotherapy (FOLFOX 4 or XELOX) is superior to chemotherapy plus placebo. The primary parameter of efficacy was progression-free survival (PFS) which resulted identical in both arms (8.5 months in the FOLFOX 4 plus placebo or bevacizumab arms, 8 months in the XELOX plus placebo or bevacizumab arms). OS was also very close (19.6 months in the FOLFOX 4 arms, 19.8 months in the XELOX arms). Capecitabine is therefore non-inferior to bolus and continuous infusion 5-FU. Regarding the second main objective, the superiority of bevacizumab to placebo, although the primary objective was met since a longer PFS was observed in the bevacizumab arms (9.4 vs. 8 months, $p = 0.023$), the results were inferior to that observed when bevacizumab was added to 5-FU/LV alone (41) (8.8 months in the FU/LV/bevacizumab group, 5.6 months in the FU/LV group; $p \leq 0.001$), to IFL (42) (10.6 months in the IFL/bevacizumab arm, 6.2 months in the IFL arm; $p < 0.001$) or when combined to FOLFOX in patients progressing following treatment with IFL (see above). Finally, ORR was identical (38%) in patients who received bevacizumab or placebo while OS was only marginally improved in patients treated with chemotherapy plus bevacizumab (21.3 vs. 19.9 months $p = 0.07$).

Cetuximab, a monoclonal antibody against the epidermal growth factor receptor, is indicated for the treatment of patients progressing after treatment with irinotecan and oxaliplatin (46). The drug is able to restore the sensitivity to irinotecan in about 20% of irinotecan-resistant patients and it is with irinotecan-containing regimens that this compound has been mostly investigated. Data with oxaliplatin-containing regimens is less abundant. In a phase II study in 43 patients, the combination of cetuximab with FOLFOX as a front-line treatment was associated with a dramatic 72% ORR, including a 9% complete remission rate (47). However, when the investigation was replicated under the more controlled rules of a randomised phase II study (The OPUS study), ORR was lower (45.6% in the cetuximab-FOLFOX arm, 35.7% in the FOLFOX only arm) (48). The addition of cetuximab to the FOLFOX or FOLFIRI regimens was also attempted in the CALGB-80203 trial. The study had planned to enrol 2,300 patients, but closed prematurely when only 224 patients were randomised because of slow accrual. In patients who received FOLFOX ($n = 58$) or FOLFOX plus cetuximab ($n = 53$) response rates were 40% and 60%, respectively (49). The concept of combining both antibodies with FOLFOX or FOLFIRI is being investigated in the CALGB Intergroup study C80405 (50). This is a 3-arm study powered for survival. The physician selects either FOLFOX or FOLFIRI, and then patients are randomly assigned to bevacizumab alone, cetuximab alone or the combination of the two. This is an important study which, if completed, will show the merits of using an anti-VEGF antibody, an anti-EGFR antibody or the combination of the two. However, a study with an identical design known with the acronym PACCE (51), sponsored by Amgen, in which cetuximab was substituted with the fully humanised monoclonal antibody panitumumab, had to be closed prematurely because the pre-planned interim analysis showed negative effect on progression-free survival.

In conclusion, in the past few years the pharmacological treatment of advanced colorectal cancer has witnessed substantial changes, with the addition to 5-FU modulated by LV of new effective drugs such as Oxaliplatin and Irinotecan and more recently with the introduction of targeted therapies such as anti-vascular and anti Epidermal Growth Factor receptor agents. As a result of the extensive clinical research in this field and of the widespread availability of new drugs for patients, the outlook of advanced colorectal cancer has improved: patients live longer and also enjoy a better quality of life. However, with five active agents, we still have to learn how best to use them.

The Adjuvant Setting

The results obtained with the addition of oxaliplatin (or irinotecan) to the 5-FU backbone in the advanced stages, prompted the launch of a series of randomised phase III studies in stage II and III colon cancer patients. In these studies patients were randomised to receive either a combination of 5-FU and LV or the same combination plus oxaliplatin (or irinotecan). The role of oxaliplatin was investigated in two studies (52, 53) while the impact of irinotecan was investigated in three (54–56). From the data summarised in Table 3 it is fair to conclude that while the addition of oxaliplatin to the regimens including 5-FU and LV is associated with a better outcome for patients, the introduction of irinotecan is either marginally effective or detrimental. Furthermore, the activity of oxaliplatin is independent from the 5-FU-LV schedule since the results initially observed in the MOSAIC trial in which oxaliplatin is given biweekly with bolus and continuous infusion 5-FU are confirmed in the NSABP C07 trial in which biweekly oxaliplatin is combined with weekly 5-FU and LV. However, the schedule issue matters in terms of toxicity, especially neurotoxicity, enteropathy and toxic deaths. The lower incidence of grade III neurotoxicity reported in the NSABP C07 trial (8%) compared to the MOSAIC trial (12.4%) is easily explained by the lower cumulative doses of oxaliplatin in the former study (765 mg/m^2 vs. 1,025 mg/m^2). The GI toxicity in the NSABP C07 was recently described in detail (57). A syndrome of bowel wall injury characterised by hospitalisation for the management of severe diarrhoea or dehydration and radiographic or endoscopic evidence of bowel wall thickening or ulceration happened in 79 out of 1,857 patients (4.3%). The majority of these patients (65%) had received bolus 5-FU-LV and oxaliplatin. Besides this syndrome, not observed in the MOSAIC trial, the incidence of grade III and IV diarrhoea was also higher in the oxaliplatin containing arm of the NSABP C07 trial (38% vs. 10.8%). Finally treatment related deaths were 0.5% in the

Table 3 Randomised studies evaluating oxaliplatin-based and irinotecan-based combinations as adjuvant treatment for colon cancer

Drug	Reference	No. of patients	Disease stage	Treatment arms	3-year disease-free, relapse-free survival (%)	Δ (%)	p value
Oxaliplatin	MOSAIC (52)	1,123	II-III	LV5-FU2	72.9		
				FOLFOX	78.2	5.3	0.002
	NSABP C07 (53)	1,207	II-III	Roswell Park	71.8		
				Roswell Park + Oxaliplatin	76.1	4.3	<0.004
Irinotecan	FNCLCC ACCORD 02 (54)	400	III high risk	LV5-FU2	60		
				FOLFIRI	51	−9	
	CALGB 89803 (55)	1,264	III	Roswell Park	69		
				Roswell Park + Irinotecan (IFL)	66	−3	
	PETACC 3 (56)	2,111	III	LV5-FU2	60.3		
				FOLFIRI	63.3	3	

MOSAIC trial and 1.2% in the NSABP C07. In conclusion, FOLFOX should be the preferred regimen in the adjuvant setting although the lower incidence of grade III neurotoxicity, the ease of administration of bolus delivery and the avoidance of the central catheter, could make FLOX preferable in some cases, with the warning that enteric toxicity should be carefully managed.

The positive results of the MOSAIC trial, which enrolled 40% of stage II patients, led the regulatory Authorities Food and Drug Administration in the USA and the European Medicine Agency to approve this protocol for the adjuvant treatment of only stage III patients. These decisions were criticised in a commentary by Grothey and Sargent (58) published in the Journal of Clinical Oncology, for the main reasons that were based upon a sub group analysis. The recently reported improved OS observed only in stage III patients (59), with an absolute difference of 4.4% ($p = 0.029$) in favour of the oxaliplatin-containing arm could, however, lend support to the conservative approach applied by the Regulatory Agencies.

The role of both bevacizumab and cetuximab is being actively investigated in the adjuvant setting. The AVANT (AVastin adjuvANT) trial is a 3-arm European trial in which 3,451 stage III and high risk stage II patients were randomised to receive: (1) FOLFOX 4 alone for 12 cycles, (2) FOLFOX 4 plus bevacizumab 5 mg/kg for 12 cycles followed by bevacizumab alone at the dose of 7.5 mg/kg every 3 weeks for eight additional cycles or (3) XELOX (capecitabine oxaliplatin) plus bevacizumab 7.5 mg/kg every 3 weeks for 8 cycles followed by bevacizumab alone at the same dose and interval for eight additional cycles. The accrual of this study was completed in 30 months (from December 2004 to June 2007). This study addresses not only the value of bevacizumab in this population but also the possibility of substituting capecitabine to bolus and PVI 5-FU, thus avoiding the need of the central catheter. In the NSABP C08 study conducted in the USA stage II and III colon cancer patients were randomised to either FOLFOX6 alone (an evolution of FOLFOX4 in which the bolus of 5-FU on day 2 is taken off while 5-FU PVI is given at the dose of 2,400 mg/m^2 over 46 h starting on day 1) or to the same combination plus bevacizumab 5 mg/kg for 12 cycles followed by bevacizumab alone at the same dose for 12 additional cycles. The addition of cetuximab to FOLFOX4 is being investigated in a randomised study performed by the Pan European Trials in Adjuvant Colon Cancer (PETACC 8) in stage III patients (60).

The results of all these studies are eagerly awaited with the hope that a further improvement in the cure rate of colon cancer will be shown. In this case the search for the best regimen to propose to radically resected stage II and III colon cancer patients will have to continue performing direct comparisons between the best bevacizumab-containing or cetuximab-containing regimens. Furthermore, it will be interesting to evaluate the results of the CALGB Intergroup study C80405, since positive findings from the strategy of blocking VEGF along with EGFR will open the way to their evaluation in the adjuvant setting.

To summarise, in less than two decades the 3-year disease-free survival for stage III colon cancer patients increased from 44% with surgery alone in 1990, to 62% with the 6 months combination of 5-FU and LV in 1995, to the 65% observed in the LV5-FU2 arm in the MOSAIC trial and finally to the 72% obtained in both oxaliplatin-containing arms of the MOSAIC and NSABP C07 trials. For sure, improvements in the imaging which allowed a better selection of patients contributed to these results but in this success story the majority of merits is attributable to adjuvant chemotherapy.

References

1. Kelly H, Goldberg RM. Systemic therapy for metastatic colorectal cancer: current options, current evidence. J Clin Oncol 2005;23:4553–60.
2. Sobrero AF, Aschele C, Bertino JR. Fluorouracil in colorectal cancer–a tale of two drugs: implications for biochemical modulation. J Clin Oncol 1997;15:368–81.
3. De Gramont A, Krulik M, Cady J, et al. High-dose folinic acid and 5-fluorouracil bolus and continuous infusion in advanced colorectal cancer. Eur J Cancer Clin Oncol 1988;24:1499–1503.
4. De Gramont A, Bosset JF, Milan C, et al. Randomized trial comparing monthly low-dose leucovorin and fluorouracil bolus with bimonthly high-dose leucovorin and fluorouracil bolus plus continuous infusion for advanced colorectal cancer: a French intergroup study. J Clin Oncol 1997;15:808–15.

5. Andre T, Louvet C, Raymond E, Tiurnigand C, De Gramont A. Bimonthly high-dose leucovorin, 5-fluorouracil infusion and oxaliplatin (FOLFOX3) for metastatic colorectal cancer resistant to the same leucovorin and 5-fluorouracil regimen. Ann Oncol 1998;9:1251–3.

6. Scheithauer W; Rosen H, Kornek G-V, Sebesta C, Depisch D. Randomised comparison of combination chemotherapy plus supportive care with supportive care alone in patients with metastatic colorectal cancer. BMJ 1993;306:752–5.

7. The Nordic Gastrointestinal Tumor Adjuvant Therapy Group. Expectancy or primary chemotherapy in patients with advanced asymptomatic colorectal cancer: a randomised trial. J Clin Oncol 1992;10:904–11.

8. Advanced Colorectal Cancer Meta-analysis Project. Modulation of fluoruracil by leucovorin in patients with advanced colorectal cancer: evidence in terms of response rate. J Clin Oncol 1992;10:896–903.

9. Advanced Colorectal Cancer Meta-analysis Project. Meta-analysis of randomised trials testing the biochemical modulation of fluorouracil by methotrexate in metastatic colorectal cancer. J Clin Oncol 1994;12:960–9.

10. O'Connel MJ, Laurie JA, Kahn M, et al. Prospectively randomised trial of postoperative adjuvant chemotherapy in patients with high-risk colon cancer. J Clin Oncol 1998;16:295–300.

11. Wolmark N, Rockette H, Mamounas E, et al. Clinical trial to assess the relative efficacy of fluorouracil and leucovorin, fluorouracil and levamisole, and fluorouracil, leucovorin and levamisole in patients with Dukes' B and C carcinoma of the colon: results from National Surgical Adjuvant Breast and Bowel Project C-04. J Clin Oncol 1999;17:3553–9.

12. QUASAR Collaborative Group. Comparison of fluorouracil with additional levamisole, higher-dose folinic acid, or both, as adjuvant chemotherapy for colorectal cancer: a randomised trial. Lancet 2000;355:1588–96.

13. Grothey A, Goldberg RM. A review of oxaliplatin and its clinical use in colorectal cancer. Expert Opin Pharmacoter 2004;5:2159–70.

14. Rothenberg ML, Oza AM, Bigelow RH, et al. Superiority of oxaliplatin and fluorouracil-leucovorin compared with either therapy alone in patients with progressive colorectal cancer after irinotecan and fluorouracil-leucovorin: interim results of a phase III trial. J Clin Oncol 2003;21:2059–69.

15. Yeh KH, Cheng AL, Wan JP, Lin CS, Liu CC. Down-regulation of thymidylate synthase expression and its steady-state mRNA by oxaliplatin in colon cancer cells. Anticancer Drugs 2004;15:71–6.

16. De Gramont A, Figer A, Seymour M, et al. Leucovorin and fluorouracil with or without oxaliplatin as first-line treatment in advanced colorectal cancer. J Clin Oncol 2000;18:2938–47.

17. Saltz LB, Cox JV, Blanke C, et al. Irinotecan plus fluorouracil and leucovorin for metastatic colorectal cancer. N Engl J Med 2000;343:905–13.

18. Douillard JY, Cunningham D, Roth AD, et al. Irinotecan combined with fluorouracil alone as first-line treatment for metastatic colorectal cancer: a multicentre randomised trial. Lancet 2000;355:1041–7.

19. Tournigand C, Andrè T, Achille E, et al. FOLFIRI followed by FOLFOX6 or the reverse sequence in advanced colorectal cancer: a randomised GERCOR study. J Clin Oncol 2004;22:229–37.

20. Goldberg RM, Sargent D, Morton RF, et al. A randomised controlled trial of fluorouracil plus leucovorin, irinotecan and oxaliplatin combinations in patients with previously untreated metastatic colorectal cancer. J Clin Oncol 2004;22:23–30.

21. Comella P, Massidda B, Filippelli G, et al. Oxaliplatin plus high-dose folinic acid and 5-fluorouracil i.v. bolus (OXAFAFU) versus irinotecan plus high-dose folinic acid and 5-fluorouracil i.v. bolus (IRIFAFU) in patients with metastatic colorectal carcinoma: a Southern Italy cooperative group phase III trial. Ann Oncol 2005;16:878–86.

22. Kalofonos HP, Aravantinos G, Kosmidis P, et al. Irinotecan or oxaliplatin combined with leucovorin and 5-fluorouracil as first-line treatment in advanced colorectal cancer: a multicenter, randomized, phase II study. Ann Oncol 2005;16:869–77.

23. Colucci G, Gebbia V, Paoletti G, et al. Phase III randomised trial of FOLFIRI versus FOFOX4 in the treatment of advanced colorectal cancer: a multicenter study of the Gruppo Oncologico dell'Italia Meridionale. J Clin Oncol 2005;23:4866–75.

24. Rothenberg ML, Meropol NJ, Poplin A, Van Cutsem E, Wadler S. Mortality associated with irinotecan plus bolus fluorouracil/leucovorin: summary findings of an independent panel. J Clin Oncol 2001;19:3801–7.

25. Grothey A, Sargent D, Goldberg RM, Schmoll HJ. Survival of patients with advanced color-ectal cancer improves with availability of fluorouracil-leucovorin, irinotecan, and oxaliplatin in the course of treatment. J Clin Oncol 2004;22:1209–14.

26. Souglakos J, Mavroudis D, Kakolyris S, et al. Triplet combination with irinotecan plus oxali-platin plus continuous infusion fluorouracil and leucovorin as first-line treatment in metastatic colorectal cancer: a multicenter phase II trial. J Clin Oncol 2002;20:2651–7.

27. Comella P, Casaretti R, De Rosa V, et al. Oxaliplatin plus irinotecan and leucovorin-modulated 5-fluorouracil triplet regimen every other week: a dose-finding study in patients with advanced gastrointestinal malignancies. Ann Oncol 2002;13:1874–81.

28. Calvo E, Cortes J, Rodriguez J, et al. Irinotecan, oxaliplatin, and 5-fluorouracil/leucovorin combination chemotherapy in advanced colorectal carcinoma: a phase II study. Clin Colorectal Cancer 2002;2:104–10.

29. Calvo E, Cortes J, Gonzalez-Cao M, et al. Combined irinotecan, oxaliplatin, and 5-fluorouracil in patients with advanced colorecatl cancer: a feasibility pilot study. Oncology 2002;63:254–65.

30. Falcone A, Masi G, Allegrini G, et al. Biweekly chemotherapy with oxaliplatin, irinotecan, infusional fluorouracil, and leucovorin: a pilot study in patients with metastatic colorectal cancer. J Clin Oncol 2002;19:4006–14.

31. Ychou M, Conroy T, Seitz JF, et al. An open phase I study assessing the feasibility of the triple combination: oxaliplatin plus irinotecan plus leucovorin/5-fluorouracil every 2 weeks in patients with advanced solid tumors. Ann Oncol 2003;14:481–9.

32. Goetz MP, Erlichman C, Windebank AJ, et al. Phase I and pharmacokinetic study of two dif-ferent schedules of oxaliplatin, irinotecan, fluorouracil, and leucovorin in patients with solid tumors. J Clin Oncol 2003;20:3761–9.

33. Cals L, Rixe O, Francois E, et al. Dose-finding study of weekly 24-h continuous infusion of 5-fluoruracil associated with alternating oxaliplatin or irinotecan in advanced colorectal cancer. Ann Oncol 2004;15:1018–24.

34. Masi G, Allegrini G, Cupini S, et al. First-line treatment of metastatic colorectal cancer with irinotecan, oxaliplatin and 5-fluorouracil/leucovorin (FOLFOXIRI): results of a phase II study with a simplified biweekly schedule. Ann Oncol 2004;15:1766–72.

35. Seium Y, Stupp R, Rushtaller T, et al. Oxaliplatin combined with irinotecan and 5-fluorouracil/-leucovorin (OCFL) in metastatic colorectal cancer: a phase I-II study. Ann Oncol 2005;16: 762–6.

36. Bonetti A, Zaninelli M, Durante E, et al. Multiple-target chemotherapy (LV-modulated 5-FU bolus and continuous infusion, oxaliplatin, CPT11) in advanced, 5-FU refractory, colorectal cancer: MTD definition and efficacy evaluation. A phase I-II study. Tumori 2006;92:389–95.

37. Souglakos A, Androulakis N, Syrigos K, et al. FOLFOXIRI (folinic acid, 5-fluorouracil, oxaliplatin and irinotecan) as first-line treatment in metastatic colorectal cancer (MCC): a multicentre randomised phase III trial from the Hellenic Oncology Research group (HORG). Br J Cancer 2007;94:798–805.

38. Falcone A, Ricci S, Brunetti I, et al. Phase III trial of infusional fluorouracil, leucovorin, oxaliplatin and irinotecan (FOLFOXIRI) compared with infusional fluoruracil, leucovorin, and irinotecan (FOLFIRI) as first-line treatment for metastatic colorectal cancer: the Gruppo Oncologico Nord Ovest. J Clin Oncol 2007;25:1670–6.

39. Kim KJ, Li B, Winer J, et al. Inhibition of vascular endothelial growth factor-induced angio-genesis suppresses tumour growth in vivo. Nature 1993;362:841–4.

40. Presta LG, Chen H, O'Connor SJ, et al. Humanization of an anti-vascular endothelial growth factor monoclonal antibody for the therapy of solid tumors and other disorders. Cancer Res 1997;57:4593–9.

41. Kabbinavar FF, Hambleton J, Mass RD, Hurwitz HI, Bergsland E, Sarkar S. Combined analysis of efficacy: the addition of bevacizumab to fluoruracil/leucovorin improves survival for patients with metastatic colorectal cancer. J Clin Oncol 2005;23:3706–12.
42. Hurwitz H, Feherenbacher L, Novotny W, et al. Bevacizumab plus irinotecan, fluorouracil, and leucovorin for metastatic colorectal cancer. N Engl J Med 2004;350:2335–42.
43. Giantonio BJ, Catalano PJ, Meropol NJ, et al. Bevacizumab in combination with oxaliplatin, fluoruracil, and leucovorin (FOLFOX4) for previously treated metastatic colorectal cancer: results from the Eastern cooperative oncology group study E3200. J Clin Oncol 2007;25:1539–44.
44. Cassidy J, Clarke S, Diaz-Rubio E, et al. XELOX vs. FOLFOX4: survival and response results from XELOX-1/NO16966, a randomised phase III trial of first-line treatment for patients with metastatic colorectal cancer (MCRC). Proc Am Soc Clin Oncol 2007;25:171:4030 (abstract).
45. Saltz L, Clarke S, Diaz-Rubio E, et al. Bevacizumab (Bev) in combination with XELOX or FOLFOX-4: updated efficacy results from XELOX-1/NO16966, a randomised phase III trial in first-line metastatic colorectal cancer. Proc Am Soc Clin Oncol 2007;25:170:4028 (abstract).
46. Cunningham D, Humblet Y, Siena S, et al. Cetuximab monotherapy and cetuximab plus irinotecan in irinotecan-refractory metastatic colorectal cancer. N Engl J Med 2004;351:337–45.
47. Diaz Rubio E, Tabernero J, Van Cutsem E, et al. Cetuximab in combination with oxaliplatin/5-fluorouracil (5-FU)/folinic acid (FA) (FOLFOX-4) in the first-line treatment of patients with epidermal growth factor receptor (EGFR)-expressing metastatic colorectal cancer: An international phase II study. Proc Am Soc Clin Oncol 2005;23:3535 (abstract).
48. Bokemeyer C, Bondarenko I, Makhson A, et al. Cetuximab plus 5-FU/FA/oxalplatin (FOLFOX 4) versus FOLFOX 4 in the fist-line treatment of metastatic colorectal cancer (mCRC): OPUS, a randomized phase II study. Proc Am Soc Clin Oncol 2007;25:4035 (abstract).
49. Venook A., Niedzwiecki D., Hollis D. et al. Phase III study of irinotecan/5FU/LV (FOLFIRI) or oxaliplatin/5FU/LV (FOLFOX) ± cetuximab for patients (pts) with untreated metastatic adenocarcinoma of the colon or rectum (MCRC): CALGB 80203 preliminary results. Proc Am Soc Clin Oncol 2006;24:3509 (abstract).
50. CALGB/SWOG C80405: A phase III trial of FOLFIRI or FOLFOX with bevacizumab or cetuximab or both for untreated metastatic adenocarcinoma of the colon or rectum. Clin Adv Hematol Oncol. 2006;4:452–3.
51. PACCE: A randomized, Open-label, controlled, clinical trial of chemotherapy and bevacizumab with and without panitumumab in the first-line treatment of subjects with metastatic colorectal cancer. (Accessed 3 May 2008, at http://www.amgen.com/media/media_pr_detail.jsp?releaseID = 977186 – 20k.)
52. Andrè T, Boni C, Monudeji-Boudiaf L, et al. Oxaliplatin, Fluorouracil, and Leucovorin as adjuvant treatment for colon cancer. N Engl J Med 2004;350:2343–51.
53. Kuebler JP, Wieand S, O'Connel MJ, et al. Oxaliplatin combined with weekly bolus fluorouracil and leucovorin as surgical adjuvant chemotherapy for stage II and III colon cancer: results from NSABP C-07. J Clin Oncol 2007;25:2198–204.
54. Ychou M, Raoul JL, Douillard JY, et al. A phase III randomised trial of LV5FU2 + CPT11 vs LV5FU2 alone in adjuvant high risk colon cancer (FNCLCC Accord02/FFCD9802). Proc Am Soc Clin Oncol 2005;23:3502 (abstract).
55. Saltz L, Niedzwiecki D, Hollis D, et al. Irinotecan fluorouracil plus leucovorin is not superior to fluorouracil alone as adjuvant treatment for stage III colon cancer: results of CALGB 89803. J Clin Oncol 2007;25:3456–61.
56. Van Cutsem E, Labianca R, Hossfeld D, et al. Randomised phase III trial comparing infused irinotecan/5-fluorouracil (5-FU)/folinic acid (IF) versus 5-FU/FA (F) in stage III colon cancer patients (pts). (PETACC 3). Proc Am Soc Clin Oncol 2005;23:8 (abstract).
57. Kuebler JP, Colangelo L, O'Connel MJ, et al. Severe enteropathy among patients with stage II/III colon cancer treated on a randomised trial of bolus 5-fluorouracil/leucovorin plus or minus oxaliplatin. A prospective study. Cancer 2007;110:1945–50.

58. Grothey A, Sargent DJ. FOLFOX for stage II colon cancer? A commentary on the recent FDA approval of oxaliplatin for adjuvant therapy of stage III colon cancer. J Clin Oncol 2005;23:3311–3.
59. de Gramont A, Boni C, Navarro M, et al. Oxaliplatin/5FU/LV in adjuvant colon cancer: updated efficacy results of the MOSAIC trial, including survival, with a median follow-up of six years. Proc Am Soc Clin Oncol 2007;25:4007 (abstract).
60. Taieb J, Puig PL, Bedenne L. Cetuximab plus FOLFOX-4 for fully resected stage III colon carcinoma: scientific background and the ongoing PETACC-8 trial. Expert Rev Anticancer Ther 2008;8:183–9.

First-Line Systemic Chemotherapy with Folfoxiri Followed by Radical Surgical Resection of Metastases for the Treatment of Unresectable Metastatic Colorectal Cancer Patients

Enrico Vasile, Gianluca Masi, Fotios Loupakis, Samanta Cupini, Giacomo Giulio Baldi, Lorenzo Fornaro, Irene Stasi, Lisa Salvatore, and Alfredo Falcone

Abstract Prognosis of patients with initially unresectable metastatic colorectal cancer (MCRC) can be improved if chemotherapy induces a significant down-sizing of metastatic disease thus allowing a radical (R0) surgical resection of metastases (mts). Moreover, it has been demonstrated that there is a clear correlation between the activity of the regimen used and the rate of secondary R0 resections.

We studied the triple drug combination FOLFOXIRI (irinotecan 165 mg/m^2 on day 1, oxaliplatin 85 mg/m^2 on day 1, 1-leucovorin 200 mg/m^2 on day 1, 5-fluorouracil 3,200 mg/m^2 48-h flat continuous infusion starting on day 1, repeated every 2 weeks) in phase II and III trials. Overall 196 patients with initially unresectable MCRC not selected for a neoadjuvant strategy were treated. This regimen was associated with a good activity (response rate ranging from 60 to 72%) and 37 patients (19%) underwent to a secondary R0 surgery on metastases after chemotherapy.

Characteristics of the 37 radically resected patients were: median age 64 years (45–73), ECOG PS ≥ 1 in 11 patients (30%), median CEA 10 ng/ml (1–288), liver involvement ≥25% in 18 patients (49%). Sites of disease were: liver only 25 patients (68%), lung only 4 patients (11%), liver + lymphnodes 5 patients (13%), liver + peritoneum 1 patient (3%), liver + lung 2 patients (5%). Mts were synchronous in 24 patients (65%) and metachronous in 13 patients (35%). There was no perioperative mortality. After a median follow up of 61 months, median OS is 40.8 months. The actuarial 5-year survival from the onset of chemotherapy is 45%. In 11 patients who showed progression of disease after surgery, a surgical re-resection and/or radiofrequency ablation was performed.

These data indicate that FOLFOXIRI allows an R0 surgical resection in about 1 out of 5 patients with initially unresectable MCRC not selected for a neoadjuvant approach. Long term survival of resected patients is significant and comparable with

E. Vasile, (✉) G. Masi, F. Loupakis, S. Cupini, G. Baldi, L. Fornaro,
I. Stasi, L. Salvatore, and A. Falcone
Division of Medical Oncology, Azienda USL 6, Livorno, Istituto Toscano Tumori
e-mail: envasile@tin.it

A. Bonetti et al. (eds.), *Platinum and Other Heavy Metal Compounds in Cancer Chemotherapy*, DOI: 10.1007/978-1-60327-459-3_32,
© Humana Press, a part of Springer Science + Business Media, LLC 2009

the survival of patients resectable up-front. This FOLFOXIRI regimen should be considered as neoadjuvant treatment in initially unresectable metastatic colorectal cancer patients.

Keywords Metastatic colorectal cancer; Neoadjuvant chemotherapy; FOLFOXIRI; Surgical resection of metastases

Colorectal cancer represents the second most frequent cause of cancer-related deaths in Western countries (1).

Approximately 25% of colorectal cancer patients have metastases at diagnosis, and an additional 25–35% of patients will develop metastases during the course of their disease. Significantly, between 20 and 30% of patients with metastatic colorectal cancer (MCRC) have liver only disease, and ~50% of recurrences following resection of the primary tumour are confined to the liver (2, 3).

The treatment of MCRC has achieved considerable progresses in the last decade with the median survival of patients reaching almost 2 years thanks to the use of novel cytotoxic and biological agents coupled with an increased use of surgery of metastases (4).

Chemotherapy remains the cornerstone for the treatment of almost all MCRC patients. For decades 5-fluorouracil (5FU) has been the only available agent (5). In the last years, irinotecan (CPT-11) and oxaliplatin (LOHP) have demonstrated good anti-tumour activity in MCRC. The combinations of CPT-11 + 5FU/leucovorin (LV) (FOLFIRI) and LOHP + 5FU/LV (FOLFOX) have shown increased activity and efficacy compared with 5FU/LV alone in several phase III randomized studies (6–10). A randomized study conducted by GERCOR have demonstrated that a treatment with two sequential doublets (first-line FOLFIRI followed by FOLFOX-6 at progression or the reverse sequence) achieved considerable activity and efficacy with an interesting median survival of ~21 months (11). It also suggests the importance for MCRC patients of receiving all the three active cytotoxic drugs available (5FU, LOHP and CPT-11). These results are strengthened by a pooled analysis of seven phase III trials demonstrating that MCRC patients receiving all the three active drugs in the course of their disease have better survival (12). Moreover this analysis showed that 20–50% of patients who progress after first-line chemotherapy are not able to receive second-line treatment, mainly because of deterioration of their performance status and liver function, and therefore cannot be exposed to the three agents.

Despite recent advances in first-line chemotherapy strategies for the treatment of MCRC patients, the resection of metastases offers the only chance of cure for these patients; in fact, 5-year survival rate following surgical resection ranges between 25 and 40% and is superior to the only 0–5% reported for patients who did not undergo resection of metastases at the same institutions (13–19). Moreover, surgical resection can offer good opportunities for long-term survival also for patients with pulmonary metastases or limited extra-hepatic disease (20, 21). However, ~85% of patients with MCRC, referred to specialist centres, have metastatic disease considered as unresectable at presentation (22).

Following the first retrospective trial published by Bismuth in 1996 (23), indicating that patients who were initially unresectable could be treated with systemic chemotherapy and, in case of a good response, radically resected in about 16% of cases, the role of pre-operative, neoadjuvant, chemotherapy for the treatment of MCRC was largely studied. In fact, the availability of more active first-line chemotherapy regimens that can increase the response rate could facilitate the downsizing of metastases from colorectal cancer contributing to render resectable some initially unresectable patient (22–24). Moreover, the prognosis of patients who become resectable and are radically resected after response to chemotherapy could be similar to that of patients resected at the onset (25).

In the last years, some prospective studies conducted with combination chemotherapy such as the FOLFOX or FOLFIRI regimens (24–26) confirmed that an active first-line chemotherapy in initially unresectable patients can allow, in case of response, a radical resection of metastatic disease in a subgroup of patients and that 20–40% of these patients can achieve long-term survival. The resection rates largely range from 10 to 40% among these different studies mainly because of the various selection criteria used for unresectability more than for the chemotherapy regimen. However, Folprecht et al. confirmed in a pooled analysis that there is a strong correlation between the response rate to first-line chemotherapy and the post-chemotherapy radical resection rate of metastatic disease and indicated that patients with metastases that might become resectable following chemotherapy should preferably be treated with a regimen that induces high response rates (27).

On these bases, of a higher rate of complete surgical removal of metastases with a more active first-line regimen and of a better outcome with the exposure to all the three cytotoxic drugs, the Italian collaborative group G.O.N.O. (namely Gruppo Oncologico del Nord-Ovest) developed from phase I to phase III a first-line regimen of combination of infusional 5FU/LV, CPT-11 and LOHP (FOLFOXIRI) with a biweekly schedule (Table 1) with the aim of improving the activity of the treatment and potentially to achieve an increased rate of secondary resection of metastases in MCRC patients.

Table 1 Schedules used and results of the FOLFOXIRI trials by G.O.N.O

	FOLFOXIRI	S-FOLFOXIRI	S-FOLFOXIRI
	Phase I–II ($N = 42$)	Phase II ($N = 32$)	Phase III ($N = 122$)
CPT-11 mg/m² in 1-h, d1	175	165	165
L-OHP mg/m² in 2-h, d1	100	85	85
l-LV mg/m² in 2-h, d1	200	200	200
5-FU mg/m² in 48-h, d1 → 3	3,800 chronomodulated	3,200 continuous	3,200 continuous
Overall response rate	71%	72%	60%
Complete response rate	12%	13%	7%
Radical surgery rate	26%	25%	15%
Median PFS	10.4 months	10.8 months	9.9 months
Median OS	26.5 months	28.4 months	23.6 months

CPT-11 irinotecan; *LOHP* oxaliplatin; *LV* leucovorin; *5FU* 5-fluorouracile; *d* day; *PFS* progression free survival; *OS* overall survival; *S-FOLFOXIRI* simplified FOLFOXIRI

In the initial phase I–II study (28), 42 MCRC patients were treated with CPT-11 125–175 mg/m^2 1-h infusion on day 1, LOHP 100 mg/m^2 2-h infusion on day 1, LV 200 mg/m^2 2-h infusion on day 1, 5FU 3,800 mg/m^2 48-h chronomodulated continuous infusion starting on day 1, obtaining a response rate of 71% and a complete response rate of 12%; median progression-free and overall survival resulted in 10.4 and 26.5 months, respectively.

In the subsequent phase II study performed in 32 MCRC patients (29) the FOLFOXIRI regimen was modified to become more feasible in clinical practice, by using a flat continuous, not chronomodulated, 48-h infusion of 5FU (3,200 mg/m^2 starting on day 1 with LV 200 mg/m^2 2-h infusion on day 1) with slightly reduced doses of CPT-11 (165 mg/m^2 1-h infusion on day 1) and LOHP (85 mg/m^2 2-h infusion on day 1). This regimen produced a lower incidence of both haematological and non-haematological toxicities, maintaining an elevated activity with an overall response rate of 72% and a median progression free survival of 10.8 months; median overall survival was 28.4 months.

On the basis of these results, a multicentre randomized phase III trial comparing the simplified FOLFOXIRI regimen to a standard doublet combination as FOLFIRI was performed (30, 31); a total of 244 patients were enrolled, 122 in each arm, demonstrating that the triple drug combination was associated with an improved activity and efficacy and, in particular, with a gain in the rate of radical surgery of metastases (15 vs.6%, $p = 0.03$ in the overall population and 36 vs.12%, $p = 0.01$ in patients with isolated liver disease).

A total of 196 unresectable MCRC patients not selected for a neoadjuvant strategy were treated with the FOLFOXIRI regimen in these three studies; in 72 of these patients (36%) a surgical resection of metastases was evaluated after chemotherapy: 25 patients were considered already unresectable, 5 patients underwent an explorative surgery alone, 5 patients were operated but the resection was not radical. The remaining 37 patients (19% of the total) underwent a radical surgical resection of all metastatic sites or a resection of metastases combined with intraoperative radiofrequency ablation of small residual hepatic nodules (in 8 patients).

The characteristics of these 37 patients are reported in Table 2; 65% of patients had synchronous metastases, with multiple sites of disease in 22% of patients; only 68% of patients had metastases confined to the liver. Main reasons of initial unresectability classified according to the OncoSurge criteria were extensive liver involvement (51% of cases) and unresectable extra-hepatic disease (16%) (Table 3).

The median number of cycles of pre-operative FOLFOXIRI administered to the 37 resected patients was 11, obtaining 5 complete and 28 partial responses (overall response rate: 85%); 4 patients remained stable during the treatment. The median time from the end of chemotherapy to the operation was 1.9 months. Post-operative chemotherapy was not planned but was allowed and received by 10 patients.

The local treatments performed in the 37 patients were: a major hepatectomy in 19 patients (52%), a minor hepatectomy in 14 patients (38%), a multiple segmental lung resection in 4 patients (10%); surgical removal of circumscribed extrahepatic disease was also performed in 8 patients with liver metastases (abdominal lymph nodes in 4 patients, peritoneum in 1 and lung in 2 patients).

Table 2 Patients' characteristics

Median age (range)	64 (45–73) years
ECOG Performance status	
0	70%
1	30%
Timing of metastases	
Synchronous	65%
Metachronous	35%
Sites of disease	
Single	78%
Multiple	22%
Sites of disease	
Liver only	68%
Liver + lymphnodes	14%
Liver + peritoneum	3%
Liver + lung	5%
Lung only	10%
Median number of metastases	5 (1–12)
Liver involvement ≥25%	49%
Median CEA (range)	10 (1–288) ng/ml

Table 3 Main reasons of initial unresectability

Extensive liver involvement	51 (%)
6 segments involved	19
70% liver parenchyma involved	27
All three hepatic veins involved	5
Unresectable extra-hepatic disease	16
Patient unfit for surgery	3
Immediate resection not appropriate	30
Inadequate radiological margins	11
Portal lymph nodes involvement	8
Number of mts >4 or ≤4 but bilobar	11

There was no intraoperative/post-operative mortality within 3 months of surgery. The post-operative complications were: transient liver failure (3 patients), biliary fistula (2 patients), wound infection (2 patients), bilioma (1 patient) and pneumonia (1 patient), all resolved without sequelae.

After a median follow up of 61 months, 31 patients have progressed after surgery; in 11 of these patients a surgical re-resection and/or radiofrequency ablation of metastases was performed. Twenty-seven progressed patients received a second-line chemotherapy with FOLFOXIRI in 9 cases, FOLFIRI in 12, FOLFOX in 5 and Cetuximab in 1 case.

The median time to progression after first resection of metastases was 17.8 months with 16% of patients free of progression at 5 years; considering also those patients who underwent a second complete re-resection or ablation of metastases after the progression of disease, 29% of the patients remained free of the disease at 5 years (Fig. 1).

The median overall survival was 40.8 months with an actuarial 5- and 8-year survival rate from the onset of chemotherapy of 45 and 33%, respectively (Fig. 2).

These data indicate that FOLFOXIRI allows a radical surgical resection of metastases in about 1 out of 5 patients with initially unresectable MCRC not selected for a neoadjuvant approach. Long-term survival of resected patients is significant and comparable with the survival of patients resectable up-front; although the 5-year survival is not dissimilar to those reported in other trials conducted with oxaliplatin or irinotecan/fluoropyrimidine doublets (24–26, 32–33), the results obtained with FOLFOXIRI seem particularly interesting because in the studies with doublets patients were usually selected for having a limited liver-only disease.

Moreover, these data support the importance of achieving a complete resection of metastases by combining chemotherapy and surgery even if the disease is initially unresectable and a minimal extra-hepatic disease is present.

This FOLFOXIRI regimen seems of particular interest in the neoadjuvant treatment of initially unresectable MCRC patients due to its elevated activity coupled with a manageable toxicity profile.

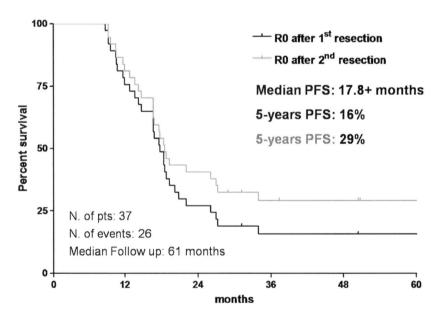

Fig. 1 Kaplan-Meier estimates of progression free survival (PFS) of radically resected and re-resected MCRC patients treated with FOLFOXIRI before surgery

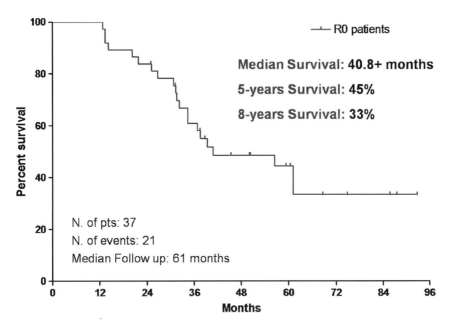

Fig. 2 Kaplan-Meier estimates of overall survival (OS) of radically resected MCRC patients treated with FOLFOXIRI before surgery

References

1. Jemal A, Siegel R, Ward E, et al. Cancer statistics 2008. CA Cancer J Clin 2008;58:71–96.
2. Van Cutsem E, Nordlinger B, Adam R, et al. Towards a pan-European consensus on the treatment of patients with colorectal liver metastases. Eur J Cancer 2006;42:2212–21.
3. Kemeny N. Presurgical chemotherapy in patients being considered for liver resection. Oncologist 2007;12:825–39.
4. Saunders M, Iveson T. Management of advanced colorectal cancer: state of the art. Br J Cancer 2006;95:131–8.
5. Jonker DJ, Maroun JA, Kocha W. Survival benefit of chemotherapy in metastatic colorectal cancer: a meta-analysis of randomised controlled trials. Br J Cancer 2000;82:1789–94.
6. Douillard JY, Cunningham D, Roth AD, et al. Irinotecan combined with fluorouracil compared with fluorouracil alone as first-line treatment for metastatic colorectal cancer: a multicentre randomised trial. Lancet 2000;355:1041–7.
7. Saltz LB, Cox JV, Blanke C, et al. Irinotecan plus fluorouracil and leucovorin for metastatic colorectal cancer. N Engl J Med 2000;343:905–14.
8. Kohne CH, van Cutsem E, Wils J, et al. Phase III study of weekly high-dose infusional fluorouracil plus folinic acid with or without irinotecan in patients with metastatic colorectal cancer: European Organisation for Research and Treatment of Cancer Gastrointestinal Group Study 40986. J Clin Oncol 2005;23:4856–65.
9. Giacchetti S, Perpoint B, Zidani R, et al. Phase III multicenter randomized trial of oxaliplatin added to chronomodulated fluorouracil-leucovorin as first-line treatment of metastatic colorectal cancer. J Clin Oncol 2000;181:136–47.

10. De Gramont A, Figer A, Seymour M, et al. Leucovorin and fluorouracil with or without oxali-platin as first-line treatment in advanced colorectal cancer. J Clin Oncol 2000;18:2938–47.
11. Tournigand C, Andre T, Achille E, et al. FOLFIRI followed by FOLFOX6 or the reverse sequence in advanced colorectal cancer: a randomized GERCOR study. J Clin Oncol 2004; 22:229–37.
12. Grothey A, Sargent D, Goldberg RM, Schmoll HJ. Survival of patients with advanced colorec-tal cancer improves with the availability of fluorouracil-leucovorin, irinotecan, and oxaliplatin in the course of treatment. J Clin Oncol 2004;22:1209–14.
13. Stangl R, Altendorf-Hofmann A, Charnley RM, Scheele J. Factors influencing the natural history of colorectal liver metastases. Lancet 1994;343:1405–10.
14. Fong Y, Cohen AM, Fortner JG, et al. Liver resection for colorectal metastases. J Clin Oncol 1997;15:938–46.
15. Registry of Hepatic Metastases. Resection of the liver for colorectal carcinoma metastases: a multi-institutional study of indications for resection. Surgery 1988;103:278–88.
16. Adson MA. Resection of liver metastases – when is it worthwhile? World J Surg 1987;11: 511–20.
17. Scheele J, Stang R, Altendorf-Hofmann A, Paul M. Resection of colorectal liver metastases. World J Surg 1995;19:59–71.
18. Scheele J, Altendorf-Hofmann A, Grube T, Hohenberger W, Stangl R, Schmidt K. Resection of colorectal liver metastases. What prognostic factors determine patient selection? Chirurg 2001;72:547–60.
19. Jaeck D, Bachellier P, Guiguet M, et al. Long-term survival following resection of colorectal hepatic metastases. Association Francaise de Chirurgie. Br J Surg 1997;84:977–80.
20. Shah SA, Haddad R, Al-Sukhni W, et al. Surgical resection of hepatic and pulmonary metas-tases from colorectal carcinoma. J Am Coll Surg 1006;202:468–75.
21. Elias D, Sideris L, Pocard M, et al. Results of R0 resection for colorectal liver metastases associated with extrahepatic disease. Ann Surg Oncol 2004;11:274–80.
22. Adam R. Chemotherapy and surgery: new perspectives on the treatment of unresectable liver metastases. Ann Oncol 2003;14(Suppl. 2):ii13–6.
23. Bismuth H, Adam R, Levi F, et al. Resection of nonresectable liver metastases from colorectal cancer after neoadjuvant chemotherapy. Ann Surg 1996;224:509–20.
24. Giacchetti S, Itzhaki M, Gruia G, et al. Long-term survival of patients with unresectable colorectal cancer liver metastases following infusional chemotherapy with 5-fluorouracil, leucovorin, oxaliplatin and surgery. Ann Oncol 1999;10:663–9.
25. Adam R, Avisar E, Ariche A, et al. Five-year survival following hepatic resection after neo-adjuvant therapy for nonresectable colorectal. Ann Surg Oncol 2001;8:347–53.
26. Pozzo C, Basso M, Cassano A, et al. Neoadjuvant treatment of unresectable liver disease with irinotecan and 5-fluorouracil plus folinic acid in colorectal cancer patients. Ann Oncol 2004;15:933–9.
27. Folprecht G, Grothey A, Alberts S, Raab HR, Köhne CH. Neoadjuvant treatment of unresect-able colorectal liver metastases: correlation between tumour response and resection rates. Ann Oncol 2005;16:1311–9.
28. Falcone A, Masi G, Allegrini G, et al. Biweekly chemotherapy with oxaliplatin, irinotecan, infusional Fluorouracil, and leucovorin: a pilot study in patients with metastatic colorectal cancer. J Clin Oncol 2002;20:4006–14.
29. Masi G, Allegrini G, Cupini S, et al. First line treatment of metastatic colorectal cancer with irinotecan, oxaliplatin and 5-fluorouracil/leucovorin (FOLFOXIRI): results of phase II study with a simplified biweekly schedule. Ann Oncol 2004;15:1766–72.
30. Falcone A, Ricci S, Brunetti I, et al. Phase III trial of infusional fluorouracil, leucovorin, oxaliplatin, and irinotecan (FOLFOXIRI) compared with infusional fluorouracil, leucovorin, and irinotecan (FOLFIRI) as first-line treatment of metastatic colorectal cancer: the Gruppo Oncologico Nord Ovest. J Clin Oncol 2007;25:1670–6.

31. Falcone A, Andreuccetti M, Brunetti I, et al. Updated results, multivariate and subgroups analysis confirm improved activity and efficacy for FOLFOXIRI versus FOLFIRI in the G.O.N.O. randomized phase III study in metastatic colorectal cancer (MCRC). Proc Am Soc Clin Oncol 2007 (abstract 4026).
32. Barone C, Nuzzo G, Cassano A, et al. Final analysis of colorectal cancer patients treated with irinotecan and 5-fluorouracil plus folinic acid neoadjuvant chemotherapy for unresectable liver metastases. Br J Cancer 2007;97:1035–9.
33. Leonard GD, Brenner B, Kemeny NE. Neoadjuvant chemotherapy before liver resection for patients with unresectable liver metastases from colorectal carcinoma. J Clin Oncol 2005;23:2038–48.

Color Plates

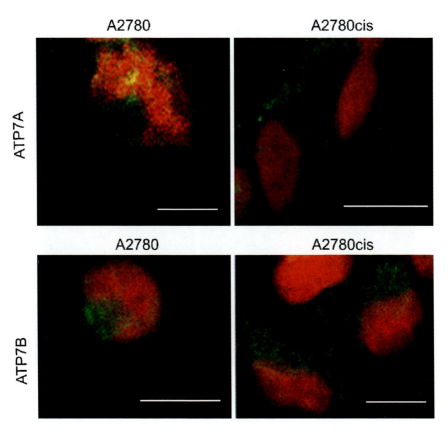

Chapter 13, Fig. 1 Immunofluorescence localization of ATP7A and ATP7B (both *green*) in A2780 and A2780cis cells. Cell nuclei were stained with propidium iodide (*red*). Scale bar, 10 μm

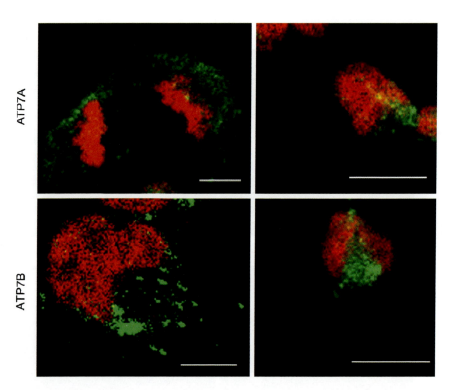

Chapter 13, Fig. 2 Immunofluorescence localization of ATP7A and ATP7B (both *green*) in A2780 cells after cisplatin exposure for 1 h (images on the *left*) and subsequent incubation of the cells in the drug-free medium for 1 h (images on the *right*). Cell nuclei were stained with propidium iodide (*red*). Scale bar, 10 μm

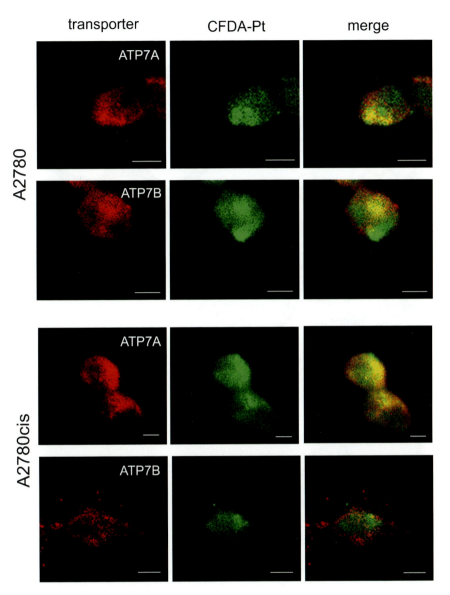

Chapter 13, Fig. 4 Co-localization of CFDA-Pt (*green*) and fluorescent markers for ATP7A and ATP7B (both *red*) in A2780 and A2780cis cells. *Yellow*, the structure is positive for both CFDA-Pt and protein markers. Scale bar, 5 μm

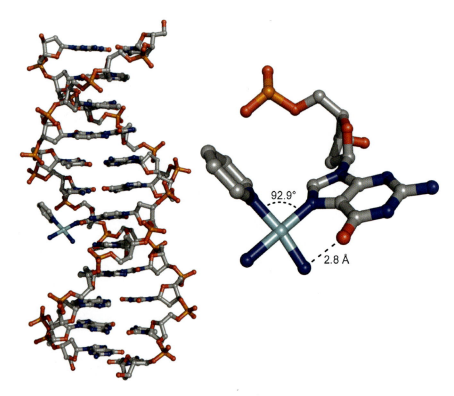

Chapter 17, Fig. 8 The structure of cDPCP -damaged DNA duplex

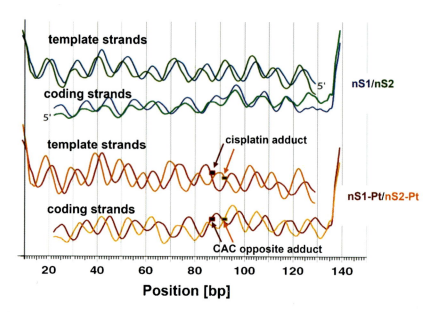

Chapter 17, Fig. 9 Cisplatin damage overrides the predefined rotational setting pattern of nucleosomes. (see Complete Caption on Page 142)

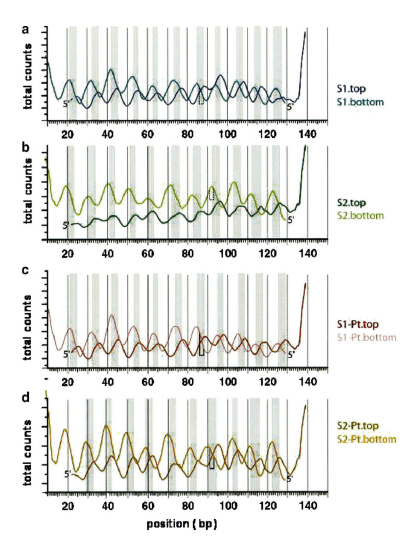

Chapter 17, Fig. 10 Cisplatin adduct faces toward histone core. Gray bars represent areas in which the minor grove is exposed to the solvent (and the major grove faces inwards to the nucleosome). (**a**) The major grove of the unplatinated d(GpTpG) site of S1 trinucleotide faces inwards, (**b**) the major grove of the unplatinated d(GpTpG) site of S2 faces to the side, (**c, d**), the major grove of the platinated d(GpTpG) sites face in both cases inwards. Modified based on Fig. 4 of (25)

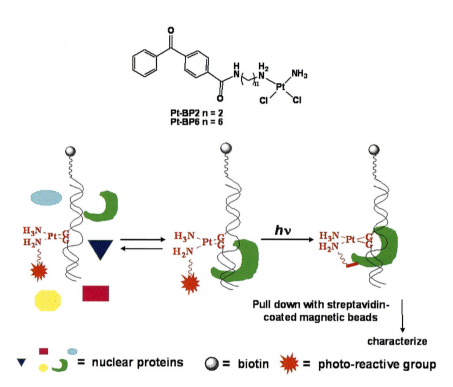

Pt-BP2 n = 2
Pt-BP6 n = 6

Pull down with streptavidin-coated magnetic beads

characterize

▼ ■ ● ● = nuclear proteins   ○ = biotin   ✺ = photo-reactive group

Chapter 17, Fig. 12 Structure of the photoactive benzophenone-modified cisplatin analogue and the methodology used to identify proteins that interact with cisplatin–DNA adducts see ref. (31)

CP-ammine-H Bonds   OX-ammine-H Bonds

5' side: A5N7   5' side: A5N7, equatorial H, axial H
3' side: G7O6   3' side: G7O6, eqatorial H only

5' side A5N7	3' side G7O6	% H bond occupancy
CP-DNA adduct		
+	−	40.2% ⎫ Total 5' = 74.2%
+	+	34.0% ⎭
−	+	13.3% ⎫ Total 3' = 47.3%
−	−	12.5%
OX-DNA adduct		
+ (ax)	−	7.7%
+ (eq)	−	6.0% ⎫ Total 5' = 58.1%
+ (ax)	+	3.5%
+ (eq)	+	40.9% ⎭ Total 3' =78.7%
−	+	34.3%
−	−	7.6%

Chapter 19, Fig. 2 Hydrogen bonds between Pt-amine hydrogens and surrounding bases in the AGGC sequence context. (See complete caption on page 164)

Chapter 19, Fig. 3 Hydrogen bonds between Pt-amine hydrogens and surrounding bases in the TGGA sequence context. Structures illustrating observed hydrogen bond formation are shown in the *upper panel*. Table indicates the percent hydrogen bond occupancy (the % of time that the hydrogen bond is observed during the trajectory) for each of those hydrogen bonds

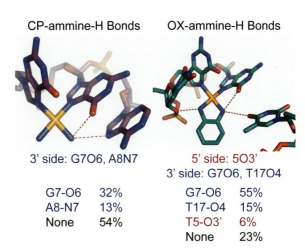

CP-ammine-H Bonds   OX-ammine-H Bonds

3' side: G7O6, A8N7   5' side: 5O3'
                        3' side: G7O6, T17O4

G7-O6	32%		G7-O6	55%
A8-N7	13%		T17-O4	15%
None	54%		T5-O3'	6%
			None	23%

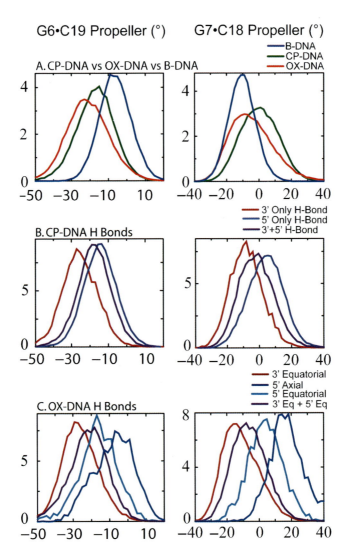

Chapter 19, Fig. 4 Effect of patterns of hydrogen bond formation on the frequency distribution of G6·C19 and G7·C18 propeller twist for CP- and OX-GG adducts in the AGGC sequence context. (**a**) Overall frequency distribution for CP-GG (*green*), OX-GG (*red*) and undamaged DNA (*blue*). (**b**) Effect of hydrogen bond pattern on the frequency distribution for CP-GG adducts (5′ A5N7 = *blue*, 3′ G7O6 = *red* & both 5′ and 3′ = *purple*). (**c**) Effect of hydrogen bond pattern on the frequency distribution for OX-GG adducts (5′ axial A5N7 = *blue*, 5′ equatorial A5N7 = *cyan*, 3′ equatorial G7O6 = *red* & both 5′ equatorial and 3′ equatorial = *purple*)

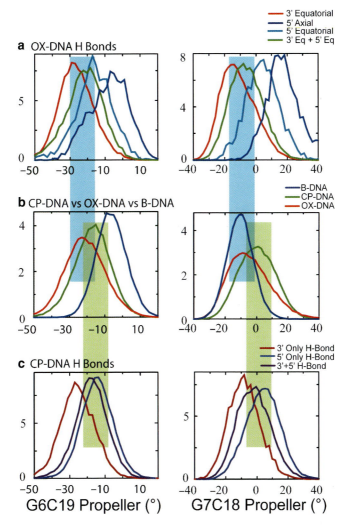

Chapter 19, Fig. 5 Correlation between patterns of hydrogen bond formation and differences in the frequency distribution of G6·C19 and G7·C18 propeller twist for CP- and OX-<u>GG</u> adducts in the A<u>GG</u>C sequence context. (**a**) Effect of hydrogen bond pattern on the frequency distribution for OX-<u>GG</u> adducts (5′ axial A5N7 = *blue*, 5′ equatorial A5N7 = *cyan*, 3′ equatorial <u>G</u>7O6 = *red* & both 5′ equatorial and 3′ equatorial = *green*). (**b**) Overall frequency distribution for CP-<u>GG</u> (*green*), OX-<u>GG</u> (*red*) and undamaged DNA (*blue*). (**c**) Effect of hydrogen bond pattern on the frequency distribution for CP-<u>GG</u> adducts (5′ A5N7 = *blue*, 3′ <u>G</u>7O6 = *red* & both 5′ and 3′ = *purple*). *Blue rectangle* indicates correlation between the frequency distribution associated with the most frequently formed hydrogen bonds for OX-<u>GG</u> (total hydrogen bond occupancy for 3′ equatorial plus 3′ and 5′ = 78.7%) and the overall frequency distribution for OX-<u>GG</u> adducts. *Green rectangle* indicates correlation between the frequency distribution associated with the most frequently formed hydrogen bonds for CP-<u>GG</u> (total hydrogen bond occupancy for 5′ A5N7 plus 5′ and 3′ = 74.2%) and the overall frequency distribution for CP-<u>GG</u> adducts

Chapter 21, Fig. 1 Central role of RPA in repair of Pt-DNA lesions and in chromosomal DNA replication. RPA is depicted as the *green heterotrimer*. In the NER complex, the nucleases are *shaded yellow*, TFIIH *orange*, XPA *red*, and the Pt-lesion as the *white circle*. The DNA polymerase and helicase are *shaded purple* and *blue* in the replication complex

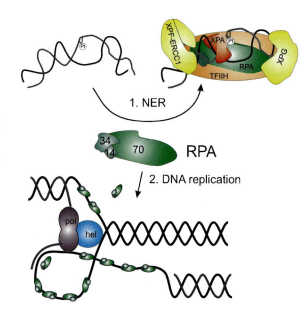

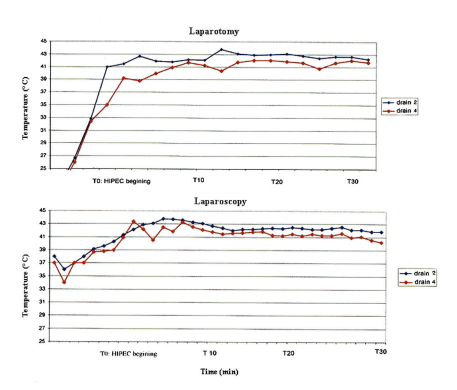

Chapter 37, Fig. 2 Temperature curve of optimal procedure in each group

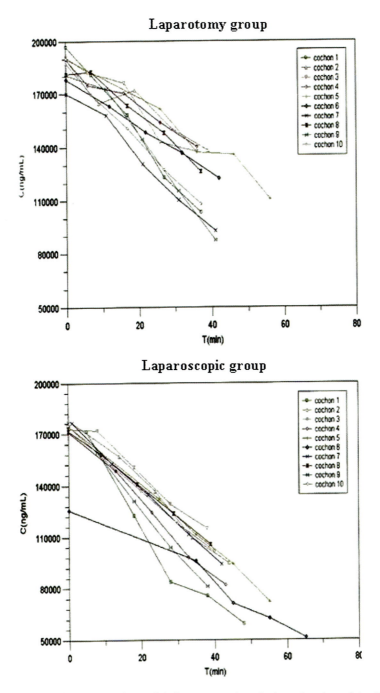

Chapter 37, Fig. 3 Decrease in oxaliplatin concentrations in heated peritoneal instillation (460 mg/m²). First point ($t = 0$ min) corresponds to concentration in the peritoneal fluid before the HIPEC (i.e. before the temperature of 43 °C was reached)

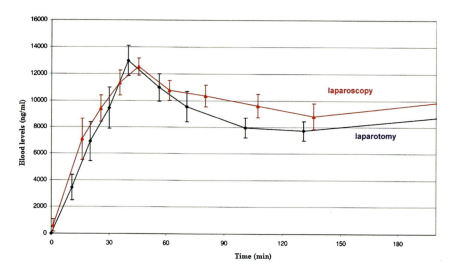

Chapter 37, Fig. 4 Oxaliplatin pharmacokinetics in plasma after heated intraperitoneal chemotherapy ($460 \, mg/m^2$)

Pre-operative Radio-Chemotherapy of Rectal Cancer: Toxicity and Preliminary Results with the Addition of Weekly Oxaliplatin

Francesco Dionisi, Daniela Musio, Gian Paolo Spinelli, Giuseppe Parisi, Nicola Raffetto, Enzo Banelli, and Giovanni Codacci-Pisanelli

Abstract The standard pre-operative treatment of rectal cancer consists of radiotherapy combined with continuous infusion of fluorouracil (FU) at a dose of $200\,mg/m^2$/day. Platinum compounds can increase the anti-tumour activity of radiotherapy and are suitable agents to be combined with FU. We report our experience with the addition of oxaliplatin to radiotherapy and FU in the pre-operative treatment of patients with rectal cancer.

Patients with locally advanced rectal cancer (cT3-T4 and/or N+) were treated with pre-operative 5-FU ($200\,mg/m^2$/day, continuous infusion) and external beam radiation ($45\,Gy$ given to large fields plus a booster dose of $5.4\,Gy$, making a total of $50.4\,Gy$ delivered in 28 daily fractions of $1.8\,Gy$). Oxaliplatin was given at a dose of $50\,mg/m^2$ in 2h once weekly. Inclusion and exclusion criteria for patients were standard and written informed consent was obtained before treatment. Surgery was planned 5 weeks after radiotherapy. Toxicity was graded using the NCI-CTC version 3. Oxaliplatin was suspended in cases of G3 haematological toxicity or G2 neurotoxicity; both oxaliplatin and FU were suspended for G3 non-haematological toxicity.

From November 2006 to January 2008, 21 patients were treated. All completed radiation treatment, and 16 received full dose chemotherapy. Chemotherapy was suspended due to G3 diarrhoea in 3 patients. We observed G2–3 proctitis in 11 patients (particularly painful in three), G1 allergic reactions in 3 of them and G1 neurotoxicity in 12. Fifteen patients were operated on. Of these, eight had a complete pathological response. The histological examination was negative in 3 patients despite the persistence of a palpable mass.

Oxaliplatin can be added to standard chemoradiation in the pre-operative treatment of rectal cancer. Toxicity is increased and requires careful monitoring. The present report and literature data indicate that the anti-tumour efficacy is promising and we look forward to the results of large randomised trials currently in progress.

F. Dionisi, D. Musio, G.P. Spinelli, G. Parisi, N. Raffetto, E. Banelli,
and G. Codacci-Pisanelli (✉)
Department of Experimental Medicine and Pathology, Sapienza University, Rome, Italy
e-mail: Giovanni.Codacci-Pisanelli@uniroma1.it

A. Bonetti et al. (eds.), *Platinum and Other Heavy Metal Compounds
in Cancer Chemotherapy*, DOI: 10.1007/978-1-60327-459-3_33,
© Humana Press, a part of Springer Science + Business Media, LLC 2009

Keywords Rectal cancer; Pre-operative treatment; Radiotherapy; Oxaliplatin

Introduction

The treatment of locally advanced rectal cancer has improved dramatically over the last few years. Surgical resection plays a major role (1), but pre-operative radiotherapy (with or without chemotherapy) is replacing post-operative regimens, which were considered standard in past decades, especially in the USA.

Pre-operative treatment of rectal cancer has several advantages when compared with the post-operative setting. From a biological point of view, poorly oxygenated neoplastic cells that remain after surgical resection are less sensitive to radiation. In terms of clinical results, the volume of bowel exposed to radiation is increased in post-operative treatments, resulting in more toxic effects. Furthermore, neoadjuvant treatments can achieve downsizing and downstaging of tumours, enhancing sphincter preservation for low-lying cancers and reducing the risk of local failure by ensuring a complete (R0) resection. Downstaging of tumours after pre-operative chemoradiation, moreover, is considered an important predictor of improved outcome in terms of better 5-year survival and local control (2).

Sauer et al. (3) showed that pre-operative treatment was associated with fewer G3–4 late complications (19 vs. 39%) and a lower rate of local recurrence (6 vs. 13%) compared with post-operative chemoradiotherapy.

Radiotherapy is generally combined with 5-fluorouracil (FU) given as a daily bolus or as a continuous infusion at a dose of 200–225 mg/m^2/day. At present there are several ongoing studies aimed at testing the role of adding different anti-cancer drugs (oxaliplatin, irinotecan) or biological agents (EGF-receptor antagonists, anti-VEGF antibodies) (4).

Platinum compounds can increase the anti-tumour activity of radiotherapy and are suitable agents for use in combination with FU. Oxaliplatin, for instance, has demonstrated high radiosensitising activity in pre-clinical observations (5) and is widely used in combination with FU in the treatment of advanced colorectal cancer and in the adjuvant treatment of colon cancer.

In this paper, we report our experience of the addition of oxaliplatin to radiotherapy and FU in the pre-operative treatment of patients with rectal cancer. The objectives of this study were the following:

- To demonstrate the feasibility of the combination of oxaliplatin, 5-FU and radiotherapy in terms of toxicity.
- To evaluate the level of downstaging of the tumours.
- To evaluate the percentage of sphincter-saving surgery for low-lying cancers.
- To evaluate the rate of pathological complete responses (pCR) after neoadjuvant treatment.

Disease-free survival (DFS) and overall survival (OS) require a longer follow-up: these are being evaluated and the results will be reported in future.

Patients and Methods

Patients with locally advanced rectal cancer (T3-T4 and/or N+) or low-lying cancers at risk for a definitive stoma were included in the study. Criteria for selection of patients for neoadjuvant treatment included: biopsy-proven adenocarcinoma located less than 12 cm from the anal verge; age ≥18 years; ECOG performance status ≤2; neutrophil count ≥1,500/mm^3; platelet count ≥100,000/mm^3; Hgb ≥10 g/dl; total bilirubin ≤1.5 mg/dl; creatinine ≤1.5 mg/dl.

Written informed consent was obtained before treatment. In the presence of previous pelvic radiotherapy, synchronous tumours, peripheral neuropathy, ischaemic heart disease, pregnancy and psychiatric disorders, patients were considered ineligible for the study. Patients treated with induction chemotherapy before concomitant RT-chemotherapy were excluded from the study, as were patients treated with other anti-neoplastic drugs in addition to 5-FU and oxaliplatin.

The pre-treatment work-up consisted in a complete medical examination, pancolonoscopy, pelvic CT/MRI scans, transrectal ultrasonography (TRUS) and abdomen-chest CT scans. 'Clinical staging' refers to the evaluation based on pre-clinical imaging studies.

Chemotherapy consisted in FU, administered as a continuous infusion at the dose of 200 mg/m^2/day for the entire duration of radiotherapy, and oxaliplatin, which was given at a dose of 50 mg/m^2 in 2 h once weekly for 5–6 weeks. The choice of administering oxaliplatin 5 or 6 times was made according to the patient's age, performance status and tumour characteristics (clinical stage and localization). Pre-medication with antiemetic drugs and corticosteroids was given to all patients.

Toxicity was graded using the NCI-CTC version 3 (6). Oxaliplatin was suspended in cases of G3 haematological toxicity or G2 neurotoxicity; both oxaliplatin and FU were suspended for G3 non-haematological toxicity.

Chemotherapy was resumed at full doses if toxicity resolved within 7 days. Otherwise, it was suspended definitively. No reduction of doses was planned.

Radiation treatment was given using high energy photons (6 MV), generated by a linear accelerator with the patient in the prone position. An immobilisation device (i.e., bellyboard) was used in all patients to reduce the radiation dose to the small bowel. A dose of 45 Gy in 25 daily fractions of 1.8 Gy each was delivered to the whole pelvis using five fields (one posterior, two oblique posterior and two lateral fields). The planned target volume included the tumour mass, all the mesorectum, the internal iliac nodes and the presacral nodes in all cases. External iliac nodes were irradiated if clinically positive and in the case of cT4 cancers. When the neoplastic mass extended into the anal canal, inguinal nodes were also included in the target volume. The L5-S1 junction was the upper border of the treatment volume, while the lower border was localised at a minimum distance of 5 cm from the lowest extent of the tumour. Lateral margins for the posterior field were 2 cm lateral to the widest extent of the bony pelvis. The posterior margin for the lateral fields was <1 cm posterior to the entire sacrum. The anterior limit for the lateral fields as the posterior margin of the symphysis for cT3 lesions and the anterior margin for cT4 tumours.

A three-field boost encompassing the tumour mass plus a 2-cm margin was given in 3 daily fractions of 1.8 Gy each, making a total dose of 50.4 Gy. In the case of cT4 tumours, two more daily fractions were added for a total dose of 54 Gy. The isodose distribution was calculated by means of a 3D treatment planning system.

Surgery was performed within 10 weeks of the end of neoadjuvant treatment. No restrictions were imposed on the technique used by the surgeons. Downstaging was defined as any reduction of stage between the clinical and pathological stage. Pathological complete response (pCR) was defined as the absence of identifiable cancer cells in the specimen after surgical resection of the tumour. In patients treated with transanal endoscopic microsurgery, where no nodes were evaluable, downstaging of the tumour and pCR rate were calculated only on T stage tumours.

Patients with pathological residual disease were encouraged to receive post-operative chemotherapy. In the case of patients with pCR, post-operative chemotherapy was administered at the discretion of the treating oncologist.

Results

From November 2006 to January 2008, 21 patients (13 men and 8 women) were enrolled into the study. Patient characteristics are described in Table 1. The median age was 63 years (range 44–76). Most of the tumours (76%) were localised in the middle-low rectum. At clinical staging, the majority of patients (57%) were classified as T3N+.

Table 1 Patient characteristics

Patient characteristics	No (%)
Male	13 (61.9)
Female	8 (38.1)
Age, median (range)	63.2 (44–76)
ECOG P. Status	
0	8 (38.1)
1	8 (38.1)
2	5 (23.8)
Tumour location	
Upper rectum (≥8 cm from a.v.)	5 (23.8)
Mid rectum (>5 < 8 cm from a.v.)	5 (23.8)
Low rectum (≤5 cm from a.v.)	11 (52.4)
TN clinical stage	
T2N+	1 (4.8)
T3N0	5 (23.8)
T3N+	12 (57.1)
T4N+	3 (14.3)

Compliance with radiotherapy was excellent. All patients were able to receive the full-planned dose (50.4–54 Gy). Radiation treatment was delayed in 4 patients (19%). Delay time varied from 4 to 21 days. Chemotherapy was delivered at full doses (5–6 courses) in 16 patients (76%). Two patients (9%) completed only two cycles of chemotherapy, another two patients completed 3 cycles of chemotherapy, and in one patient chemotherapy was stopped after four courses. Chemotherapy cycles were delayed in 6 patients (28%).

The incidence of acute toxicity is shown in Table 2. No G2 haematological toxicity occurred. We observed G2–3 proctitis (particularly painful in 3 patients) in 11 patients (52%). G3 diarrhoea occurred in 6 patients (28%). Seven patients with low-lying tumours (33%) experienced G2-G3 radiation dermatitis requiring appropriate medication. One patient developed a herpes infection associated with ≥G2

Table 2 Acute toxicity according to NCI CTC version 3.0. Number of patients ($n=21$) and percentage in brackets

Acute toxicity	G1	G2	G3	G4	G5
Blood – bone marrow					
Neutrophils – granulocytes	2 (9.5%)				
Haemoglobin					
Platelets					
Allergy – immunology					
All reaction – hypersensitivity	3 (14.3%)	1 (4.8%)			
Constitutional symptoms					
Fatigue	4 (19.0%)	1 (4.8%)			
Fever	1 (4.8%)				
Dermatology – skin					
Pruritus – itching	1 (4.8%)				
Rash – desquamation	4 (19.0%)				
Radiation dermatitis	3 (14.3%)	3 (14.3%)	4 (19.0%)		
Infection					
Opp. infection associated with ≥G2 lymphopenia		1 (4.8%)			
Gastrointestinal					
Enteritis – colitis		1 (4.8%)			
Constipation	2 (9.5%)				
Diarrhoea	4 (19.0%)	3 (14.3%)	6 (28.6%)		
Proctitis	1 (4.8%)	5 (23.8%)	6 (28.6%)		
Neurology					
Neuropathy – sensory	12 (57.1%)				
Pain					
Pelvic pain	1 (4.8%)	6 (28.6%)	6 (28.6%)		
Abdominal pain or cramping	3 (14.3%)				
Chest pain		1 (4.8%)			
Renal – genitourinary					
Dysuria – painful urination		4 (19.0%)			
Urinary frequency		4 (19.0%)			

lymphopenia; neoadjuvant treatment was immediately discontinued and resumed at full doses after complete recovery. Another patient experienced G2 allergic reaction-hypersensitivity after the first administration of chemotherapy. Chemotherapy was discontinued and resumed after 1 week. During the second administration G2 allergic reaction occurred again and chemotherapy was suspended definitively. Reversible G1 neurotoxicity related to oxaliplatin was observed in 12 (57%) patients. One patient experienced G2 chest pain at the end of neoadjuvant treatment; cardiological examinations were negative. Two weeks later he had a myocardial infarction and died.

As on February 2008, 15 of 21 patients had undergone surgery. The median time to surgery was 8 weeks. R0 resection was achieved in all patients (100%).

A sphincter-saving surgical procedure was feasible in 14 of 15 patients (93%): 11 patients underwent anterior resection; total mesorectal excision (TME) was performed in 8 (46%) patients, in the case of cancers located in the mid and distal rectum. One patient received laparoscopic TME, other 2 patients were treated with transanal endoscopic microsurgery, and in only one case did abdominoperineal resection with a permanent stoma (Miles surgery) prove necessary.

Surgical complications occurred in 4 patients (26%, consisting in one anastomotic leak, one post-operative fever, one retrorectal abscess and one case of post-operative fistula.

Tumour downstaging occurred in 13 patients (87%). One patient with a clinical T3N1 tumour completed only 2 cycles of chemotherapy owing to G3 diarrhoea and did not achieve any downstaging at surgery (pT3pN1). The other patient with no downstaging suspended chemotherapy after 3 cycles for pelvic pain–proctitis G3; he underwent abdominoperineal resection for a very low-lying cancer and examination of the pathological specimen revealed a pT3pN0 tumour.

A pathological complete response (pCR) was observed in 8 of 15 patients (53%). The two patients treated with TEM experienced a pCR and a pT2 disease, respectively, at surgery. When detected, nodes proved negative in 11 of 13 cases (85%).

Comparison of T and N stages before neoadjuvant treatment and after surgery is reported in Tables 3 and 4.

Table 3 T stage comparison before neoadjuvant treatment and after surgery ($n = 15$)

Pre-treatment	After surgery				
	pT0	pT1	pT2	pT3	pT4
T2 ($n = 1$)	1				
T3 ($n = 13$)	7	2	2	2	
T4 ($n = 1$)		1			

Table 4 N stage comparison before neoadjuvant treatment and after surgery ($n = 13^a$)

Pre-treatment	After surgery	
	pN0	pN+
N0 ($n = 3$)	3	
N+ ($n = 10$)	8	2

ᵃIn two patients nodes were not detected because of TEM surgery

Discussion

The standard treatment for locally advanced rectal cancer consists in surgery and radiotherapy. Whether radiation treatment should be given before or after tumour removal, and the dose and scheduling to be used, are still a matter of debate. Pre-operative external beam radiotherapy is generally given in 5–6 weeks, and is combined with continuous infusion of 5-FU.

The CAO/ARO/AIO-94 trial compared pre- and post-operative radiotherapy, demonstrating that neoadjuvant treatment is associated with fewer G3–G4 complications. There was, however, no significant difference in overall survival (76 vs. 74% at 5 years) and the rates of distant metastases in the two groups were similar (36 vs. 38%). These data suggest the need for intensified neoadjuvant radiochemotherapy in order to improve the prognosis of patients affected by rectal cancer.

The rationale for intensifying neoadjuvant treatment is based on the following factors:

- Potential micrometastases can be better controlled
- Improved downstaging of tumours, which the results of a number of studies (7, 8) have shown to be a good predictor of outcome and survival
- Improved local control. In the German rectal cancer study the rates of local recurrence for advanced stages of disease even in the neoadjuvant group are still high (9)
- The rate of sphincter-saving surgery for low-lying cancers can be increased
- Finally, by intensifying neoadjuvant radiochemotherapy the pCR rate can be improved. According to some studies (10), complete responders after chemoradiation have a better prognosis in terms of local recurrence and survival compared with incomplete responders

Some anti-neoplastic drugs such as irinotecan, oxaliplatin, EGF receptor antagonists and vascular EGF antibodies are being studied in various neoadjuvant protocols (11–13) to identify the best combination of drugs to be administered in new intensified neoadjuvant treatments for advanced rectal cancer.

Oxaliplatin, a third-generation platinum analogue, is a good radiosensitising agent, which has also been shown to have a synergistic anti-tumour activity with 5-FU (14).

In our study, we evaluated the addition of oxaliplatin to the standard neoadjuvant treatment for locally advanced rectal cancer. The main aim of our study was to test the feasibility of the combination of oxaliplatin and 5-FU plus radiotherapy in terms of toxicity and compliance with treatment.

Since radiation treatment combined with the continuous infusion of FU is the standard pre-operative regimen, we considered the addition of oxaliplatin acceptable only if it would not require any reduction in the dose of FU and/or of radiotherapy.

The toxic side-effects that we observed are similar to those reported in other studies in which oxaliplatin was administered once a week (15, 16). In other trials where oxaliplatin was given in different schedules (monthly, twice a month or

once every 3 weeks) the rates of neurotoxicity observed were significatively higher
(17). This difference seems to indicate that dose fractionation in weekly regimens
might result in lower toxicity.

The toxicity rates experienced by patients enrolled in our study are slightly higher
than those observed with conventional neoadjuvant treatment regimens (18), but with
careful monitoring and proper medical therapy the majority of patients were able to
complete the full pre-operative treatment. Radiotherapy, in particular, was delivered
at full doses to all patients, and radiation treatment was delayed in only four cases
(19%). Compliance with chemotherapy was also high: 16 of 21 patients (76%), in fact,
were able to receive full doses of chemotherapy. A delay in the administration of antineoplastic drugs occurred in 6 patients (28%). These compliance rates with chemotherapy are higher than those of other studies: Ryan et al. (15) reported that only 56%
of patients completed all cycles of oxaliplatin, but in their study oxaliplatin was given
once weekly 6 times at doses of $60\,mg/m^2$, making a total dose of $360\,mg/m^2$, which
is higher than the total dose in our study (250–$300\,mg/m^2$). In contrast, in the study
by Rodel et al. (19), 89% of patients received full doses of chemotherapy, but in their
case the total dose of oxaliplatin administered was only $200\,mg/m^2$. Aschele et al. (16),
in their original article published in 2005, recommended a dose of oxaliplatin that
was the same as that indicated by Ryan ($60\,mg/m^2$ for 6 cycles), but compliance with
chemotherapy was greater (84 vs. 56%).

Another aim of our present study was to evaluate the level of downstaging
induced by the combination of oxaliplatin, 5-FU and external radiotherapy. Our
preliminary results are encouraging: 15 patients underwent surgery, and downstaging occurred in 13 cases (87%). It is interesting to observe that two patients with
no evidence of downstaging at pathological examination had not completed the full
course of chemotherapy.

The prognostic relevance of downstaging after neoadjuvant treatment in terms
of local control and survival is demonstrated by several studies. Janjan et al.
(8) observed that any grade of downstaging after pre-operative treatment can
improve the rates of disease-free survival and the incidence of distant recurrences.
Valentini et al. (20), in a retrospective study of 165 patients affected by locally
advanced rectal cancer (LARC), found that patients with a pathological response
after pre-operative radiochemotherapy had a uniformly favourable long-term outcome, irrespective of their initial stage. The authors conclude that the behaviour
of downstaged cancers can be comparable to that of T1-T2 tumours treated with
surgery only. In Kaminsky-Forrett et al.'s experience (2), patients with downstaging had significantly higher cancer-specific 5-year survival rates than the group
without downstaging (100 vs. 45%, respectively). These findings justify the
efforts to improve tumour response before surgery, and intensifying radiochemotherapy with the addition of weekly oxaliplatin would appear to be a step in the
right direction.

We also evaluated the rate of sphincter preservation for low-lying cancer after
radiochemotherapy. The preliminary results indicate that this neoadjuvant treatment
is effective in allowing sphincter-saving surgery at this time. Only one of 8 patients
(12.5%) at risk for a permanent stoma underwent Miles surgery after neoadjuvant

therapy. In this case, chemotherapy was suspended after only 3 cycles for G3 anorectal pain and no downstaging was found in this patient at the pathological examination.

A pCR after neoadjuvant treatment is a crucial objective of radiochemotherapy even if the role of pCR in predicting a better outcome in terms of lower recurrence and survival is still debatable. In a study by Onaitis et al. (21), no difference was found in local recurrence, and disease-free survival between the pCR group and the non-pCR group. In other studies, opinions are different: in the study by Garcia-Aguilar et al. (22) based on 168 patients treated by neoadjuvant chemoradiation followed by total mesorectal excision, a pCR was associated with improved local control and survival. In another study, the recurrence rate and the 5-year disease-free survival rate significantly improved in patients with pCR compared with patients with residual disease in the specimen (23).

In patients treated with standard neoadjuvant treatment for LARC, the range of pCR varies from 8 to 10%. In studies which include oxaliplatin in pre-operative treatment (24–27), summarised in Table 5, the pCR rate is higher and varies from 12 to 28%.

The preliminary data of our study are quite surprising: 8 of 15 patients (53%) undergoing surgery at this time experienced a pCR. Obviously, the number of patients who underwent surgery is still small and the complete results of the entire study population must be awaited before we can consider this pCR rate as the definitive rate for our work.

However, a number of considerations are necessary. First of all, in our study the median interval between the end of chemoradiotherapy and surgery was 8.6 weeks (range 5–10) in the group of pathological complete responders. In standard neo-adjuvant treatment for LARC, resection is typically performed within 5–8 weeks of the end of radiotherapy. Increasing the RT-surgery interval can improve rates of downstaging and pathological responses, as demonstrated by recent work on this aspect (28). In this study, operative difficulty and morbidity were not increased by prolonging the RT-surgery interval and the rate of post-operative complications was 26%. Delaying surgery after pre-operative treatment appears safe, with morbidity and mortality similar to those observed in surgery performed less than 8 weeks after chemoradiotherapy (29).

Table 5 Selected phase II trials with oxaliplatin as part of pre-operative chemoradiation therapy for locally advanced rectal cancer

Trial (ref)	Oxaliplatin dose (mg/m^2)	Schedule (days)	N	Grade III/IV diarrhoea (%)	Path CR (%)
CALGB-89901 (15)	60	1, 8, 15, 22, 29, 36	32	33	25
Aschele et al. (16)	60	1, 8, 15, 22, 29, 36	25	16	28
Pinto et al. (12)	60	1, 8, 15, 22, 29, 36	26	14	12
Alonso et al. (24)	60	1, 8, 15, 22, 29, 36	52	7.5	23
Machielis et al. (25)	50	1, 8, 15, 22, 29	40	30	14
Rödel et al. (26)	50	1, 8, 22, 29	104	12	16
Rödel et al. (19)	50–60	1, 8, 22, 29	32	12.5	19
Glynne-Jones et al. (11)	130	1, 29	94	9	17
Carraro et al. (28)	25	1–4, 29–32	22	27	25

Another element of bias in our work could be that not all complete responders could be evaluated in terms of the pathological nodal stage: one patient, in fact, underwent transanal endoscopic microsurgery (TEM), and with this technique no nodes were detected. This patient experienced a complete response only in terms of T stage. The TEM procedure, introduced by Buess in 1983, is a conservative technique that allows the surgeon to perform a precise excision of a rectal tumour via a transanal approach. According to some authors (30), this procedure is justified in neoadjuvated T2 tumours without evidence of nodal spread, because rates of local recurrences and survival are similar to those of patients undergoing less conservative surgery.

Other authors are going even further, following the positive long-term results of the landmark study by Habr-Gama et al. (31) on avoidance of surgery for selected patients with radiological and clinical evidence of a complete response after radio-chemotherapy. A prospective trial (32) at the Royal Mardsen Hospital and Pelican Cancer Foundation is currently being conducted to investigate a non-operative approach for complete responders. Patients with locally advanced rectal cancer with a complete response (as evidenced by MRI 4 weeks after completion of pre-operative CRT and confirmed by MRI at 8 weeks) will avoid surgery and enter a strict programme of MRI, clinical, and endoscopic follow up.

In our opinion, surgery still remains the cornerstone in the treatment of LARC. At present there is no completely reliable imaging technique capable of diagnosing a complete response after neoadjuvant treatment. In our experience, patients were evaluated 4–6 weeks after the end of neoadjuvant treatment by means of CT scan and MRI. In patients with a pCR at surgery, MRI often registered a focal area of low signal intensity at the site of disease, but whether that residual scar actually represented absence of tumour cells could not be determined with certainty by the radiologists. A combination of PET and MRI could improve the accuracy in predicting complete response to radiochemotherapy (33). The rising pCR rates with intensified neoadjuvant radiochemotherapy and the development of modern imaging techniques could lead in future to more conservative approaches or even to 'wait and see' protocols for very selected cases.

In summary, the preliminary results of our study show that the addition of weekly oxaliplatin to the standard neoadjuvant treatment for LARC is feasible. Toxicity is increased and requires careful monitoring. The early data on downstaging and pCR rate are encouraging and we look forward to the results of two large randomised trials currently in progress, namely, the USA NSABP R-04 and the Italian STAR trials investigating the role of oxaliplatin in pre-operative treatment of rectal cancer. In the STAR study, patients are randomised to continuous 5-FU infusion concomitantly with radiotherapy up to the dose of 50.4 Gy or to the same combination plus oxaliplatin at the dose of 60 mg/m^2 administered once weekly 6 times.

The initial purpose of the NSABP R-04 study was to compare pre-operative radiation therapy and the oral fluoropyrimidine capecitabine with pre-operative radiation therapy and continuous iv infusion (CVI) of 5-FU in the treatment of patients with operable carcinoma of the rectum. As the study was about to be launched, the whole oxaliplatin issue came to head and the design of the study was changed. Patients are now randomised to four groups (5-FU-RT, 5-FU-RT and OHP, capecitabine-RT, capecitabine-RT and OHP), and the final results of the study should clarify the role of capecitabine and that of oxaliplatin.

Conclusions

The role of neoadjuvant treatment of rectal cancer is still debated, mostly because few studies have shown it to have a positive effect on overall survival. It is important to note, however, that local relapse of rectal cancer generally has a tremendous effect on the quality of life of patients and local-disease-free survival might therefore be considered a relevant endpoint. Our data, though preliminary, suggest that adding oxaliplatin to the standard treatment is feasible and results in an improvement in pCR. Longer follow-up will tell us whether this more intensive chemotherapy will also have an impact on distant metastases and survival. This would then need to be confirmed in a phase III trial.

References

1. Heald RJ, Husband EM, Rtall RDH, et al. Recurrence and survival after total mesorectal excision for rectal cancer. Lancet 1986;1:1479–82.
2. Kaminsky-Forrett M, Conroy T, Luporsi E. Prognostic implications of downstaging following preoperative radiation therapy for operable T3–T4 rectal cancer. Int J Radiat Biol Phys 1998;42:935–41.
3. Sauer R, Becker H, Hohenberger W, et al. Preoperative versus post-operative chemoradiotherapy for rectal cancer. N Eng J Med 2004;351:1731–41.
4. Fernando HF, Hurwitz IH. Targeted therapy of colorectal cancer: clinical experience with bevacizumab. Oncologist 2004;9(suppl 1):11–8.
5. Blackstock AW. Hess S, Chaney S, et al. Oxaliplatin: in vitro evidence of its radiosensitizing activity. Preclinical observations relevant to clinical trials. Int J Radiat Oncol Biol Phys 1999: 45:253–4.
6. Cancer Therapy Evaluation Program. Common Terminology Criteria for Adverse Events, Version 3.0, 9 August 2006, (http://ctep.cancer.gov).
7. Osti MF, Valeriani M, Masoni L, et al. Neoadjuvant chemoradiation for locally advanced carcinoma of the rectum. Tumori 2004;90:303–9.
8. Janjan NA, Abruzzese J, Padzur R, et al. Prognostic implications of response to preoperative infusional chemoradiation in locally advanced rectal cancer. Radiother Oncol 1999;51:153–60.
9. Kalutke G, Fietkau R. Intensified neoadjuvant radiochemotherapy for locally advancer rectal cancer: a review. Int J Colorectal Dis 2007;22:457–65.
10. Biondo S, Navarro M, Marti-Rague J, et al. Response to neoadjuvant therapy for rectal cancer: influence of long-term results. Colorectal Dis 2005;7:472–9.
11. Glynne-Jones R, Falk S, Maughan T, et al. Results of preoperative radiation and oxaliplatin in combination with 5-fuorouracil (5-Fu) and leucovorin (Lv). Proc Asco 2000;19:310a (abstract).
12. Pinto C, Gentile Al, Iacopino A, et al. Neoadjuvant therapy with oxaliplatin (oxa) and 5-fluorouracil (5-Fu) continuous infusion (Ci) combined with radiotherapy (Rt) in rectal cancer: first results of the Bologna Phase II Study. Proc Asco 2004:3557 (Abstract).
13. Harris M. Monoclonal antibodies as therapeutic agents for rectal cancer. Lancet Oncol 2004; 5:292–302.

14. Cividalli A, Ceciarelli F, Lividi E, et al. Radiosensitization by oxaliplatin in a mouse adenocarcinoma: influence of treatment schedule. Int J Radiat Oncol Biol Phys 2002;52: 1092–8.

15. Ryan DP, Niedzwiecki D, Hollid D. Phase I-II study of preoperative oxaliplatin, fluorouracil, and external-beam radiation therapy in patients with locally advanced rectal cancer: cancer and leukaemia group B 89901. J Clin Oncol 2006;24:2557–62.

16. Aschele C, Friso ML, Pucciarelli S, et al. A phase I-II study of weekly oxaliplatin, 5-fluorouracil continuous infusion and preoperative radiotherapy in locally advanced rectal cancer. Ann Oncol 2005;16:1140–1146.

17. Gerard JP, Chapet O, Nemoz C, et al. Preoperative concurrent chemoradiotherapy in locally advanced rectal cancer with high dose radiation and oxaliplatin-containing regimen: the Lyon R0–04 phase II trial. J Clin Oncol 2003;21:1119–124.

18. Chari RS, Tyler DS, Anscher MS, et al. Preoperative radiation and chemotherapy in the treatment of adenocarcinoma of the rectum. Ann Surg 1995;221:778–786.

19. Rodel C, Grabenbauer GG, Papadopoulos T, et al. Phase I-II trial of capecitabine, oxaliplatin and radiation for rectal cancer. J Clin Oncol 2003;21:3098–104.

20. Valentini V, Coco C, Picciocchi A, et al. Does downstaging predict improved outcome after preoperative chemoradiation for extraperitoneal locally advanced rectal cancer? A long-term analysis of 165 patients. Int J Radiat Biol Phys 2002;53:664–74.

21. Onaitis MW, Noone RB, Fields R, et al. Complete response to neoadjuvant chemoradiation for rectal cancer does not influence survival. Ann Surg Oncol 2001;8(10):801–806.

22. Garcia-Aguilar J, Hernandez De Anda E, Sirivongs P, et al. A pathological complete response to preoperative chemoradiation is associated with lower local recurrence and improved survival in rectal cancer patients treated by mesorectal excision. Dis Colon Rectum 2003;46:298–304.

23. Kuo L, Liu M, Jian JJ, et al. Is final TNM staging a predictor for survival in locally advanced rectal cancer after preoperative chemoradiation therapy? Ann Surg Oncol 2007;14:2766–72.

24. Alonso V, Salud A, Escudero P, et al. Preoperative chemoradiation with oxaliplatin and 5-fluorouracil in locally advanced rectal carcinoma. J Clin Oncol 2004;22(14S):3607 (abstract)

25. Machiels JP, Duck L, Honhon B, et al. Phase II study of preoperative oxaliplatin, capecitabine and external beam radiation in patient with rectal cancer: the RadioOxCape study. Ann Oncol 2005;16:1898–905.

26. Rodel C, Liersch T, Herman RM, et al. Multicenter phase II trial of chemoradiation with oxaliplatin for rectal cancer. J Clin Oncol 2007;25:110–7.

27. Carraro S, Roca LE, Cartelli C, et al. Radiochemotherapy with short daily infusion of low-dose oxaliplatin, leucovorin, and 5-Fu in T3-T4 unresectable rectal cancer. A phase II study. Int J Radiat Biol Phys 2002;54:397–402.

28. Moore GH, Gittleman AE, Minsky BD, et al. Rate of pathological complete response with increased interval between preoperative combined modality therapy and rectal cancer resection. Dis Col Rectum 2004;47:279–86.

29. Tran CL, Udani HA. Evaluation of safety of increased time interval between chemoradiation and resection for rectal cancer. Am J Surg. 2006;192:873–7.

30. Lezoche G, Baldarelli M, Paganini AM, et al. A prospective randomised study with a 5-year minimum follow-up evaluation of transanal endoscopic microsurgery versus laparoscopic total mesorectal excision after neoadjuvant therapy. Surg Endosc 2008;22:352–8.

31. Habr-Gama A, Perez RO, Nadalin W, et al. Operative versus nonoperative treatment for stage 0 distal rectal cancer following chemoradiation therapy: long term results. Ann Surg 2004;240:711–7.

32. O'Neill BDP, Brown G, Heald RJ. Non operative treatment after neoadjuvant cemoradiotherapy for rectal cancer. Lancet Oncol 2007;8:625–33.

33. Denecke T, Rau B, Hoffman K-T, et al. Comparison of CT, MRI and FDG-PET in response prediction of patients with locally advanced rectal cancer after multimodal preoperative therapy: is there a benefit in using functional imaging? Eur Radiol 2005;115:1658–66.

The Role of Platins in Newly Diagnosed Endometrial Cancer

Paul J. Hoskins

Abstract Twenty percent of women with endometrial cancer will die from it, predominantly from systemic spread. Chemotherapy is, therefore, needed both for "high risk" women at diagnosis (stages III and IV – all histologies; stage II Clear Cell or grade 3; Papillary Serous or MMMT, irrespective of stage) and for relapsers, unless grade 1, when hormones are a preferable initial option. The most active single agents are: the anthracyclines, taxanes and platins; response rates 17–37, 21–67 and 13–14%, respectively. Combinations have proven to be superior in terms of relapse but not survival. Taxane-/platin-containing regimens are the phase III proven best combinations.

The GOG is currently comparing the two "winning combinations", doxorubicin/cisplatin + paclitaxel + GCSF and carboplatin-paclitaxel. As carboplatin-paclitaxel is a more convenient and less toxic regimen, it would be preferable if equally efficacious. It is likely that other platinum doublets are equally good. Platin/vinorelbine or carboplatin-pegylated liposomal doxorubicin have similar RRs to platin/taxane in phase II studies.

Chemotherapy, predominantly cisplatin–doxorubicin, has improved survival in 3 of the 4 phase III studies conducted, in comparison to irradiation.

Progression still was seen in up to 50% (dependant upon stage). Using "platin/taxane" should improve this somewhat, but adding agents directed at molecular targets, e.g., EGFR, VEGF, AKt will be required.

Keywords Endometrial cancer; Taxanes; Combination regimens; Anthracyclines; Platins

Introduction

The role of chemotherapy in endometrial cancer, in comparison to breast and ovarian cancers, has been under appreciated by the oncology community. Reasons for this include: (1) its high curability, 80% or so, with purely local measures;

P.J. Hoskins
British Columbia Cancer Agency, Vancouver, BC, Canada
e-mail: phoskins@bccancer.bc.ca

A. Bonetti et al. (eds.), *Platinum and Other Heavy Metal Compounds in Cancer Chemotherapy*, DOI: 10.1007/978-1-60327-459-3_34,
© Humana Press, a part of Springer Science + Business Media, LLC 2009

(2) an older, less chemotherapy-tolerant population –33% are over 70 at diagnosis and (3) less pharmaceutical industry sponsorship/cooperative group interest – fewer women need chemotherapy compared to those with breast and ovary cancer and so it is of lower priority.

Despite this high cure rate, 20% of women still die from endometrial cancer: 10,000/year in the USA, 12,000/year in Europe and the survival outcomes have altered minimally over the years, a 0.2% average improvement per year from 1994 to 2003. Disseminated disease due to hematogenous, lymphatic or transcoloemic spread is the reason for this. To improve upon this outcome, effective adjuvant chemotherapy is mandatory for those with disseminated disease, be it macroscopic or microscopic.

Ideally, chemotherapy would only be given to those "high tissue" patients with disseminated disease and thus avoid the toxicity/costs in those already cured by surgery. In the future, hopefully, genomic profiling of an individual's cancer will accurately identify those whose cancer is purely localized. Until then, the less accurate standbys of stage, grade and histopathology will have to suffice for risk assessment with the resultant, inevitable over-treatment of some women. At the British Columbia Cancer Agency, we have arbitrarily chosen a risk of death of 25% or greater as mandating the use of chemotherapy. Surgical stage is the single most important predictor (Table 1). All women with spread outside the body of the uterus, i.e., stages II, III or IV, fulfill the 25% or more risk criterion (1). Grade and histopathology can further help by identifying the "at risk" within those with apparent stage I (uterine confined) disease. Then, stage Ic, grade 3 patients will be included, as their survival is 68% at 5 years. Grade also helps us to exclude stage II, grade 1 patients (survival 81–91%). Except for stage Ia, all stage I patients with papillary serous or malignant mixed Mullerian tumors (MMMTs) need chemotherapy, as their survival is 50% or less. MMMTs were earlier regarded as sarcomas but are now recognized as high grade, metaplastic adenocarcinomas (2).

Table 1 Surgical stage and outcomes (1)

Stage	Definition	Pts (%)	5-year OS (%)
IA	Endometrium only	17	90
IB	Inner 50%	36	90
IC	Outer 50%	17	81
IIA	Cervix glands	6	71
IIB	Cervix stroma	7	67
IIIA	Uterine serosa, cytology (+), adnexa	8	60
IIIB	Vagina	2	41
IIIC	Pelvic or para-aortic nodes	4	32
IVA	Bladder, bowel mucosa	1	20
IVB	Distant	3	5

OS overall survival

Table 2 Single-agent activity in endometrial cancer (3, 4)

Drug	Response rate (%)	Drug	Response rate (%)
Cisplatin	4–42	Aminothiadiazole	0
Carboplatin	13–38	Methotrexate	6
Doxorubicin	17–27	Echinomycin	5
Epirubicin	26	Irofulven	4
Pegylated liposomal doxorubicin	10–21	Piroxantrone	7
Paclitaxel	36–77	Cyclophosphamide	0–25
Docetaxel	21–31	Esorubicin	0
5FU	20–23	Idarubicin	10
Topotecan	10–20	Pirarubicin	7
Ifosfamide	15–24	6 mercaptopurine	6
VP16	0–14	Amonafide	8
Hexamethylmelamine	9–30	AMSA	5–25
AZQ	8	Fludarabine	0
Methyl GAG	14	Vincristine	0–18
Piperazinedione	5	Vinblastine	0–12
Galactitol	6	Razoxane	0
Mitoxantrone	0–9		

Single-Agent Activity

The most active drugs (response rates 20–40%) are the platin analogues, anthracyclines, taxanes and 5-fluorouracil (Table 2). Topotecan, ifosfamide and etoposide have a lower degree of activity (3, 4). There is no data with regard to some of the newer agents such as gemcitabine, capecitabine or vinorelbine.

Combination Chemotherapy

A central tenet of medical oncology is that combinations are better than single agents. Historically, drugs were combined if they had different mechanisms of action and no significant additive toxicity; more latterly if they had different mechanisms of resistance. Platin-taxane-based combinations have thus become the current regimen of choice as the result of phase III comparisons. Tables 3 and 4 outline the results of all the phase III comparisons (5–12). As with the single agent data in Table 2, these studies contained both newly diagnosed, advanced patients and those with relapsed disease, with relapsed disease predominant. Only in the taxane era, has improved survival occurred as well as improved response rates.

The current gold standard, for those physicians whose treatment decisions require phase III evidence, is: cisplatin (50 mg/m^2); paclitaxel (160 mg/m^2 over 3 h);

Table 3 Phase III studies – the winners

Reference	Regimens	No. of Patients	RR (%)	PFS (months)	OS (months)
Thigpen (5)	Doxorubicin/cyclophosphamide	144	30	4	7
	Doxorubicin	132	23	3	7
Aapro (6)	Doxorubicin/cisplatin	90	43	8	9
	Doxorubicin	87	17	7	7
Thigpen (7)	Doxorubicin/cisplatin	131	42	6	9
	Doxorubicin	150	25	4	9
Fleming (8)	Doxorubicin/cisplatin/ paclitaxel/GCSF	134	57	8*	15*
	Doxorubicin/cisplatin	129	34	5	12
Weber (9)	Carboplatin/paclitaxel	36	35	8	40(at 15)
	Doxorubicin/cisplatin	34	28	7	27%

RR response rate; *PFS* progression-free survival; *OS* overall survival
*statistically significant

Table 4 Phase III studies: equivalent regimens

Reference	Regimens	No. of Patients	RR (%)	PFS (months)	OS (months)
Gallion (10)	Doxorubicin/cisplatin	169	46	6	11
	Doxorubicin/cisplatin (circadian)	173	49	6	13
Fleming (11)	Doxorubicin/cisplatin	157	40	7	13
	Doxorubicin/paclitaxel/GCSF	160	43	6	14
Long (12)	Doxorubicin/cisplatin	15	20	4	13
(D/C Toxic +++)	MVAC	13	46	7	17

RR response rate; *PFS* progression-free survival; *OS* overall survival

doxorubicin (45 mg/m^2) and G-CSF (days 3–12). This is both a toxic and expensive regimen to deliver. 24% discontinued treatment because of toxicity, 12% had grade 3 or 4 vomiting, and grade 3 or 4 thrombocytopenia occurred in 22% (8). This parallels the experience with carboplatin/paclitaxel/epirubicin in ovarian cancer except that the rate of febrile neutropenia was then 12.5%, as routine G-CSF was not used (13). There is an alternative regimen that can be used instead: carboplatin (AUC 5–6) plus paclitaxel (175 mg/m^2 over 3 h) (14). Its efficacy seems equivalent, as it is in ovarian cancer, it is easy to deliver, and most physicians are highly experienced in its use for ovarian cancer. The GOG is comparing its use to their triplet plus GCSF but the results are a long way off. Until then, one has to make do with the comparative, but not randomized, efficacy data which are given in Table 5.

Other platin-based doublets, namely, carboplatin plus pegylated liposomal doxorubicin, and cisplatin or carboplatin plus vinorelbine have been tested in small phase II studies (Table 6). The results seem to be similar to platin-taxanes (15–19). Personally, I would stay with carboplatin-paclitaxel unless either particular side

Table 5 Comparative efficacy: carboplatin/paclitaxel vs. cisplatin/doxorubicin/paclitaxel/GCSF, modified from the references (8, 14)

Regimens	Reference	No. of Patients	RR (%)	PFS (months)	OS (months)
Cisplatin/doxorubicin/ paclitaxel/GCSF	Fleming (8)	134	57	8	15
Carboplatin/paclitaxel	Weber (9)	36	35	8	
	Scudder(29)	47	40	7	14
	Sovak (30)	85	43	5	13
	Akram (31)	18	63	24	27
	Hoskins (14)	21 (A)	78	23	36
		18 (R)	56	6	15
	Price (32)	8	63		
	Nakamura (33)	11	72		
	Trudeau (34)	8	75		

RR response rate; *PFS* progression-free survival; *OS* overall survival; *(A)* advanced disease; *(R)* recurrent disease

Table 6 Other possible platinum doublets (15–19)

Carboplatin-Pegylated liposomal doxorubicin (PLD)						
Reference	Carboplatin target AUC	PLD dose (mg/m²)	No. of Patients	RR (%)	PFS (months)	OS (months)
Le (15)	AUC = 5	35	31	32	5	11
Pignata (16)	AUC = 5	30	50	68		
Hilpert (17)	AUC = 5	40	31	44		

Cisplatin/Carboplatin–Vinorelbine						
Reference	Platin dose (mg/m²)	Vinorelbine dose (mg/m²)	No. of Patients	RR (%)	PFS (months)	OS (months)
Gebbia (18)	80 (cisplatin)	25 (day 1 + 8)	35	57	9	
Santoro (19)	300 (carboplatin)	25 (day 1 + 8)	13	69		

RR response rate; *PFS* progression-free survival; *OS* overall survival

effects need to be avoided or uncontrollable or dangerous side effects develop during carboplatin-paclitaxel treatment.

Does Combination Chemotherapy Improve Survival?

Four randomized studies have been carried out in newly diagnosed women looking at the question of "is survival improved by chemotherapy compared to irradiation" (20–23). The chemotherapy used was the less effective cisplatin–doxorubicin combination, except in the case of the Scandinavian trial in which some patients

Table 7 Survival outcomes with chemotherapy compared to irradiation in the newly diagnosed patients

Reference	FIGO Stage (grading)	Treatment	5-year PFS (%)	5-year OS (%)
Maggi (22)	I (G3); II (G3), III	Pelvic XRT	67	69
		Cisplatin/doxorubicin/ cyclophosphamide	62	66
Susumu (23)	Ic (G3), II, III	Pelvic XRT	66	74
		Cisplatin/doxorubicin/ cyclophosphamide	84	90
Randall (21)	III/IV	Whole abdomen XRT	38	42
		Cisplatin/doxorubicin	50	55
Hogberg (20)	I, II, IIIa, IIIc	Pelvic XRT	75	
		Pelvic XRT + platin combinations	82	

PFS progression-free survival; *OS* overall survival

received platin-taxane. Three of the four trials showed an absolute improvement in five year progression survival of 7–20%, with a similar improvement in overall survival (Table 7). The Italian study (22), in contrast, showed equivalence. The reasons for this are not clear but include; less total chemotherapy was delivered, it took longer, and the patients in the Italian trial were of somewhat lower risk and so a true benefit would be harder to demonstrate.

Malignant Mixed Mullerian Tumors (MMMTs)

MMMTs, otherwise known as carcinosarcomas, were traditionally recognized as sarcomas and as such treated with ifosfamide or ifosfamide combinations. Now, they are regarded as true carcinomas, albeit metaplastic and high grade (2). The experience with these tumors is essentially the same as with standard endometrial cancers, i.e., platinum doublets are amongst the best chemotherapies and their use in the newly diagnosed leads to an improvement in survival (24). The two combination regimens that are superior to ifosfamide alone are cisplatin–ifosfamide and ifosfamide-paclitaxel-GCSF (25, 26): response rates improved to 56% and 45%, respectively (*versus* 29–34% with ifosfamide); progression-free survival increased to six months from four months in both the studies, and with an improved survival in the ifosfamide-paclitaxel study (14 vs. 8 months). As with "standard" endometrial cancers, carboplatin-paclitaxel is another option. Ifosfamide-containing regimens are more costly, inconvenient (3–5 days in patient care) and toxic; especially, the cisplatin–ifosfamide combination. Ifosfamide-paclitaxel plus GCSF is not overly toxic, in fact, similar to carboplatin–paclitaxel, and so would be the better choice of the ifosfamide regimens. Our experience, albeit with limited numbers, was a response rate of 60% in the newly diagnosed, 55% in the recurrent and a median progression-free survival of 12–16 months with carboplatin-paclitaxel, certainly not inferior to the ifosfamide doublets (27).

The GOG compared whole abdominal irradiation to cisplatin–ifosfamide in the newly diagnosed, optimally debulked women. The relapse rate was lower with chemotherapy (52% vs. 58% at 5 years, $p = 0.2$) with a borderline increased survival (45% vs. 35% at 5 years, $p = 0.08$) (24).

Future Directions

Chemotherapy using platin-based combinations has improved the outcome for high-risk, newly diagnosed women. However, many still relapse and merely adding more chemotherapeutic agents is unlikely to improve upon this, as has already been proven in ovarian and lung cancer. Different approaches are mandatory. Chemotherapy remains the cornerstone to which other approaches should be added. Modulating platinum resistance is one obvious additional route to be tried. Targeting pathways, involved in endometrial cancer, is another. Examples of pathways/ targets of interest are the PTEN-P13k-AkT-mTOR axis, EGFR/Her2-neu, and Bcr-Abl (28).

References

1. FIGO. Annual report on the results of treatment in gynecologic cancers – vol 23. J Epidemiol Biostat 1998;3:335–61.
2. McCluggage WG. Uterine carcinosarcomas (malignant mixed Mullerian tumors) are metaplastic carcinomas. Int J Gynecol Cancer 2002;12:687–90.
3. Fleming GF. Systemic chemotherapy for uterine carcinoma: metastatic and adjuvant. J Clin Oncol 2007;25:2983–90.
4. Elit L, Hirte H. Novel strategies for systemic treatment of endometrial cancer. Expert Opin Investig Drugs 2000;9: 2831–53.
5. Thigpen JT, Blessing JA, DiSaia PJ, Yordan E, Carson LF, Evers C. A randomized comparison of doxorubicin alone versus doxorubicin plus cyclophosphamide in the management of advanced or recurrent endometrial carcinoma: a Gynecologic Oncology Group study. J Clin Oncol 1994;12:1408–14.
6. Aapro MS, van Wijk FH, Bolis G, et al. Doxorubicin versus doxorubicin and cisplatin in endometrial carcinoma: definitive results of a randomised study (55872) by the EORTC Gynaecological Cancer Group. Ann Oncol 2003;14:441–8.
7. Thigpen JT, Brady MF, Homesley HD, et al. Phase III trial of doxorubicin with or without cisplatin in advanced endometrial carcinoma: a gynecologic oncology group study. J Clin Oncol 2004;22:3902–8.
8. Fleming GF, Brunetto VL, Cella D, et al. Phase III trial of doxorubicin plus cisplatin with or without paclitaxel plus filgrastim in advanced endometrial carcinoma: a Gynecologic Oncology Group Study. J Clin Oncol 2004;22:2159–66.
9. Weber B, Mayer F, Bougnoux P, et al. What is the best chemotherapy regimen in recurrent or advanced endometrial carcinoma? Preliminary results. Proc Am Soc Clin Oncol 2003;22:453 (abstract).
10. Gallion HH, Brunetto VL, Cibull M, et al. Randomized phase III trial of standard timed doxorubicin plus cisplatin versus circadian timed doxorubicin plus cisplatin in stage III and IV or recurrent endometrial carcinoma: a Gynecologic Oncology Group Study. J Clin Oncol 2003;21:3808–13.

11. Fleming GF, Filiaci VL, Bentley RC, et al. Phase III randomized trial of doxorubicin + cisplatin versus doxorubicin + 24-h paclitaxel + filgrastim in endometrial carcinoma: a Gynecologic Oncology Group study. Ann Oncol 2004;15:1173–8.

12. Long HJ, Nelimark RA, Cha SS. Comparison of methotrexate, vinblastine, doxorubicin and cisplatin (MVAC) vs doxorubicin and cisplatin (AC) in advanced endometrial carcinoma. Proc Am Soc Clin Oncol 1995;12:1408–14 (abstract).

13. Kristensen GB, Vergote I, Eisenhauer E, et al. First line treatment of ovarian/tubal/ peritoneal cancer FIGO stage II or without epirubicin (TEC vs. TC). A Gynecologic Cancer Intergroup and NCIC CTG. Results on progression free survival. Proc Am Soc Clin Oncol 2004;23:A5003 (abstract).

14. Hoskins PJ, Swenerton KD, Pike JA, et al. Paclitaxel and carboplatin, alone or with irradiation, in advanced or recurrent endometrial cancer: a phase II study. J Clin Oncol 2001;19: 4048–53.

15. Le LH, Swenerton KD, Elit L, et al. Phase II multicenter open-label study of carboplatin and pegylated liposomal doxorubicin in uterine and cervical malignancies. Int J Gynecol Cancer 2005;15:799–806.

16. Pignata S, Scambia G, Savarese A, et al. Carboplatin plus paclitaxel versus carboplatin plus Stealth liposomal doxorubicin in patients with ovarian cancer (AOC): preliminary activity results o the MITO-2 randomized trial. Proc Am Soc Clin Oncol 2007;A5532 (abstract).

17. Hilpert F, Loibi S, Huober J, et al. Combination therapy with pegylated liposomal doxorubicin and carboplatin in malignant gynecologic tumors: a prospective multicenter phase II trial of the AGO-OVAR and the AGO Kommission Uterus (AGO-K-Ut). J Clin Oncol 2006;24:279s (abstract).

18. Gebbia V, Testa A, Borsellino N, Ferrera P, Tirrito M, Palmeri S. Cisplatin and vinorelbine in advanced and/or metastatic adenocarcinoma of the Endometrium: a new highly active chemotherapeutic regimen. Ann Oncol 2001;12:767–72.

19. Santoro A. Carboplatin and vinorelbine combination for treatment of advanced endometrial cancer. Proc Am Soc Clin Oncol 1998;17:A1444 (abstract).

20. Hogberg T, Rosenberg P, Kristensen G, et al. A randomized phase III study on adjuvant treatment with radiation (RT) ± chemotherapy in early stage high risk endometrial cancer. Proc Am Soc Clin Oncol 2007:A5503.

21. Randall ME, Filiaci VL, Muss H, et al. Randomized phase III trial of whole abdominal irradiation versus doxorubicin and cisplatin chemotherapy in advanced endometrial carcinoma: A Gynecologic Oncology Group study. J Clin Oncol 2006;24:36–44.

22. Maggi R, Lissoni A, Spina F, et al. Adjuvant chemotherapy vs. radiotherapy in high-risk endometrial carcinoma: results of a randomized trial. Br J Cancer 2006;95:266–71.

23. Susumu N, Sagae S, Udagawa Y, et al. Randomized phase III trial of pelvic radiotherapy versus cisplatin-based combined chemotherapy in patients with intermediate and high-risk endometrial cancer: a Japanese Gynecologic Oncology Group study. Gynecol Oncol 2008;108: 226–33.

24. Wolfson AH, Brady MF, Rocereto T, et al. A gynecologic oncology group randomized phase III trial of whole abdominal irradiation (WAI) vs cisplatin–ifosfamide and mesna (CIM) as post-surgical therapy in stage I-IV carcinosarcoma (CS) of the uterus. Gynecol Oncol 2007;107:177–85.

25. Sutton G, Brunetto VL, Kilgore L, et al. A phase III trial of ifosfamide with or without cisplatin in carcinosarcoma of the uterus: a Gynecologic Oncology Group Study. Gynecol Oncol 2000;79:147–53.

26. Homesley HD, Filiaci V, Markman M, et al. Phase III trial of ifosfamide with or without paclitaxel in advanced uterine carcinosarcoma: a Gynecologic Oncology Group Study. J Clin Oncol 2007; 25:526–31.

27. Hoskins PJ, Le N, Ellard S, et al. Carboplatin plus paclitaxel for advanced or recurrent uterine malignant mixed mullerian tumors. The British Columbia Cancer Agency experience. Gynecol Oncol 2008;108:58–62.

28. Gadducci A, Cosio S, Genazzani AR. Old and new perspectives in the pharmacological treatment of advanced or recurrent endometrial cancer: hormonal therapy, chemotherapy and molecularly targeted therapies. Crit Rev Oncol Hematol 2006;58:242–56.
29. Scudder SA, Liu PY, Wilcynski SP, Smith HO, Jiang C, Hallum III AV, Smith GB, Hannigan EV, Markman M, Alberts DS. Paclitaxel and carboplatin with amifostine in advanced, recurrent, or refractory endometrial adenocarcinoma: a phase II study of SWOG. Gynecologic Oncology 2005;96:610–615.
30. Sovak MA, Dupont J, Hensley ML, et al. Paclitaxel and carboplatin in the treatment of advanced or recurrent endometrial cancer: a large retrospective study. Int J Gynecol Cancer 2007;17:197–203.
31. Akram T, Maseelall P, Fanning J. Carboplatin and paclitaxel for the treatment of advanced or recurrent endometrial cancer. Am J Obstet Gynecol 2005;192:1365–1367.
32. Price FV, Edwards RP, Kelley JL et al. A trail of outpatient paclitaxel and carboplatin to advanced, recurrent, and histologic high risk endometrial carinoma: a preliminary report. Seminars in Oncology 1997;24:S15–78–S15–82.
33. Nakamura T, Onishi Y, Yamamoto F, et al. Evaluation of paclitaxel and carboplatin in patients with endometrial cancer. Gan To Kagaku Ryoho 2000;27:257–262.
34. Trudeau M, Stanmir G, Langleben G, Letendre E, Gagne G. Paclitaxel and cisplatin: an active regimen in metastatic cancer of the endometrium. Int J Gynecol Cancer 1999;9(suppl 1):69.

Platinum Compounds: Key Ingredients in Ovarian Cancer Treatment and Strategies

Franco M. Muggia

Abstract Epithelial ovarian cancer and other cancer of Mullerian epithelial origin are adenocarcinomas with remarkable sensitivity to platinum drugs: the introduction of cisplatin revolutionized treatment approaches to this disease, and the development of carboplatin markedly enhanced the acceptance of these drugs by patients. In spite of this initial sensitivity, the majority of patients treated recur, and it may be most useful to understand reasons for the emergence of drug resistance. Clues may emerge from preclinical models and from studies in hereditary cancers, where defects in DNA repair likely predict for enhanced sensitivity to platinums. Future steps in improving the outcome from this disease, in addition to developing better methods for screening and detection, should involve understanding mechanisms of platinum cytotoxicity and resistance.

Keywords Cisplatin; Carboplatin; Drug resistance; Intraperitoneal therapy; BRCA mutations; Stem cells

Introduction and Overview of Ovarian Cancer Treatment

Data from the Princess Margaret Hospital from 1970 to 1980 estimated that 95% of patients diagnosed with ovarian cancer were candidates for adjuvant chemotherapy (1). After the studies of Wiltshaw and colleagues at the Royal Marsden (2, 3) established the activity of platinum compounds (first cisplatin and then the better tolerated carboplatin) against this most lethal gynecologic cancer of women, the exposure to systemic chemotherapy has risen and the survival of patients presenting with this advanced stage of the disease has slowly improved (4). However, a continued challenge that these patients face is our inability to fully eradicate the disease through surgery and platinum-based chemotherapy. While other cytotoxic drug classes such as anthracyclines, taxanes, topoisomerase I inhibitors,

F.M. Muggia
Division of Medical Oncology, New York University School of Medicine and NYU
Cancer Institute, NY, USA
e-mail: Franco.Muggia@nyumc.org

A. Bonetti et al. (eds.), *Platinum and Other Heavy Metal Compounds in Cancer Chemotherapy*, DOI: 10.1007/978-1-60327-459-3_35,
© Humana Press, a part of Springer Science + Business Media, LLC 2009

and antimetabolites (gemcitabine) (5) have anti-tumor activity with a reasonable therapeutic index, their contribution is confined to prolongation of remission and only exceptionally leading to tumor eradication. Notwithstanding these ultimately unsatisfactory results, one should not lose sight of the remarkable activity of cisplatin and carboplatin even in the most advanced presentations, with the development of intraperitoneal (IP) local dose-intensification, and the possibility that insight into the mechanisms of resistance to these drugs will lead to other substantial advances. Diagnosing the disease at lower tumor burden will undoubtedly lead to more dramatic alterations in vital statistics.

Epithelial ovarian cancer is not one disease, and there is evidence that the high grade papillary serous cancer may originate in the Fallopian tube fimbriae, possibly contributing to its late discovery. These papillary serous cancers typically carry mutations in p53, and coupled with abnormalities in BRCA1 and BRCA2 genes (seen in hereditary forms) have been associated with pre-malignant lesions in the fimbriae of patients undergoing risk-reducing surgery (6). Endometrioid cancers are also associated with the hereditary forms, and both these histologic subtypes make up about 80% of these cancers, with the remainder being mucinous, clearcell and mixed types. Clinical trials have lumped all of these together in reporting results for the most advanced presentations, i.e. when surgery is unable to achieve a "favorable" less than one centimeter residuum (Table 1) (7–10). Analysis by the

Table 1 Paclitaxel/platinum combinations in randomized first-line advanced ovarian cancer trials. Adapted from Physician Data Query - NCI's Comprehensive Cancer Database (http://www.cancer.gov/cancertopics/pdq)

Trial (ref)	Treatment regimens	No. of patients	Early crossover (%)	Progression-free survival (mo)	Overall survival (mo)
GOG-132 (7)	Paclitaxel (135 mg/m^2, 24 h) and cisplatin (75 mg/m^2)	201	22	14.2	26.6
	Cisplatin (100 mg/m^2)	200	40	16.4	30.2
	Paclitaxel (200 mg/m^2, 24 h)	213	23	11.2*	26
MRC-ICON3 (8)	Paclitaxel (175 mg/m^2, 3 h) and carboplatin AUC 6	478	23	17.3	36.1
	Carboplatin AUC 6	943	25	16.1	35.4
	Paclitaxel (175 mg/m^2, 3 h) and carboplatin AUC 6	232	23	17	40
	Cyclophosphamide (750 mg/m^2) and doxorubicin (75 mg/m^2) and cisplatin (75 mg/m^2)	421	20	17	40
GOG-111 (9)	Paclitaxel (135 mg/m^2, 24 h) and cisplatin (75 mg/m^2)	184	None	18	38
	Cyclophosphamide (750 mg/m^2) and cisplatin (75 mg/m^2)	202	None	13*	24*
OV-10 (10)	Paclitaxel (175 mg/m^2, 3 h) and cisplatin (75 mg/m^2)	162	None	15.5	35.6
	Cyclophosphamide (750 mg/m^2) and cisplatin (75 mg/m^2)	161	4	11.5*	25.8*

* statistically significant inferior result

Gynecologic Oncology Group (GOG) indicates that the outcome is more favorable for the papillary serous and endometrioid types (11), presumably as a result of the sensitivity to platinums. Curiously, in patients diagnosed in stages I and II, the histologic subtype distribution is considerably different with low grade papillary and endometrioid cancers, mucinous, and clear cell cancers making up the majority of the histologies (12). Molecular features point towards a different etiology than the high grade papillary serous cancer, and different treatment strategies may be required (13).

First-Line Treatment of Ovarian Cancer

Early Stage Disease

When ovarian cancer is diagnosed in its early stages (mostly as a coincidental occurrence), as noted above,the histologic subtypes play a role in determining the need for treatment and its outcome. After excluding subtypes and a stage I with low probability of relapse, studies randomizing chemotherapy versus observation have strongly pointed to the efficacy of cisplatin, and by pooling data, European studies have provided indications that survival is improved (14–16). A disputed point is whether the chemotherapy is in part making up for inadequate surgical staging.

Chemotherapy for the Advanced Stages

The GOG and groups from Europe and Canada through a series of studies have established the standard "platinum-based" ovarian cancer treatment. GOG-111 proved that the prior combination with cyclophosphamide yielded inferior results to a taxane-containing regime, and OV-10 confirmed this finding. However, the GOG-132 and ICON-3 trials (that were started before a mature data from these two studies was available) pointed to a relatively minor, if any, effect of taxanes in the progression-free survival (PFS) and responses achieved by either cisplatin or carbo-platin as single agents. This finding, and the subsequent lack of effect on the outcome by other drugs given up front in the 5-arm, 2,000 patient trial, GOG-182, point to the dominant effect of the platinum drugs, in determining the initial outcome. While other drugs may contribute to the overall survival (OS), it may make little difference if they are added up-front in combination or sequentially. Once there is some plati-num resistance, such as in the recurrent setting, the trial ICON-4 indicates that the addition of paclitaxel to carboplatin is superior to carboplatin as a single agent (17). A focus on determinants of platinum sensitivity of recently diagnosed ovarian cancer would seem amply justified by these data.

Intraperitoneal (IP) Cisplatin Studies

The pharmacologic basis for the delivery of anticancer drugs by the IP route was established in the late 1970s and early 1980s, and is covered elsewhere in this volume/chapter. Of the many drugs studied, mostly, in the setting of minimal residual disease at reassessment after patients had received their initial chemotherapy, cisplatin alone and in combination received the most attention. Favorable outcomes from IP cisplatin were most often seen when tumors had shown responsiveness to platinums and with small-volume tumors (usually defined as tumors < 1 cm) (18). The use of IP cisplatin as part of the initial up-front approach in patients with stage III optimally debulked ovarian cancer, is now supported principally by the results of three randomized clinical trials (GOG-104, GOG-14, and GOG-172) (19–21). These studies tested the role of IP drugs (IP cisplatin in all three studies and IP paclitaxel in the last study) against the standard IV regimen. In the three studies, superior progression-free survival (PFS) and overall survival (OS) favoring the IP arm was documented. A Cochrane-sponsored meta-analysis of all randomized IP versus IV trials shows a hazard ratio of 0.79 for disease-free survival and 0.79 for OS, favoring the IP arms (22). In another meta-analysis of seven IP versus IV randomized trials that were conducted by Cancer Care of Ontario, the relative ratio (RR) of progression at 5 years based on the three trials that reported this endpoint was 0.91 (95% confidence interval [CI], 0.85–0.98) and the RR of death at 5 years based on six trials was 0.88 (95% CI, 0.81–0.95) (23). Recent Consensus Statements by the National Cancer Institute making IP therapy the standard treatment following initial "optimal" or "favorable" debulking have met with resistance (24). However, the studies provide another signal that maneuvers to enhance platinum drug delivery may play a key role in the outcome of ovarian cancer.

"Biological" or "Targeted" Agents

Contrasting it with breast, lung, and colon cancers, a role for "targeted" drugs in the first-line of ovarian cancer has not been established. Although this may seem surprising based on the molecular pathways that are known to be deranged in epithelial ovarian cancer, plausible explanations include the relative rarity of ovarian cancer compared to the others, and the dominant role of the platinums obscuring other interventions when the disease is far-advanced. The mouse model developed by Dinulescu and co-workers (25) supports the remarkable effects of cisplatin in nearly the end-stage of the disease, and the lesser effects through the targeting of various deranged pathways. Current clinical trials are seeking to study the effect of adding bevacizumab to the carboplatin + paclitaxel first-line regimen, based on the known activity of this antibody to the vascular endothelial growth factor (VEGF) in patients with recurrent disease (26–29).

Recurrent Ovarian Cancer

The majority of patients (likely as high as 85% over 5 years) with advanced-stage ovarian cancer recur with serum marker (CA125), or imaging (PET/CT) evidence of the disease after a variable period after completion of first-line chemotherapy (5). Within a few months of such detection, if untreated, the women go on to manifest signs and symptoms of the disease. The time to recurrence after platinum-based chemotherapy is close to one-and-a-half years for patients who have had "suboptimal" or "unfavorable" debulking (see PFS duration in Table 1) and in excess of two years in patients with "optimal" debulking. The treatment of recurrent disease is based on how effective the platinums were on first-line, leading to operational definitions of "platinum resistant" (evidence of recurrence within 6 months), or of "platinum sensitive" if the interval was 6 months or more.

Treatment Options for "Platinum Sensitive" Recurrences

Carboplatin was approved in 1987 for the treatment of patients with ovarian cancer whose disease recurred after treatment with cisplatin, based on improved survival when compared with etoposide or 5-fluorouracil (30). In a randomized phase II of a currently used second-line drug, paclitaxel, the cisplatin-containing combination CAP yielded a superior survival outcome (31). These, and subsequent studies (32–35) (see Table 2) have reinforced using carboplatin as the treatment core for patients with "platinum-sensitive" recurrences. Cisplatin is occasionally used, particularly in combination, because of its lesser myelosuppression, but this advantage over carboplatin is counterbalanced by its greater intolerance (34). Oxaliplatin, initially introduced with the hope that it would overcome platinum resistance, has

Table 2 Trials in "platinum-sensitive" ovarian cancer recurrence

Eligibility	Platinum regimen	No. of Patients	Comparator	Comments on outcome (ref)
Platinum sensitive	Cisplatin + doxorubicin + cyclophosphamide	97	Paclitaxel	Randomized phase II; CAP superior PFS, OS (31)
Platinum sensitive	Carboplatin + epirubicin	190	Carboplatin	Powered for response differences; OS 17 vs. 15 m (32)
Platinum sensitive	Carboplatin + gemcitabine	356	Carboplatin	PFS 8.6 m vs. 5.8 m OS 18 m vs. 17 m (33)
Platinum sensitive	Cisplatin or carboplatin + paclitaxel	802	Single or non-taxane + platinums	PFS 11 m vs. 9 m OS 24 m vs. 19 m (34)
Platinum sensitive	Carboplatin + pegylated liposomal doxorubicin	104	None	PFS 9 m, median OS 32 m (35)

activity mostly in "platinum-sensitive" patients (36) but has not been compared with carboplatin alone or in combinations. The outcome is generally better with all platinums the longer is the initial interval without recurrence from the initial platinum-containing regimens (33). Therefore, on occasions, patients with platinum-sensitive recurrences relapsing within one year have been included in trials of non-platinum drugs. In one such trial, comparing the pegylated liposomal doxorubicin (PLD) to topotecan, the subset of patients who were platinum-sensitive had better outcomes with both drugs (and in particular with PLD) relative to the platinum-resistant cohort (37).

Second-Line Drugs for "Platinum-Resistant" Disease

The long list of studies (26–29, 38–47) in Table 3 underscores both, the reasonable therapeutic index for those drugs in common use, as well as the often transient or marginal benefit from drug regiments used. Patients with platinum-resistant disease should be encouraged to enter clinical trials. Treatment with paclitaxel historically provided the first agent with consistent activity in patients with platinum-refractory or platinum-resistant recurrences (39). Subsequently, randomized studies have indicated that the use of topotecan achieved results that were comparable to those achieved with paclitaxel (40). More recently, topotecan was compared with pegylated liposomal doxorubicin in a randomized trial of 474 patients, and demonstrated similar response rates, PFS and OS with no differences in the "platinum resistant" subset (37). Lengthening the "platinum-free" may restore sensitivity, but this hypothesis has not been formally tested.

The Rationale for Maintenance

Following a clinical complete response to the initial induction treatment, 9 additional monthly paclitaxel doses over the 3 additional ones for the control group, led to highly significant lengthening of PFS in a GOG/Southwest Oncology Group study (48). Although other trials, yet to be published beyond abstract form, may not fully confirm this result, it suggests that maintenance with a non-platinum drug may be an even more reasonable strategy to test where responses are likely to be shorter (i.e., for treatment at recurrence).

When platinums cease to lead to dramatic reductions in tumor burden in the majority of patients as they do at the initial induction, the more obvious becomes the need for some "maintenance" chemotherapy. Although the term has been denigrated as denying patients the chance for aggressive treatment alternating with "treatment holidays", it may be the most realistic strategy to date given the late presentations and the reasonable therapeutic index of some of the drugs used. In fact, our experience with the pegylated liposomal doxorubicin indicates that very

Table 3 Drugs for platinum-resistant ovarian cancer

Drugs	Drug class/target	Major toxicities	Comments (ref)
Paclitaxel	Mitotic inhibitor	Alopecia, neuropathy	(39)
Docetaxel	Mitotic inhibitor	Alopecia, fatigue, myelosuppression	(41)
Topotecan	Topoisomerase I	Myelosuppression	(40)
Pegylated liposome doxorubicin	Topoisomerase II	Skin and mucosal toxicities	(42)
Gemcitabine	Antimetabolite	Myelosuppression, short "flu" symptoms	(43)
Bevacizumab	Antibody to VEGF	Hypertension, proteinuria	(26–29)
Etoposide	Topoisomerase II inhibitor	Myelosuppression; alopecia	Oral; rare leukemia dampens interest (38)
Cyclophosphamide, ifosfamide and other alkylating agents	Alkylating agents	Myelosuppression; alopecia (only the oxazaphosphorines)	Leukemia and cystitis; uncertain activity after platinums (38)
Hexamethylmelamine (Altretamine)	Unknown but probably alkylating prodrugs	Emesis and neurotoxicity	Oral; uncertain activity after platinums (44)
Irinotecan	Topoisomerase I inhibitor	Diarrhea and other gastrointestinal symptoms	Cross-resistant to topotecan (45)
Oxaliplatin	Platinum	Neuropathy, emesis, myelosuppression	Cross resistant to usual platinums, but less so (36)
Vinorelbine	Mitotic inhibitor	Myelosuppression	Erratic activity (46)
Fluorouracil and capecitabine	Fluoropyrimidine antimetabolites	Gastrointestinal symptoms and myelosuppression	Capecitabine is oral; may be useful in mucinous tumors (38)
Pemetrexed	Folic acid antagonist	Myelosuppression, rash	Under study in combinations with carboplatin (47)
Tamoxifen	Antiestrogen	Thromboembolism	Oral; minimal activity, perhaps more in subsets (38)

bolded are those in common use

long term maintenance (in excess of 4 years) is acceptable to patients (49). Other non-platinum drugs may be suitable for maintenance, but are less practical because of requiring dosing at shorter intervals or having some less acceptable toxicities, even if non-cumulative. Platinums are not suitable for long-term maintenance because of cumulative effects primarily on the bone marrow, but also because of their high emetic potential. Anti-angiogenesis strategies have been recently built on this concept.

The other factor encouraging the use of maintenance relates to the shorter remissions that one encounters upon retreatment. Two different groups have shown that a second remission from the same regimen is likely to be shorter and is only exceptionally longer – even though the second treatment is often applied at a time when the tumor burden is less. Such an experience is best explained by the emergence of a platinum-resistant population; lesser tolerance by the host the second time around may contribute to this in some instances.

Future Steps

This overview has highlighted reasons for devoting more research towards optimizing the role of platinum compounds: (1) cisplatin and/or carboplatin are the key drugs in the induction of long-lasting remissions (an observation that became obvious in the 1970s when cisplatin joined a cluttered pharmacopeia, in retrospect, of marginally active combinations; (2) intraperitoneal platinums have provided a signal in three randomized trials of improved survival when given as first-line treatment; (3) upon recurrence there is clear evidence that these drugs are again the most useful, but in this instance are best used in combination with other drugs such as taxanes leading to survival; and (4) lengthening the platinum-free interval by the use of the many drugs used for recurrence may restore sensitivity to the platinum (but its value is limited by subsequent development of resistance, possibly by selecting out further a resistant "stem cell" population). Integration of such strategies may continue to improve the outcome.

Preclinical Models

The model by Dinulescu et al, mentioned earlier (25), provides some indications of questions that may be addressed from their experimental observations. For example, one may begin to characterize a platinum-resistant subset not only as a population that currently defeats our treatment, but also perhaps to define a "tumor stem cell". In any event, these studies could lead to testing novel therapeutic strategies for their elimination. Another consequence of work on this animal model has been the identification of serum markers of platinum resistance.

Models incorporating p53 and BRCA1 conditional knockouts in breast tissue, have given rise to breast tumors that are exquisitively sensitive to cisplatin (50). Here, as in the preceding model, eventually, if not cured, the animals succumb to platinum-resistant disease. Anthracyclines are also effective, although somewhat less than cisplatin in this model. Strategies to improve therapeutic results include the use of PARP-1 inhibitors that were shown to be more cytotoxic to cells that had mutations in BRCA1 and BRCA2. A combination of cisplatin with a PARP-1 inhibitor appeared encouraging in this animal model.

Clinical Clues from Hereditary Ovarian Cancer

Most patients with hereditary ovarian cancers carry deleterious germ-line mutations in either BRCA1 or BRCA2. The tumors arising in this background of mutations may be hypersensitive to platinums (51, 52). Conversely, a recent report in Nature 2008 has linked platinum resistance to the restoration of function of BRCA2 in patients where additional mutations bypass the message for an inactive protein from the original mutation (53). Accumulating evidence supports the premise that ovarian cancers arising in BRCA mutation carriers have longer responses to platinum-based chemotherapy; in addition, some studies support a better outcome to pegylated liposomal doxorubicin therapy. Studies with PARP-1 inhibitors alone and in combination are ongoing and the results are eagerly awaited.

These clinical clues are prompting a greater study of DNA repair pathways in ovarian cancer, and the role of epigenetic changes in silencing BRCA genes. The occurrence of DNA repair defects among sporadic cases of ovarian cancer may provide an explanation for the efficacy of platinums in this disease. Identifying how these occur has both etiologic and therapeutic significance and represents an important path for future clinical investigations seeking to improve the outcome of patients with ovarian cancer.

References

1. Dembo AJ, Bush RS, Beale FA, et al. The Princess Margaret Hospital Study of ovarian cancer: stage I, II and asymptomatic III presentations. Cancer Treat Rep 1979;63:249–54.
2. Wiltshaw E, Subramanian S, Alexopoulos C, Baker GH. Cancer of the ovary: a summary of experience with cis-platinum diamminedichloride (II) in the Royal Marsden Hospital. Cancer Treat Rep 1979;63:1546–8.
3. Rozencweig M, Martin M, Beltangady M, et al. Randomized trials of carboplatin versus cisplatin in advanced ovarian cancer. In: Bunn PA Jr, Canetta R, Ozols RF, Rozencweig M, eds. Carboplatin (JM-8) current perspectives and future directions. Philadelphia, US: WB Saunders, 1990:175–92.
4. Oksefhell H, Sandstad B, Trope C. Improved survival for stage IIIC ovarian cancer patients treated at the Norwegian Eaium Hospital between 1984 and 2001. Eur J Gynaecol Oncol 2007;28:256–62.
5. Muggia FM, Hazarika M. Ovarian cancer: rationale and strategies beyond first line treatment. In: Angioli R, Panici PB, Kavanagh JJ, Pecorelli S, Penalver M, eds. Chemotherapy for gynecological neoplasms: current therapy and novel approaches. New York, USA: Marcel Dekker, 2004:471–82.
6. Folkins AK, Jarboe EA, Saleemuddin A, et al. A candidate precursor to pelvic serous cancer (p53 signature) and its prevalence in ovaries and fallopian tubes from women with BRCA mutations. Gynecol Oncol 2008;109:168–73.
7. Muggia FM, Braly PS, Brady MF, et al. Phase III randomized study of cisplatin versus paclitaxel versus cisplatin and paclitaxel in patients with suboptimal stage III or IV ovarian cancer: a Gynecologic Oncology Group study. J Clin Oncol 2000;18:106–15.
8. The ICON Collaborators. Paclitaxel plus carboplatin versus standard chemotherapy with either single-agent carboplatin or cyclophosphamide, doxorubicin, and cisplatin in women with ovaraian cancer: the ICON3 randomized trials. Lancet 2002;360:505–15.

9. McGuire WP, Hoskins WJ, Brady MF, et al. Cyclophosphamide and cisplatin compared with palcitaxel and cisplatin in patients with stage III and stage IV ovarian cancer. N Eng J Med 1996;334:1–6.
10. Piccart MJ, Bertelsen K, James K, et al. Randomized intergroup trial of cisplatin-paclitaxel versus cisplatin-cyclophosphamide in women with advanced epithelial ovarian cancer: three-year results. J Natl Cancer Inst 2000;92:699–708.
11. Omura GA, Brady MF, Homesley HD, et al. Long-term follow-up and prognostic factor analysis in advanced ovarian carcinoma: the Gynecologic Oncology Group experience. J Clin Oncol 1991;9:1138–50.
12. Bell J, Brady MF, Young RC. Randomized phase III trial of three versus six cycles of adjuvant carboplatin and paclitaxel in early stage epithelial ovarian carcinoma: a Gynecologic Oncology Group study. Gynecol Oncol 2006;102:432–9.
13. Ueda M, Toji S, Noda S. Germ line and somatic mutations of B-raf V599E in ovarian carcinoma. Int J Gynecol Cancer 2007;17:794–7.
14. Trimbos JB, Parmar M, Vergote I, et al. International collaborative ovarian neoplasm trial 1 and adjuvant chemotherapy in ovarian neoplasm trial: two parallel randomized phase III trials of adjuvant chemotherapy in patients with early-stage ovarian carcinoma. J Natl Cancer Inst 2003;95:105–12.
15. Trimbos JB, Vergote I, Bolis G, et al. Impact of adjuvant chemotherapy and surgical staging in early-stage ovarian carcinoma: European organisation for research and treatment of cancer-adjuvant chemotherapy in ovarian neoplasm trial. J Natl Cancer Inst 2003;95: 113–25.
16. Colombo N, Guthrie D, Chiari S, et al. International collaborative ovarian neoplasm trial 1: a randomized trial of adjuvant chemotherapy in women with early-stage ovarian cancer. J Natl Cancer Inst 2003;95:125–32.
17. Parmar MK, Ledermann JA, Colombo N, et al. Paclitaxel plus platinum-based chemotherapy versus conventional platinum-based chemotherapy in women with relapsed ovarian cancer: the ICON4/AGO-OVAR-2.2 trial. Lancet 2003;361:2099–106.
18. Alberts DS, Markman M, Armstrong D, Rothenberg ML, Muggia F, Howell SB. Intraperitoneal therapy for stage III ovarian cancer: a therapy whose time has come! J Clin Oncol 2002;20:3944–6.
19. Alberts DS, Liu PY, Hannigan EV, et al. Intraperitoneal cisplatin plus intravenous cyclophosphamide versus intravenous cisplatin plus intravenous cyclophosphamide for stage III ovarian cancer. N Engl J Med 1996;335:1950–5.
20. Markman M, Bundy BN, Alberts DS, et al. Phase III trial of standard-dose intravenous cisplatin plus paclitaxel versus moderately high-dose carboplatin followed by intravenous paclitaxel and intraperitoneal cisplatin in small-volume stage III ovarian carcinoma: an intergroup study of the Gynecologic Oncology Group, Southwestern Oncology Group, and Eastern Cooperative Oncology Group. J Clin Oncol 2001;19:1001–7.
21. Armstrong DK, Bundy B, Wenzel L, et al. Intraperitoneal cisplatin and paclitaxel in ovarian cancer. N Engl J Med 2006;354:34–43.
22. Jaaback K, Johnson N. Intraperitoneal chemotherapy for the initial management of primary epithelial ovarian cancer. Cochrane Database Syst Rev 2006;(1):CD005340.
23. Elit L, Oliver TK, Covens A, et al. Intraperitoneal chemotherapy in the first-line treatment of women with stage III epithelial ovarian cancer: a systematic review with metaanalyses. Cancer 2007;109:692–702.
24. National Cancer Institute Consensus Statement on Intraperitoneal Therapy. January 2006.
25. Dinulescu DM, Ince TA, Quade BJ, Shafer SA, Crowley D, Jacks T. Role of K-ras and Pten in the development of mouse models of endometriosis and endometrioid ovarian cancer. Nature Med 2005;11:63–70.
26. Burger RA, Sill M, Monk BJ, et al. Phase II trial of bevacizumab in persistent or recurrent epithelial ovarian cancer or primary peritoneal cancer: a Gynecologic Oncology Group study. J Clin Oncol 2007;25:5615–71.

27. Cannistra SA, Matulonis U, Penson R, et al. Phase II study of bevacizumab in patients with platinum-resistant ovarian cancer or peritoneal serous cancer. J Clin Oncol 2007;25: 5180–6.
28. Garcia AA, Hirte J, Fleming G, et al. Phase II clinical trial of bevacizumab and low-dose metronomic oral cyclophosphamide in recurrent ovarian cancer: a trial of the California, Chicago, and Princess Margaret Hospital Phase II consortia. J Clin Oncol 2008;26: 76–82.
29. Aghajanian C. The role of bevacizumab in ovarian cancer: an evolving story. Gynecol Oncol 2006;102:131–3.
30. Muggia FM. Overview of carboplatin: replacing, complementing and extending the therapeutic horizons of cisplatin. Semin Oncol 1989;16(suppl 5):1–7.
31. Cantù MG, Buda A, Parma G, et al. Randomized controlled trial of single-agent paclitaxel versus cyclophosphamide, doxorubicin, and cisplatin in patients with recurrent ovarian cancer who responded to first-line platinum-based regimens. J Clin Oncol 2002;20:1232–7.
32. Bolis G, Scarfone G, Giardina G, et al. Carboplatin alone vs carboplatin plus epidoxorubicin as second-line therapy for cisplatin- or carboplatin-sensitive ovarian cancer. Gynecol Oncol 2001;81:3–9.
33. Pfisterer J, Plante M, Vergote I, et al. Gemcitabine plus carboplatin compared with carboplatin in patients with platinum-sensitive recurrent ovarian cancer: an intergroup trial of the AGO-OVAR, the NCIC CTG, and the EORTC GCG. J Clin Oncol. 2006;24:4699–707.
34. Parmar MK, Ledermann JA, Colombo N, et al. Paclitaxel plus platinum-based chemotherapy versus conventional platinum-based chemotherapy in women with relapsed ovarian cancer: the ICON4/AGO-OVAR-2.2 trial. Lancet 2003;361:2099–106.
35. Ferrero JM, Weber B, Geay JF, et al. Second-line chemotherapy with pegylated liposomal doxorubicin and carboplatin is highly effective in patients with advanced ovarian cancer in late relapse: a GINECO phase II trial. Ann Oncol 2007;18:263–8.
36. Stordal B, Pavlakis N, Davey R. Oxaliplatin for the treatment of cisplatin-resistant cancer: a systematic review. Cancer Treat Rev 2007;33:347–57.
37. Gordon AN, Tonda M, Sun S, et al. Long-term survival advantage for women treated with pegylated liposomal doxorubicin compared with topotecan in a phase 3 randomized study of recurrent and refractory epithelial ovarian cancer. Gynecol Oncol 2004;95:1–8.
38. Gore M. Treatment of relapsed epithelial ovarian cancer. In: ASCO Educational Book Spring. Philadelphia, US: Lippincott Williams and Wilkins, 2001:468–76.
39. Trimble EL, Adams JD, Vena D, et al. Paclitaxel for platinum-refractory ovarian cancer: results from the first 1,000 patients registered to National Cancer Institute Treatment Referral Center 9103. J Clin Oncol 1993;11:2405–10.
40. ten Bokkel Huinink W, Gore M, Carmichael J, et al. Topotecan versus paclitaxel for the treatment of recurrent epithelial ovarian cancer. J Clin Oncol 1997;15:2183–93.
41. Berkenblit A, Seiden MV, Matulonis UA, et al. A phase II trial of weekly docetaxel in patients with platinum-resistant epithelial ovarian, primary peritoneal serous cancer, or fallopian tube cancer. Gynecol Oncol 2004;95:624–31.
42. Muggia FM, Hainsworth JD, Jeffers S, et al. Phase II study of liposomal doxorubicin in refractory ovarian cancer: antitumor activity and toxicity modification by liposomal encapsulation. J Clin Oncol 1997;15:987–93.
43. Lund B, Hansen OP, Theilade K, et al. Phase II study of gemcitabine (2',2'-difluorodeoxycytidine) in previously treated ovarian cancer patients. J Natl Cancer Inst 1994;86:1530–3.
44. Muggia F, Norris K Jr. Hexamethylmelamine in platinum-resistant ovarian cancer: how active? Gynecol Oncol 1992;47:279–81.
45. Matsumoto K, Katsumata N, Yamanaka Y, et al. The safety and efficacy of the weekly dosing of irinotecan for platinum- and taxanes-resistant epithelial ovarian cancer. Gynecol Oncol 2006;100:412–6.
46. George MJ, Heron JF, Kerbrat P, et al. Navelbine in advanced ovarian epithelial cancer: a study of the French oncology centers. Semin Oncol 1989;16(Suppl 4):30–2.

47. Smith I. Phase II studies of pemetrexed in metastatic breast and gynecologic cancers. Oncology (Williston Park) 2004;18(Suppl 8):63–5.
48. Markman M, Liu PY, Wilczynski S, et al. Phase III randomized trial of 12 versus 3 months of maintenance paclitaxel in patients with advanced ovarian cancer after complete response to platinum and paclitaxel-based chemotherapy: a Southwest Oncology Group and Gynecologic Oncology Group trial. J Clin Oncol 2003;21:2460–5.
49. Andreopoulou E, Gaiotti D, Kim E, et al. Pegylated liposomal doxorubicin HCL (PLD; Caelyx/Doxil): experience with long-term maintenance in responding. Ann Oncol 2007;18:716–21.
50. Liu X, Holstege H, van der Gulden H et al. Somatic loss of BRCA1 and p53 in mice induces mammary tumors with features of human BRCA1-mutated basal-like breast cancer, PNAS 2007;104:1217–1222.
51. Bhattacharyya A, Ear US, Koller BH, Weichselbaum RR, Bishop DK. The breast cancer susceptibility gene BRCA1 is required for subnuclear assembly of Rad51 and survival following treatment with the DNA cross-linking agent cisplatin. J Biol Chem 2000;275:23899–903.
52. Kauff ND. Is it time to stratify for BRCA mutation status in therapeutic trials in ovarian cancer? J Clin Oncol 2008;26:9–10.
53. Sakai W, Swisher EM, Karlan BY, et al. Secondary mutations as a mechanism of cisplatin resistance in BRCA2-mutated cancers. Nature 2008;451:1116–20.

Intraperitoneal Chemotherapy: An Important Strategy in Ovarian Cancer Treatment

Franco M. Muggia

Abstract Three trials by the Gynecologic Oncology Group (GOG), adequately powered, utilizing an intraperitoneal (IP) platinum-based regimen versus a standard intravenous (IV) regimen yielded results favorable to the IP regimen, with the last two trials having median survivals exceeding five years. However, only the first trial was a direct comparison of IP vs. IV cisplatin at the same dose (both combined with cyclophosphamide); the tolerances of the two regimens were quite similar. The conclusion that IP administration of cisplatin yields superior results to IV should not be discounted solely on the asymmetry of the two subsequent regimens, and on the tolerance issues that differ substantially among the 3 IP regimens used.

Keywords Intraperitoneal chemotherapy; Cisplatin; Paclitxel; Neurotoxicity

In 2005, the National Cancer Institute (NCI) issued a clinical alert to call attention to the latest trial by the Gynecologic Oncology Group (GOG) showing a significant impact of an intraperitoneal (IP) arm of the study over IV cisplatin + paclitaxel. These alerts are issued by the governmental agency when thoroughly analyzed scientific findings could have an impact on the care of U.S. citizens. In contrast to the adoption of a particular new regimen, lack of familiarity with an IP strategy has resulted in an intense focus on all aspects of the last study (GOG 172). After an overview of the randomized IP vs. IV studies in ovarian cancer, various components of the IP strategy are reviewed and the rationale for adopting an IP strategy is discussed.

The pharmacologic basis for the delivery of anticancer drugs by the IP route was established in the late 1970s and early 1980s (and is reviewed by Howell in this book). When several drugs were studied, mostly in the setting of minimal residual disease at reassessment after patients had received their initial chemotherapy, cisplatin alone and in combination received the most attention. Favorable outcomes

F.M. Muggia
Division of Medical Oncology, New York University School of Medicine and NYU
Cancer Institute, NY, USA
e-mail: Franco.Muggia@nyumc.org

A. Bonetti et al. (eds.), *Platinum and Other Heavy Metal Compounds in Cancer Chemotherapy*, DOI: 10.1007/978-1-60327-459-3_36,
© Humana Press, a part of Springer Science + Business Media, LLC 2009

from IP cisplatin were most often seen when tumors had shown responsiveness to platinums and with small-volume tumors (usually defined as tumors < 1 cm) (1). Accordingly, in the 1990s, randomized trials were conducted to evaluate whether the IP route would prove superior to the IV route in such an optimally debulked population, and prior to exposure to any platinum. IP cisplatin was the common denominator of the IP arm in these randomized trials. The IV arm evolved over various trials since the standard has evolved from cisplatin + cyclophosphamide, to cisplatin + paclitaxel and eventually to carboplatin + paclitaxel.

The use of IP cisplatin as part of the initial up-front approach in patients, with stage III optimally debulked ovarian cancer, is supported principally by the results of three randomized clinical trials by the GOG (GOG-104, GOG-14, and GOG-172), that are also the largest studies (546, 523, and 429 patients, respectively) (2–4). These studies tested the role of IP drugs (IP cisplatin in all the three studies and IP paclitaxel in the last study) against the standard IV regimen. In the three studies, superior progression-free survival (PFS) and overall survival (OS) favoring the IP arm was documented. Specifically, the most recent study, GOG-172, resulted in a median survival rate of 66 months for patients on the IP arm vs. 50 months for patients who received IV administration of cisplatin and paclitaxel ($P = .03$) (4). Toxic effects were greater in the IP arm, contributed in large part by the cisplatin dose per cycle ($100\,\mathrm{mg/m^2}$) and by sensory neuropathy from the additional IP as well as from the IV administration of paclitaxel. The rate of completion of six cycles of treatment was also less frequent in the IP arm (42% vs. 83%) because of the toxic effects and catheter-related problems (5). Efforts are under way by the GOG and individual institutions to examine some modifications of the IP regimen used in GOG-172 to improve its tolerability (e.g., to reduce the total 3-hour amount of cisplatin given by at least 25%; and to shift from the less practical 24-hour IV administration of paclitaxel to a 3-hour IV administration). A Cochrane-sponsored meta-analysis of all randomized IP vs. IV trials shows a hazard ratio of 0.79 for disease-free survival and 0.79 for OS, favoring the IP arms (6). These studies mostly reflect the GOG, since three other studies randomized studies from Taiwan, Greece, and Italy entered 132, 90, and 113 patients, respectively. In another meta-analysis of seven IP (seventh trial is a California study closed early) vs. IV randomized trials conducted by Cancer Care of Ontario, the relative risk (RR) of progression at 5 years based on the three trials that reported this endpoint was 0.91 [95% confidence interval (CI), 0.85–0.98] and the RR of death at 5 years based on six trials was 0.88 (95% CI, 0.81–0.95) (7).

GOG-104: A Direct Comparison of IV vs. IP Cisplatin

This study, run by the Southwest Oncology Group and later joined by GOG is remarkable because it represents the "pure" direct comparison of the route of administration of cisplatin utilizing in both arms the same dose: $100\,\mathrm{mg/m^2}$

every 3 weeks, both in combination with IV cyclophosphamide. The RR for the IP arm in PFS and OS were both significant with median survivals of 49 and 41 m, respectively, for the IP and IV arms. The completion of 6 cycles was the same in the two groups (58%), the discontinuation rate for toxic effects being greater in the IV arm. A total of 297 patients with no clinical evidence of disease at the end of chemotherapy underwent adequate second-look surgery. The rate of complete pathological responses was 36% in the IV group (complete responses in 57 of 158 patients) and 47% in the IP group (complete responses in 66 of 139) (2).

Since paclitaxel had by then made an impact on GOG trials, the IP arm was not adopted, but another IP vs. IV had begun (GOG-114). Moreover, skepticism had arisen because the study was modified to include more patients with small volume disease; yet this subset did not appear to benefit any more than the other patients with volumes up to 2 cm (no longer considered "minimal residual disease").

GOG-114: A Complex Design Including an IV vs. IP Cisplatin Randomization

Because of the complexity in design, the study results favoring IP cisplatin were not promulgated for adoption and a third study was planned by the GOG. Initially, this study included a randomization to an IV cisplatin + cyclophosphamide comparator but it closed early when the IV cisplatin + 24 h paclitaxel was declared superior in the suboptimally debulked trial GOG-111 in PFS (8). However, two major confounders were added to these comparisons: (1) the IV arm by now was using $75 \, mg/m^2$ of cisplatin, a reasonable extrapolation from other trial data, but the IP arm persisted with $100 \, mg/m^2$, and (2) the IP arm was preceded by a strategy of "chemical debulking" (advanced by the Memorial Sloan-Kettering group) for two cycles – carboplatin AUC 9 was adopted for such pre-treatment. Although 96% of the patients completed those two cycles, IV carboplatin exposure likely contributed to the high rate of hematologic toxicities in the IP arm, and a completion rate of only 71% (compared to 86% for the control). Pathologic responses were not assessed but 22.6% in the IP arm refused reassessment, compared to 15% in the IV. If one considers the numbers completing to be eligible for second-look these would represent only 129 patients eligible for such reassessment in the IP arm vs. 176 in the IV arm; because any results from such large difference in the denominators were deemed subject to bias, the analysis was not carried out.

The results in PFS significantly favored the IP regimen: a median of 27.9 m compared to 22.2 m for the IV regimen. It should be noted that the long PFS median associated with the IP regimen is an outlier relative to other trials in optimally debulked stage III. OS of 63.2 m vs. 52.2 m gave a one-tail p value of 0.05 and has been regarded by critics as "non-significant."

GOG-172: Adding IP Paclitaxel in the IP Comparator

GOG-172 gave a clear survival superiority signal in favor of the IP regimen: 65.6 m compared to 49.7 m to the cisplatin + 24 h paclitaxel IV control. The toxicity problems in GOG-114 should have alerted the investigators to seek at least a dose equivalence of cisplatin in the IV vs. IP comparison. However, based on a pilot study by the Southwest Oncology Group, not only was the dose not reduced but the addition of IV paclitaxel on day 8 was certain to add further to toxicity differences, particularly in the neurotoxicity. In fact, thrombocytopenia grade 3 and 4 were lower in this protocol than in GOG-114 (12 vs. 49%) because of the absence of the pretreatment with carboplatin AUC 9. The completion rate of the IV regimen was maintained at 83%, but it fell drastically in this protocol (as compared to GOG-114) to 42%. The PFS in the IP arm was 23.8 m, while in the IV arm it was 18.3, and the rates of pathologic complete responses were 46 of 81 patients (57%) following the IP regimen and 35 of 85 patients (41%) following the IV regimen. In addition to neurologic and gastrointestinal toxicities, the IP arm was associated with a number of catheter complications. As in the other studies, treatment-related deaths were similarly distributed (4 in IV and 5 in IP arms), but were twice the number relative to the preceding studies.

Discussion

The sequential GOG studies are very informative in several aspects: (1) once gynecologic oncologists are trained in IP port placement, treatment may be accomplished safely and accrual has not been a major problem; (2) except for the first study (GOG-104), the comparison of IP vs. IV is confounded by dose difference in cisplatin. The adoption of 75 mg/m^2 of cisplatin in both arms could have resolved this problem (IV carboplatin is now the standard, but the dose reduction would still be reasonable); and (3) the IP paclitaxel on day 8 of each cycle has added greatly to the complexity and it is not clear that it adds to the therapeutic effects. In particular, it should be noted that the PFS was the longest in the second trial.

Going forward, it is important that the controversial aspects of the trials do not negate the consistent signals observed from IP administration of platinum compounds. *Additional trials urgently needed are*: (1) toxicity reduction including substitution of IP carboplatin for IP cisplatin; (2) strong consideration of omitting IP paclitaxel until a reasonable regimen is adopted with greater tolerance, less neurotoxicity, and fewer catheter complications; (3) studies comparing a variable number of cycles (do we need 6 cycles? The poor record of completion but continued advantage would not suggest); (4) studies following chemical debulking in suboptimal or neoadjuvant situations; and (5) studies with the addition of biological agents such as bevacizumab.

In spite of the problems raised by the studies, one should not loose sight of the variable nature of the studies that reinforces the most likely biological principle leading to this therapeutic advantage: IP administration of cisplatin or carbo-platin has the potential of more efficiently eliminating large number of tumor cells on the peritoneal surfaces than IV administration. My interpretation of the findings is that this better efficiency leads to slower development of peritoneal recurrences that are life-threatening because of the small-bowel dysfunction they precipitate.

References

1. Howell SB, Zimm S, Markman M, et al. Long-term survival of advanced refractory ovarian carcinoma patients with small-volume disease treated with intraperitoneal chemotherapy. J Clin Oncol 1987;5:1607–12.
2. Alberts DS, Liu PY, Hannigan EV, et al. Intraperitoneal cisplatin plus intravenous cyclophosphamide versus intravenous cisplatin plus intravenous cyclophosphamide for stage III ovarian cancer. N Engl J Med 1996;335:1950–5.
3. Markman M, Bundy BN, Alberts DS, et al. Phase III trial of standard-dose intravenous cisplatin plus paclitaxel versus moderately high-dose carboplatin followed by intravenous paclitaxel and intraperitoneal cisplatin in small-volume stage III ovarian carcinoma: an intergroup study of the Gynecologic Oncology Group, Southwestern Oncology Group, and Eastern Cooperative Oncology Group. J Clin Oncol 2001;19:1001–7.
4. Armstrong DK, Bundy B, Wenzel L, et al. Intraperitoneal cisplatin and paclitaxel in ovarian cancer. N Engl J Med 2006;354:34–43.
5. Walker JL, Armstrong DK, Huang HQ, et al. Intraperitoneal catheter outcomes in a phase III trial of intraperitoneal versus intravenous chemotherapy in optimal stage III ovarian and primary peritoneal cancer: a Gynecologic Oncology Group study. Gynecol Oncol 2006;100:27–32.
6. Elit L, Oliver TK, Covens A, et al. Intraperitoneal chemotherapy in the first-line treatment of women with stage III epithelial ovarian cancer: a systematic review with metaanalyses. Cancer 2007;109:692–702.
7. Jaaback K, Johnson N. Intraperitoneal chemotherapy for the initial management of primary epithelial ovarian cancer. Cochrane Database Syst Rev (1): CD005340, 2006.
8. McGuire WP, Hoskins WJ, Brady MF, et al. Assessment of dose-intensive therapy in suboptimally debulked ovarian cancer: a Gynecologic Oncology Group study. J Clin Oncol 1995;13:1589–99.

Novel Strategies for Enhancing the Efficacy of Intraperitoneal Chemotherapy for Patients with Ovarian Cancer

Stephen B. Howell

Abstract Intraperitoneal chemotherapy with cisplatin and paclitaxel-based programs improves survival of women with small volume ovarian cancer. The challenge now is to further improve efficacy and reduce toxicity of this approach. Limited penetration of drug from the surface of tumor nodules is a major challenge. Drug gradients, tumor nodule blood flow, capillary permeability and drug reactivity all play important roles in determining depth of penetration. Several different approaches to pharmacologically manipulating these parameters have demonstrated increased efficacy in pre-clinical animal models. Additional strategies for directing drugs to the surface of tumor nodules are also under development. There is now a firm basis for the expectation that efficacy and safety of IP therapy can be substantially improved in the future.

Keywords Intraperitoneal chemotherapy; Cisplatin; Paclitaxel; Ovarian cancer

Introduction

Intraperitoneal (IP) chemotherapy has now been shown to improve survival of ovarian cancer patients with small volumes of disease in multiple randomized clinical trials (1). These trials have established that the basic pharmacologic principles of intraperitoneal therapy developed by Dedrick and his colleagues based on work in animal models (2) can improve therapeutic outcomes when applied in women. However, incremental benefit of IP therapy is not great. In addition, IP therapy is associated with new kinds of adverse events including abdominal pain and catheter complications, and this treatment is technically demanding to administer. The challenge now is to determine whether these basic pharmacologic principles can inform the development of new strategies that will further enhance efficacy and safety of IP therapy.

S.B. Howell
Department of Medicine and the Moores Cancer Center,
University of California, San Diego, La Jolla, CA, USA
e-mail: showell@ucsd.edu

A. Bonetti et al. (eds.), *Platinum and Other Heavy Metal Compounds in Cancer Chemotherapy*, DOI: 10.1007/978-1-60327-459-3_37,
© Humana Press, a part of Springer Science + Business Media, LLC 2009

The therapeutic promise of IP therapy is based on the concept that if one can deliver more drug to tumor cells without delivering more drug to dose-limiting normal tissues, one can kill more of the tumor for the same amount of systemic toxicity. This principle is well-established for cytotoxic drugs acting against tumor cells in vitro where the amount of drug getting access to the tumor cell is proportional to drug concentration. However, in vivo incremental increases in drug exposure do no always result in equivalent increases in the amount of drug reaching all tumor cells. In part, this is related to the heterogeneity of vascular supply to tumors which almost always contain regions into which the drug does not penetrate well. However, it is now clear that there is also great heterogeneity in the sensitivity of individual malignant cells within the tumor. The dose-response curves may be quite steep for many tumor cells but very flat for cells that make up the progenitor compartment of the tumor. Nevertheless, large increases in selective delivery of drug to the tumor are generally associated with significant improvements in tumor response rate in experimental models of malignancy. This concept underlies the practice of high-dose chemotherapy followed by hematologic stem cell transplant that has been successfully utilized in patients with acute leukemias and some types of lymphoma and myeloma.

Pharmacologic Principles of Intraperitoneal Therapy

To identify additional strategies for improving the efficacy of IP therapy it is useful to review the basic pharmacologic principles that determine how much drug reaches the tumor relative to the amount delivered to sensitive normal tissues. As IP therapy is currently practiced, drugs are typically diluted in 1–2 liters of saline solution and instilled rapidly into the peritoneal cavity. The exposure for the peritoneal cavity relative to that of the blood is determined by measuring drug concentrations in the two compartments and determining the area under the concentration times time curves (AUC). The ratio of the AUC in the two compartments provides a measure of the pharmacologic advantage of the IP approach. The major route of absorption of chemotherapeutic agents from the peritoneal cavity is via the visceral peritoneum that drains into the portal circulation. The ideal drug of IP therapy would be one that is very slowly absorbed from the peritoneal cavity, is extensively inactivated in the liver before it gets to the systemic circulation and that is immediately removed once it reaches the blood. Drugs that have extensive first-pass metabolism in the liver, such as cytarabine, 5-fluorouracil, 6-thioguanine and floxuridine have very much higher AUC ratios than drugs with little or relatively slow hepatic metabolism such as cisplatin and carboplatin. A basic principle of IP therapy is to give enough drug by the IP route so that exposure to the systemic circulation is equivalent to that which could be produced if the drug was given IV. This requires that the drug not cause a lot of peritoneal toxicity and eliminates drugs such as the anthracyclines and mitoxantrone that produce peritoneal sclerosis.

Clinical trials that have demonstrated a survival advantage in women with ovarian cancer have utilized various combinations of IP cisplatin and paclitaxel. Table 1

Table 1 Pharmacokinetic parameters of intraperitoneally administered cisplatin, carboplatin and paclitaxel

	Cisplatin	Carboplatin	Paclitaxel
$T_{1/2peritoneum,}$ h	0.88		73.4
$Cl_{peritoneum}$ (L/m²/h)	1.4		0.0175
V_d (L/m²)	NR[a]	NR	1.9
AUC ratio	15[b]	17[b]	996
Bioavailability	100%	100%	46–53%

[a]Not reported; [b]Filtrable Pt

summarizes the pharmacokinetic parameters for intraperitoneally administered cisplatin, carboplatin and paclitaxel as reported by representative studies drawn from among the many that have been done (3–6). While not all parameters are available for carboplatin, the AUC ratio appears to be similar for cisplatin and carboplatin. Paclitaxel is of particular interest because its AUC ratio is ~60-fold greater than that of cisplatin or carboplatin.

While it is clear that IP administration of several classes of chemotherapeutic agents can produce very high peritoneal/plasma AUC ratios, effective killing of the tumor requires that the drug be able to penetrate deeply into tumor nodules growing on the peritoneal surface. Inadequate penetration is a major problem for both IP and IV therapy (7). Although drug is driven into the nodule by very steep concentration gradient between the nodule surface and the blood, it faces a number of obstacles as it diffuses inward. First, the interstitial pressure of tumor nodules is generally greater than the pressure in the peritoneal cavity and there is substantial convective flow of fluid from the center of the nodule outward that thwarts the inward diffusion of drug. Second, since the drug concentration in the plasma is much lower than that at the nodule surface, tumor capillaries can function like a heat sink sweeping drug out of the tumor. The greater the permeability of the capillaries, and greater the tumor blood flow, the more will be the limitation of further penetration of the drug. Third, as the drug penetrates the nodule, some of it is taken up into the tumor cells, and becomes irreversibly bound to extracellular matrix or is inactivated by metabolism in the extracellular fluid. This serves to reduce concentration of free drug available to penetrate into the next layer of cells. As a result of these factors, even if the peritoneal concentration is maintained at a steady level, one can anticipate that there will be a gradient of drug concentration with the tumor nodule such that the tumor cells near the surface will be exposed to substantially higher concentrations than those deep within the nodule.

Current studies suggest that key determinants of drug penetration are the area of the capillaries within the tumor, permeability of these capillaries and blood flow within the nodule, and diffusion coefficient of the drug (8). It is now clear that there is substantial variation in each of the first three of these determinants, not only between different patients, but also between different nodules within the same patient and even within a single nodule. The interaction of these determinants leads to some counter-intuitive predictions regarding tumor penetration. For example, one would predict that drug penetration would be better; (1) in poorly vascularized nodules; (2) for large drugs that have difficulty getting into capillaries and thus will not be swept out of the nodule as readily; (3) for non-reactive drugs that do not bind extensively to extracellular matrix; (4) for drugs that are not rapidly transported into tumor cells; and, (5) drugs that are not metabolized to inactive forms either in the extracellular matrix or inside tumor cells. It is manipulation of these determinants that hold the greatest promise for improving the efficacy of IP therapy.

The importance of inadequate penetration as a factor that limits efficacy of IP therapy is borne out by clinical observations and experimental measurements. IP therapy can produce significant increases in survival for a patient whose largest tumor nodule is less than 2 cm, but is less effective in patients with larger amount of residual tumor following primary surgery (9). There are very few studies in which cisplatin levels in tumor nodules have been measured, and none in ovarian cancer models. A study done in a rat colon carcinoma model suggested that the advantage of an intraperitoneal over an intravenous injection was limited to the first ~1.5 mm depth into the tumor, that a peritoneal to plasma AUC ratio of 12–15 was associated with a 1.7-fold increase in drug delivery in millimeter sized tumors and there was marked heterogeneity of drug levels in different parts of the same nodule (10).

Strategies for Improving Drug Penetration

Several groups have undertaken studies in model systems exploring whether manipulations of the key determinants of concentration gradients within a tumor nodule actually enhanced drug penetration. Esquis et al. (11) reported that increasing the intra-abdominal pressure to 22 mgHg during a 1 h exposure to IP cisplatin increased Pt levels in colon carcinoma serosal 0.5–3 mm nodules by a factor of ~1.6-fold. This approach may be difficult to implement in patients due to the effect of increased abdominal pressure on venous return to the right heart. In principle, tumor nodule blood flow might be reduced by administering IP epinephrine. Studies to date of this approach in a colon carcinomatosis model have demonstrated that IP epinephrine can increase the levels of Pt in small tumor nodules (2–5 mm) in a concentration-dependent manner up to 3.7-fold (12). In a subsequent phase 1 trial, 100 gm of cisplatin was given IP over 2 h in fluid containing increasing concentrations of epinephrine (13). An epinephrine concentration of even 5 mg/L was well tolerated in terms of cardiovascular adverse events, and produced a peritoneal/plasma concentration ratio of >3,000 at the end of the instillation. Further randomized trials are now needed to assess the efficacy of this approach. Bevacizumab can markedly alter the permeability of tumor capillaries and tumor blood flow; it will be particularly interesting to determine whether this antibody can enhance drug penetration into ovarian cancer tumor nodules.

Another approach to enhancing drug penetration is to maintain extremely high concentrations of the chemotherapeutic agent in the peritoneal cavity for very prolonged periods of time. This can only be done with drugs that have extensive hepatic metabolism and/or very high rates of plasma clearance such that levels in the blood never reach intolerable levels. Phase 1 and 2 trials of this strategy utilizing cytarabine and fluordeoxyuridine were reported a number of years ago and produced promising results that have not been adequately investigated further (14–16). Recent early stage clinical trials have shown gemcitabine also has very high peritoneal/plasma AUC ratio (791–847) (17, 18), making it a candidate for use in this strategy.

Instead of flooding the peritoneal cavity with free drug, several groups are attempting to increase drug penetration by producing particles that slowly release a chemotherapeutic agent that might get randomly distributed to the surface of tumor nodules by the same diaphragmatic motion that distributes tumor cells throughout the peritoneal cavity. The first of these paclitaxel-loaded particle formulations to reach clinical testing failed in phase 1 due to a foreign body reaction to the particle (19). However, two other paclitaxel-loaded particles (20, 21) and a cisplatin-loaded particle (22) have shown promise in pre-clinical tumor models.

An even more sophisticated approach would be to produce extremely high drug concentrations at the surface of the tumor nodule but not elsewhere in the peritoneal cavity or systemic circulation. A number of peptides have now been identified that bind quite selectively to ovarian cancer cells (23) or to integrins expressed on these cells. Despite the fact that these have limited affinity as free molecules, promising results have been reported for an RGD peptide that binds to integrins conjugated to a chelating group capable of carrying ^{111}In to the tumor in an experimental model of ovarian cancer (24). Since the avidity of such peptides to tumor cells can be increased when they are multimerized on the surface of particles (25), truly tumor selective peptides hold substantial promise for the development of tumor targeting toxins for intraperitoneal use.

Recent studies of transporters that mediate the uptake of cisplatin and carboplatin into ovarian cancer cells have identified another potential strategy for enhancing the tumor cell uptake of these drugs. The major copper influx transporter, CTR1, plays an important role in the initial influx of cisplatin and carboplatin (26, 27). It has been know for some time that high levels of Cu trigger degradation of CTR1, thus limiting further influx of this toxin. It has now been shown that even very low concentrations of cisplatin initiate very rapid down-regulation of CTR1 which limits the amount of cisplatin that can enter the cells (28). Degradation of CTR1 occurs through action of the proteosome, and drugs that inhibit proteosome activity can prevent this from occurring (29). Thus, there is now substantial interest in determining whether, by maintaining CTR1 on the plasma membrane for longer periods of time, proteosome inhibitors can increase the uptake of cisplatin and enhance ovarian cell kill.

Summary

Intraperitoneal chemotherapy with cisplatin and paclitaxel-based programs can improve survival in women with small volume ovarian cancer. The challenge now is to build on these achievements to further improve efficacy and reduce toxicity.

Strategies based around manipulation of the basic determinants of drug penetration into tumor nodules are of particular interest because pharmacologic agents that can influence parameters such as capillary permeability and tumor nodule blood flow are readily available. In addition, several new drug delivery technologies offer promise of maintaining extremely high drug concentrations at the surface of tumor nodules in a highly selective manner.

References

1. Trimble E, Christian M. Intraperitoneal chemotherapy for women with advanced epithelial ovarian cancer. Gynecol Oncol 2006;100:3–4.
2. Dedrick RL, Myers CE, Bungay PM, DeVita VT, Jr. Pharmacokinetic rationale for peritoneal drug administration in the treatment of ovarian cancer. Cancer Treat Rep 1978;62:1–11.
3. Howell SB, Pfeifle CL, Wung WE, et al. Intraperitoneal cisplatin with systemic thiosulfate protection. Ann Intern Med 1982;97:845–51.
4. Howell SB, Pfeifle CE, Wung WE, Olshen RA. Intraperitoneal cis-diamminedichloroplatinum with systemic thiosulfate protection. Cancer Res 1983;43:1426–31.
5. Markman M, Rowinsky E, Hakes T, et al. Phase I trial of intraperitoneal taxol: a gynecoloic oncology group study. J Clin Oncol 1992;10:1485–91.
6. Elferink F, van der Vijgh WJ, Klein I, ten Bokkel Huinink WW, Dubbelman R, McVie JG. Pharmacokinetics of carboplatin after intraperitoneal administration. Cancer Chemother Pharmacol 1988;21:57–60.
7. Minchinton AI, Tannock IF. Drug penetration in solid tumours. Nat Rev Cancer 2006;6:583–92.
8. Dedrick RL, Flessner MF. Pharmacokinetic problems in peritoneal drug administration: tissue penetration and surface exposure. J Natl Cancer Inst 1996;89:480–7.
9. Howell SB, Zimm S, Markman M, et al. Long term survival of advanced refractory ovarian carcinoma patients with small-volume disease treated with intraperitoneal chemotherapy. J Clin Oncol 1987;5:1607–12.
10. Los G, Mutsaers PH, Lenglet WJ, Baldew GS, McVie JG. Platinum distribution in intra-peritoneal tumors after intraperitoneal cisplatin treatment. Cancer Chemother Pharmacol 1990;25:389–94.
11. Esquis P, Consolo D, Magnin G, et al. High intra-abdominal pressure enhances the penetration and antitumor effect of intraperitoneal cisplatin on experimental peritoneal carcinomatosis. Ann Surg 2006;244:106–12.
12. Favoulet P, Magnin G, Guilland JC, et al. Pre-clinical study of the epinephrine-cisplatin association for the treatment of intraperitoneal carcinomatosis. Eur J Surg Oncol 2001;27:59–64.
13. Molucon-Chabrot C, Isambert N, Benoit L, et al. Feasibility of using intraperitoneal epine-phrine and cisplatin in patients with advanced peritoneal carcinomatosis. Anticancer Drugs 2006;17:1211–7.
14. King ME, Pfeifle CE, Howell SB. Intraperitoneal cytosine arabinoside therapy in ovarian carcinoma. J Clin Oncol 1984;2:662–9.
15. Kirmani S, Zimm S, Cleary SM, Mowry J, Howell SB. Extremely prolonged continuous intra-peritoneal infusion of cytosine arabinoside. Cancer Chemother Pharmacol 1990;25:454–8.
16. Muggia FM, Jeffers S, Muderspach L, et al. Phase I/II study of intraperitoneal floxuridine and platinums (cisplatin and/or carboplatin). Gynecol Oncol 1997;66:290–4.
17. Morgan RJ, Jr., Synold TW, Xi B, et al. Phase I trial of intraperitoneal gemcitabine in the treatment of advanced malignancies primarily confined to the peritoneal cavity. Clin Cancer Res 2007;13:1232–7.
18. Sabbatini P, Aghajanian C, Leitao M, et al. Intraperitoneal cisplatin with intraperitoneal gemcitabine in patients with epithelial ovarian cancer: results of a phase I/II Trial. Clin Cancer Res 2004;10:2962–7.

19. Armstrong DK, Fleming GF, Markman M, Bailey HH. A phase I trial of intraperitoneal sustained-release paclitaxel microspheres (Paclimer) in recurrent ovarian cancer: a Gynecologic Oncology Group study. Gynecol Oncol 2006;103:391–6.
20. Vassileva V, Grant J, De Souza R, Allen C, Piquette-Miller M. Novel biocompatible intraperitoneal drug delivery system increases tolerability and therapeutic efficacy of paclitaxel in a human ovarian cancer xenograft model. Cancer Chemother Pharmacol 2007;60:907–14.
21. Tsai M, Lu Z, Wang J, Yeh TK, Wientjes MG, Au JL. Effects of carrier on disposition and antitumor activity of intraperitoneal Paclitaxel. Pharm Res 2007;24:1691–701.
22. Xu P, Van Kirk EA, Murdoch WJ, et al. Anticancer efficacies of cisplatin-releasing pH-responsive nanoparticles. Biomacromolecules 2006;7:829–35.
23. Aina OH, Marik J, Liu R, Lau DH, Lam KS. Identification of novel targeting peptides for human ovarian cancer cells using "one-bead one-compound" combinatorial libraries. Mol Cancer Ther 2005;4:806–13.
24. Dijkgraaf I, Kruijtzer JA, Frielink C, et al. Alpha v beta 3 integrin-targeting of intraperitoneally growing tumors with a radiolabeled RGD peptide. Int J Cancer 2007;120:605–10.
25. Carlson CB, Mowery P, Owen RM, Dykhuizen EC, Kiessling LL. Selective tumor cell targeting using low-affinity, multivalent interactions. ACS Chem Biol 2007;2:119–27.
26. Safaei R, Howell SB. Regulation of the cellular pharmacology and cytotoxicity of cisplatin by copper transporters. In: Beverly A, Teicher PD, eds. Cancer Drug Discovery and Development. Totowa, New Jersey, US: Humana Press, 2006:309–27.
27. Holzer AK, Samimi G, Katano K, et al. The copper influx transporter human copper transport protein 1 regulates the uptake of cisplatin in human ovarian carcinoma cells. Mol Pharmacol 2004;66:817–23.
28. Holzer AK, Katano K, Klomp LW, Howell SB. Cisplatin rapidly down-regulates its own influx transporter hCTR1 in cultured human ovarian carcinoma cells. Clin Cancer Res 2004;10:6744–9.
29. Holzer AK, Howell SB. The internalization and degradation of human copper transporter 1 following cisplatin exposure. Cancer Res 2006;66:10944–52.

Laparoscopically Assisted Heated Intra-Operative Intraperitoneal Chemotherapy (HIPEC): Technical Aspect and Pharmacokinetics Data

Gwenaël Ferron, Amélie Gesson-Paute, Laurence Gladieff,
Fabienne Thomas, Etienne Chatelut, and Denis Querleu

Abstract Hyperthermic intraperitoneal chemotherapy (HIPEC) is being evaluated for patients with minimal residual or no residual disease after complete cytoreductive surgery. An experimental study on the porcine model was carried out to demonstrate the feasibility of the laparoscopic approach and to compare oxaliplatin pharmacokinetics during a laparoscopic assisted vs. the "coliseum" technique for HIPEC.

In the first step, feasibility of the peritonectomy procedure followed by HIPEC was evaluated in five adult pigs. In the second step, ten adult pigs were selected to receive laparoscopic assisted HIPEC procedure and ten pigs were selected for standard HIPEC in laparotomy. The HIPEC procedure was based on $460\,mg/m^2$ of oxaliplatin for 30 min with a heated perfusate at 41–43 °C. HIPEC drains were placed in the upper and lower quadrants of the abdomen. Peritoneal fluid and blood samples were collected every 10 min during the procedure and the pharmacokinetics of oxaliplatin was studied.

For the first step, the procedure was successfully completed with an adequate intrabdominal temperature and distribution. For the second step, no major technical problems were encountered. At the end of the HIPEC, 41.5% of the chemotherapy was absorbed in the laparoscopic group compared to 33.4% in the laparotomy group ($p = 0.0543$). The peritoneal oxaliplatin half-life ($T_{1/2}$) was significantly shorter in the laparoscopic procedure (median value of 37.5 min vs. 59.3 min, $p = 0.02$). The area under the curve ratio for peritoneal/plasma reflects a faster oxaliplatin absorption through the peritoneal barrier in the laparoscopic procedure (ratio: 16.4 in the laparoscopic group vs. 28.1 in the laparotomy group, $p = 0.03$).

This study confirms the technical feasibility and reliability of the laparoscopic approach for HIPEC, and improves understanding of peritoneal drug absorption. Oxaliplatin absorption is significantly higher with laparoscopy, regarding time course in the peritoneal perfusion. Clinical application in selected patients may be expected after further experimental investigation designed to define adequate drug dosage.

G. Ferrron (✉), A. Gesson-Paute, L. Gladieff, F. Thomes, E. Chatelut, and D. Querleu
Department of Surgical Oncology, Institut Claudius Regaud, 20-24 Rue du Pont Pierre,
31052 Toulouse Cedex, France
e-mail: ferron.gwenael@claudiusregaud.fr

A. Bonetti et al. (eds.), *Platinum and Other Heavy Metal Compounds in Cancer Chemotherapy*, DOI: 10.1007/978-1-60327-459-3_38,
© Humana Press, a part of Springer Science + Business Media, LLC 2009

343

Keywords Hyperthermia; Intraperitoneal chemotherapy; Laparoscopy; Oxaliplatin; Pharmacokinetics

Introduction

Hyperthermic intraperitoneal chemotherapy (HIPEC) based on platinum compounds administration is being evaluated in patients with peritoneal carcinomatosis and sometimes in patients with previous intravenous chemotherapy. HIPEC has been proposed following advantage of IP vs. IV in randomized trials in patients with colorectal, gastric, peritoneal and ovarian cancer (1). We assume that HIPEC can be applied without performing a laparotomy, particularly when no bulky disease is present especially as a consolidation treatment after standard adjuvant chemotherapy or in cases of high risk of peritoneal recurrence. This may be applicable during a second look laparoscopy in high risk cases. In addition, laparoscopic surgery is adapted for adhesiolysis and comprehensive examination of the peritoneal cavity with acceptable accuracy and morbidity (2, 3).

To reinforce this approach, we performed a two step experimental study on the porcine model. The first step demonstrates the feasibility of laparoscopic peritonectomy and heated intraperitoneal chemohyperthermia (HIPEC) (4). The second step compares the pharmacokinetics of oxaliplatin between an open vs. a laparoscopically assisted intraperitoneal hyperthermic chemotherapy (5).

Materials and Methods

A total of twenty five adult pigs were used. During the first step we performed five laparoscopic procedures to evalue the feasibility of peritonectomy followed by HIPEC. A 12 mm trocar was placed in the umbilical area to accommodate the endoscope. Four additional 12 mm Versastep® (Tyco Healthcare Group LP, Norwalk, Connecticut USA) trocars were placed in each quadrant of the abdomen (Fig. 1). The positioning of trocars in the four quadrants was planned to perform a complete peritonectomy and later to place the HIPEC drains. The umbilical trocar was then replaced by a Lapdisc® (Ethicon Endo Surgery Inc, Cincinnati, USA) allowing placement of the hand and forearm in the abdomen without any gas or liquid leakage. Four drains were placed under laparoscopic guidance: in the right and left upper quadrants with an inflow and an outflow circuit respectively. For the lower abdomen, the outflow drain was placed in the pelvis. The hand of the surgeon manipulated the inflow drain in order to evenly distribute the flow within the abdominal cavity. For the first step, no anticancer drug was used. At the end of the procedure, methylene blue was injected in order to check the completeness of peritoneal exposure to the heated fluid.

Twenty adult pigs were used for the second step. Half of the group underwent HIPEC via laparotomy as previously described by Elias et al. (6) using the

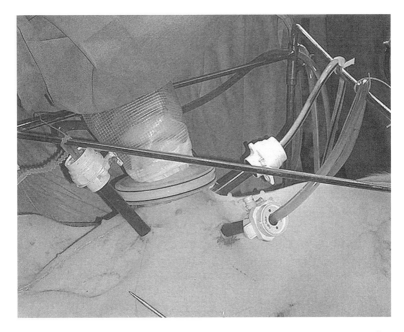

Fig. 1 Positioning of HIPEC drains with the surgeon's right hand through the Lapdisc®

"coliseum" technique. The other group of pigs underwent laparoscopically assisted HIPEC featuring the same dosage and physical parameters. Oxaliplatin was delivered at a dose of 460 mg/m² filled heated (43 °C) in the abdominal cavity with a fixed volume (dextrose 5%–2L/m²) during 30 min (7). Knowing that the therapeutic index is optimal at 41–43 °C, the goal for achieving the adequate intraabdominal temperature was fullfilled using a perfusate heated at 46–52 °C, with a 1,360 mL/min flow that resulted in outflow temperature at 41–43 °C.

Blood and Peritoneal Fluid Sampling

Nine blood samples were collected from each animal at different times: before HIPEC, at time zero (T0) when the peritoneal fluid reached 43 °C, and every 10 min during the procedure. Blood samples were then collected after the HIPEC at 45 min, 1 h, 1.5 h and 2 h after T0. Samples were immediately centrifuged at +4 °C, for 10 min at 1,500 g. For samples collected at the end of the procedure (i.e. 30 min after T0), at 1 and 2 h after the HIPEC beginning, an aliquot of plasma was ultrafiltered by centrifugation at +4 °C for 20 min at 2,000 × g through a Amicon MPS1 micropartition system with YMT membranes (cut-off 30,000 Da).

Five 5 ml samples of peritoneal fluid were collected from each animal at different time points: before the temperature reached 43 °C, at the beginning of the HIPEC and then every 10 min during the procedure. All samples were frozen at −20 °C until assay.

Platinum Determination

Platinum levels in the plasma and in the plasma ultrafiltrate were measured by means of flameless atomic absorption spectrophotometric analysis according to a previously described method. Nominal values of platinum controls were 21, 105 and 210 ng/mL for plasma ultrafiltrate and 20.9, 104.7 and 209.3 ng/mL for plasma samples. Platinum determination in samples was validated when measured control values were comprised within 10% for the medium and high level control and 20% for the low level control.

Results

In the first step, the peritonectomy procedure was successfully completed in all five animals. Active permanent manipulation of the bowel and viscera, and manual adaptation of the direction of the inflow by the surgeon's hand, allowed us to obtain a homogeneous intraabdominal temperature. The distribution of blue dye was even in the abdominal cavity in all the pigs. Exposure of all peritoneal surfaces to heated perfusate, including the root of the mesentery and the omental bursa, was achieved.

In the second step, no noticeable technical problems were encountered in the laparotomy group as a result of our experience in human clinical practice. The most frequently encountered complication during laparoscopic procedures was circuit obstruction by the contact of small bowel and omentum with the tips of the drains in three procedures. As a result, target temperature was reached after 8 min (median value) in the laparotomy group vs. 12.5 min in the laparoscopic group ($p = 0.03$) (Fig. 2).

Pharmacokinetics of Heated Intraoperative Intraperitoneal Oxaliplatin

A decrease in platinum concentration was observed in the peritoneal perfusion during HIPEC in both groups (Fig. 3). Analysis of $T_{1/2}$ of the drug showed a significantly faster tissue absorption of oxaliplatin in the laparoscopic group (median value: 37.5 min vs. 59.3 min, $p = 0.02$), giving evidence that the "closed" technique seemed to influence and raise platinum absorption through the peritoneal barrier. At the time of completion of HIPEC, 41.5% of the chemotherapy was absorbed in the laparoscopic group, compared to 33.4% in the laparatomy group ($p = 0.05$).

Time Course of Oxaliplatin in the Peripheral Blood

Peak plasma concentration of platinum was observed on average 30 min after starting HIPEC in the laparotomy group whereas peak plasma concentration was

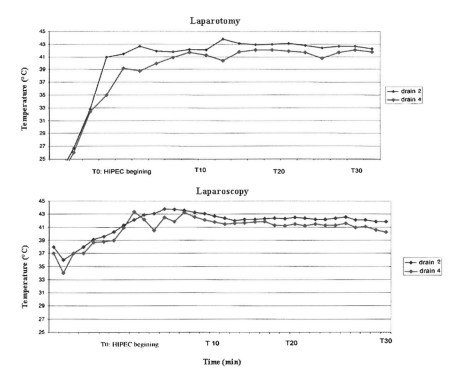

Fig. 2 Temperature curve of optimal procedure in each group (*see Color Plates*)

obtained after 46.4 min ($p = 0.87$) in the laparoscopic group (Fig. 4). Platinum concentration then dropped rapidly in both groups, resulting in a limited systemic area under the curve (AUC). The AUC_{2h} was higher for the laparoscopic procedure, as was C_{2h} in ultrafiltrat (Table 1). The AUC ratio peritoneal/plasma (at 30 min) was larger in the laparotomy group (28.1 vs. 16.4, $p = 0.03$), reflecting the fact that oxaliplatin was kept in the abdominal cavity with less penetration through the peritoneal barrier to the blood compartment compared to the laparoscopic group. During HIPEC, oxaliplatin was more rapidly absorbed in the laparoscopic group: 41.5% of oxaliplatin was absorbed in the laparoscopic group, compared to 33.4% in the laparotomy group at the end of the HIPEC procedure ($p = 0.0543$).

Discussion

Development of intraperitoneal drug therapy is one of the main areas of research to improve the long-term survival for patients with peritoneal carcinomatosis. Encouraging results of a randomized controlled study of HIPEC in the management of peritoneal carcinomatosis in colorectal cancer patients have been published (8). HIPEC has also been proposed in ovarian cancers, mesothelioma and pseudomyxoma peritonei (9, 10). Laparoscopic techniques may prove to be an optimal route

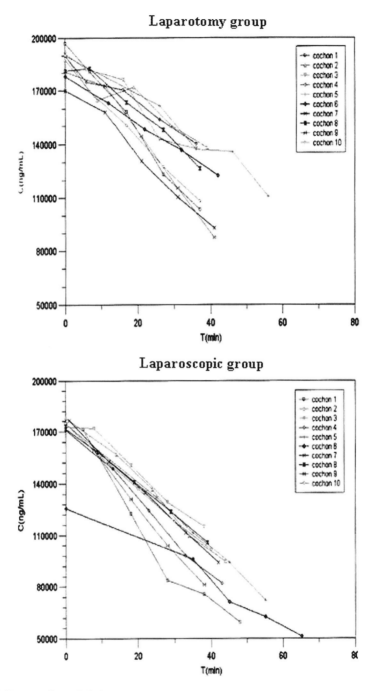

Fig. 3 Decrease in oxaliplatin concentrations in heated peritoneal instillation (460 mg/m²). First point ($t = 0$ min) corresponds to concentration in the peritoneal fluid before the HIPEC (i.e. before the temperature of 43 °C was reached) (*see Color Plates*)

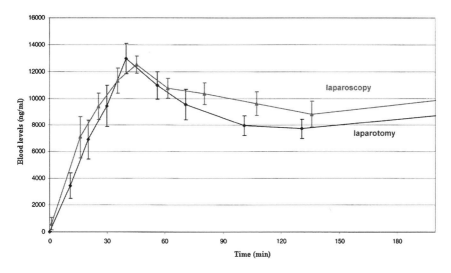

Fig. 4 Oxaliplatin pharmacokinetics in plasma after heated intraperitoneal chemotherapy (460 mg/m²) (*see Color Plates*)

Table 1 Oxaliplatin concentrations after heated intraperitoneal chemotherapy (460 mg/m²)

	Laparotomy	Laparoscopy	p
Mean ultrafiltrate C_{2h} (ng/ml)	2295.26	2994.17	0.04
Mean plasma AUC_{2h} (ng/ml × min)	1102.01	1292.65	0.23
Median peritoneal $T_{1/2}$ (min)	59.3	37.5	0.02

AUC Area under the plasma concentration-time curve; $T_{1/2}$ Half life elimination

to administer intraperitoneal chemotherapy especially after complete cytoreductive surgery and adjuvant chemotherapy as a consolidation treatment. This approach can also be utilised in cases at high risk of peritoneal recurrence in patients with colorectal cancer or gastric cancer. HIPEC administered in only one session, under direct surgical monitoring, might be more applicable in clinical practice than sequential intraperitoneal chemotherapy using permanent catheters.

The possibility of using a closed technique, while manipulating the viscera using the hand-assisted technique and/or laparoscopic instruments, combines advantages of both laparotomy techniques.

In this study, we developed techniques to overcome the limitations of a "closed" HIPEC procedure in terms of intraabdominal temperature homogeneity and complete exposure of all peritoneal surfaces, including the root of the mesentery and the omental bursa, to heated perfusate. Considering that manual mobilisation of the bowel by the surgeon's hand is an essential component of even distribution of the drug and complete exposure of the bowel (6), the use of hand-assisted technique has proved to be useful. Xiphopubic laparotomy is no longer required. In this regard, the laparoscopic hand-assisted HIPEC is superior to standard "closed" HIPEC procedure that has been proposed for palliation of debilitating malignant ascites in a series of 14 patients (11). Hand-assisted surgery mimicks the Sugarbaker modification of the "coliseum" technique using an impermeable disposable drape covering the entire operative field with a cruciate cut in its central portion to open the access site to the surgeon's arm (12). In addition, the laparoscopic technique avoids exposure of the operative room staff from droplets of chemotherapy and aerosols that may escape into the environment (13). This study provides evidence that laparoscopic HIPEC is feasible, and was successfully completed in all animals after resolution of minor technical problems (15 cases with a laparoscopic approach). The minimal additional time to reach target temperature is likely to disappear with experience.

From the pharmacokinetic point of view we demonstrated that laparoscopic HIPEC provides equivalent exposure of the peritoneum compared to an open one. Evidence is given that high intraabdominal pressure facilitates drug penetration into the blood compartment. A massive crossing of the molecule through the peritoneal barrier has been observed, but these results must be interpreted with caution, as they are significant only for ultrafiltrat values. Further experimental studies are required, to investigate tissue concentrations of platinum in the peritoneum, liver and omentum, assess the role of peritoneal pressure, and define appropriate dosage of drug, taking into account higher blood concentrations of drug during laparoscopic procedures.

Conclusions

This experimental study provides further evidence of the feasibility and reliability of HIPEC laparoscopic approach. We obtained optimal conditions in terms of temperature and agent distribution in the laparoscopy group as well as the laparotomy group. The hand-assisted concept is revolutionary compared to classic "closed" techniques and matched the requirements of the open approach from the technical point of view. In addition, the "closed" procedure avoids drug exposure to the staff present in the operative room. The results of this study favours further investigation of the role of laparoscopic HIPEC as an innovative application of laparoscopic surgery in surgical oncology, with the aim of reducing surgical morbidity and hopefully improving the quality of life of patients.

Acknowledgments This study was supported by the research program of the Institut Claudius Regaud Cancer Centre, Comprehensive cancer center by Sanofi-Aventis who provided the drug and Karl Storz INC. who provided the laparoscopic equipment. All experiments were carried out in the surgery laboratory of the Rangueil university Hospital in Toulouse, France.

References

1. Armstrong DK, Bundy B, Wenzel L, et al. Intraperitoneal cisplatin and paclitaxel in ovarian cancer. N Engl J Med 2006;354:34–43.
2. Leblanc E, Querleu D, Narducci F, Occelli B, Papageorgiou T, Sonoda Y. Laparoscopic restaging of early stage invasive adnexal tumors: a 10-year experience. Gynecol Oncol ;94:624–9.

3. Paraskeva PA, Purkayastha S, Darzi A. Laparoscopy for malignancy: current status. Semin Laparosc Surg 2004;11:27–36.
4. Ferron G, Gesson-Paute A, Classe JM, Querleu D. Feasibility of laparoscopic peritonectomy followed by intra-peritoneal chemohyperthermia: an experimental study. Gynecol Oncol 2005;99:358–61.
5. Gesson-Paute A, Ferron G, Thomas F, de Lara EC, Chatelut E, Querleu D. Pharmacokinetics of oxaliplatin durin open versus laparoscopically assisted heated intraoperative intraperitoneal chemotherapy (HIPEC): an experimental study. Ann Surg Oncol 2008;15:339–44.
6. Elias D, Bonnay M, Puizillou JM, et al. Heated intra-operative intraperitoneal oxaliplatin after complete resection of peritoneal carcinomatosis: pharmacokinetics and tissue distribution. Ann Oncol 2002;13:267–72.
7. Elias D, Antoun S, Raynard B et al. Treatment of peritoneal carcinomatosis using complete excision and intraperitoneal chemohyperthermia. A phase I-II study defining the best technical procedures. Chirurgie 1999;124:380–9.
8. Verwall VJ, van Ruth S, de Bree E, et al. Randomized trial of cytoreduction and hyperthermic intraperitoneal chemotherapy versus systemic chemotherapy and palliative surgery in patients with peritoneal carcinomatosis of colorectal cancer. J Clin Oncol 2003;21:3737–43.
9. Sugarbaker PH. New standard of care for appendiceal epithelial neoplasms and pseudomyxoma peritonei syndrome? Lancet Oncol 2006;1:69–76.
10. Elias D, Blot F, Otmany A, et al. Curative treatement of peritoneal carcinomatosis arising from colorectal cancer by complete resection and intraperitoneal chemotherapy. Cancer 2001;92:71–6.
11. Garofalo A, Valle M, Garcia J, Sugarbaker PH. Laparoscopic intraperitoneal hyperthermic chemotherapy for palliation of debilitating malignant ascites. Eur J Surg Oncol 2006;32:682–5.
12. Sugarbaker PH. An instrument to provide containment of intraoperative intraperitoneal chemotherapy with optimized distribution. J Surg Oncol 2005;92:142–6.
13. Stuart OA, Stephens AD, Welch L, Sugarbaker PH. Safety monitoring of the coliseum technique for heated intraoperative intraperitoneal chemotherapy with mitomycin C. Ann Surg Oncol 2002;9:186–91.

Organic Cation Transporters 2 as Mediators of Cisplatin Nephrotoxicity

Giuliano Ciarimboli

Abstract Cisplatin is an effective but highly nephrotoxic antineoplastic agent. Though many aspects of cisplatin interactions with DNA and cellular proteins are well described, specific systems for cisplatin transport across the cell membrane have only recently been identified. In this paper our findings on this topic are illustrated and reviewed in relation to studies conducted by other groups. The human organic cation transporter 2 (hOCT2) would appear to be a critical transporter for cisplatin nephrotoxicity, since it mediates the accumulation of cisplatin in renal tubular cells. However, the less nephrotoxic platin derivative oxaliplatin shares the same transporter to enter renal proximal tubule cells. Its lower nephrotoxicity could be due to its substantial excretion in urine mediated by the apical hMATE1 and hMATE2-K transporters. Conversely, cisplatin is not a good substrate for these apical transporters and accumulates at a higher level in renal cells. Cisplatin transport competition at hOCT2 offers a potential mechanism to reduce nephrotoxicity in clinical practice. However, the feasibility of such an approach needs to be tested in an in-vivo model and the expression of hOCT2 in cisplatin-sensitive tumour cells needs to be investigated. Screening of hOCT2 polymorphisms and their association with resistance to cisplatin nephrotoxicity should also be investigated.

Keywords Cisplatin; Organic cation transporters; Nephrotoxicity; Proximal tubules

Cisplatin is one of the most effective and potent anticancer drugs for the treatment of epithelial malignancies such as lung, head and neck, ovarian and bladder cancer (1). When combined with bleomycin and etoposide, cisplatin is considered to be a curative treatment for testicular cancer (2). However, its use is limited by serious side effects such as nephrotoxicity, emetogenesis, ototoxicity and peripheral neuropathy (1). Though the antineoplastic effect of cisplatin is dosc-dependent, nephrotoxic risks preclude the use of higher doses to maximise the therapeutic effect (3).

G. Ciarimboli
Universitätsklinikum Münster, Medizinische Klinik und Poliklinik D,
Experimentelle Nephrologie, Münster, Germany
e-mail: gciari@uni-muenster.de

A. Bonetti et al. (eds.), *Platinum and Other Heavy Metal Compounds in Cancer Chemotherapy*, DOI: 10.1007/978-1-60327-459-3_39,
© Humana Press, a part of Springer Science + Business Media, LLC 2009

Many aspects of cisplatin's interaction with DNA and cellular proteins have been described in detail (4). However, the uptake route of cisplatin across the plasma membrane is not yet completely understood. This topic is of great importance, because an exact knowledge of cisplatin transport systems in tumour and normal cells would contribute, on the one hand, to the design of platin derivatives with better uptake in, or slower release from, tumour cells and, on the other hand, to establishing suitable therapeutic protocols to protect renal cells against cisplatin toxicity. This paper describes our findings on cisplatin transport systems in renal cells and discusses them in relation to those reported by other groups.

The existence of a specific renal transport system for cisplatin has been suggested by studies demonstrating its active secretion in renal tubules (5). A vectorial polarised transport of cisplatin has been demonstrated in epithelial cells derived from proximal tubules of the opossum (OK cell line), where basolateral-to-apical transport of cisplatin is higher than apical-to-basolateral transport (6). In these cells, co-incubation of cisplatin with tetraethylammonium (TEA, a model substrate for organic cation transporters [OCT]) significantly decreased the accumulation and transport of cisplatin from the basolateral medium (6), in a manner similar to that observed in rabbit isolated proximal tubules (7). Moreover, TEA uptake by NIH3T3 cells (a mouse embryonic fibroblast cell line) stably transfected with rat OCT2 was competitively inhibited by cisplatin (8). Other indications for the importance of OCTs in the uptake of cisplatin by proximal tubule cells are provided by studies with the C7 clone of Madin-Darby canine kidney (MDCK) cells. These cells have been shown to express the isoform 2 of OCT and to be more sensitive to cisplatin toxicity when cisplatin is added to the basolateral vs. luminal side (3). This toxicity could be decreased by incubation with cimetidine, a substrate of OCT (3). Taken together, these results suggest that OCT could be a specific renal transport system for cisplatin that mediates its accumulation in renal cells.

OCTs are classified as uniporters (transporters where a single species is transported by facilitated diffusion) belonging to the Major Facilitator Superfamily (MFS) and have been assigned to the SLC22A transporter family. In addition to OCTs, this family also includes electroneutral organic cation transporters (OCTNs, OCTN1–3) and a large group of transporters involved in organic anion transport (OATs, OAT1–5 and urate transporters, URAT1) (9). Since many of these proteins are expressed in the intestines, liver and kidney, transporters of the SLC22A family play a pivotal role in drug absorption and excretion (9). Transport mediated by OCTs has been characterised as polyspecific, electrogenic, voltage-dependent and bidirectional, but pH- and Na^+-independent (10). Three isoforms of OCTs have been identified in the rat, mouse and man: OCT1, OCT2 and OCT3 (10). The different isoforms of these transporters have a species- and tissue-specific distribution: for example, OCT2 is the main OCT of the human kidney, while in rat kidney the principal OCT is OCT1; in man, OCT1 is the main hepatic isoform (11). Interaction of a substance with a particular isoform of OCT does not necessarily predict interaction with other OCTs, because the affinity of these transporters for different substrates is species- and isoform-specific (for a review see (12)). In humans, hOCT2 has been shown to be expressed on the basolateral side in all three segments of the proximal tubule (13).

In a previous study, we showed for the first time that cisplatin directly interacts with hOCT2, the renal OCT isoform in humans (14). Cisplatin inhibited, in a concentration-dependent manner, the uptake of the fluorescent organic cation 4-(4-(dimethyl-amino) styril)-methylpyridinium (ASP) in HEK293 cells stably transfected with hOCT2 with an IC_{50} of 1.5 µM. A cisplatin concentration of 100 µM, which gave rise to significant inhibition of ASP-uptake by hOCT2, failed to inhibit ASP-uptake by hOCT1, the human hepatic OCT isoform. The less nephrotoxic platin derivatives carboplatin and oxaliplatin at a concentration of 100 µM, showed no significant effect on ASP-uptake by hOCT2. These experiments demonstrated for the first time that cisplatin interacts with hOCT2, but not with hOCT1. Since hOCT2 is the renal isoform of OCTs and hOCT1 is the hepatic one in humans (11), these results could explain the high kidney-specific toxicity of cisplatin. Carboplatin and oxaliplatin, which are less nephrotoxic analogues of cisplatin, presented no interaction with hOCT2 in this work. It is important to note that cisplatin inhibited ASP-uptake in a concentration-dependent manner via hOCT2 with 40% maximal inhibition. This result can be explained by taking into account the recently proposed structure-function properties of OCTs. These transporters appear to have a large binding pocket with overlapping interaction domains for different substrates (15, 16). For example, it has been suggested that rOCT1 contains a large substrate binding region within a large cleft capable of binding several substrates and/or inhibitors simultaneously (16). Transport of ASP or cisplatin may therefore require simultaneous or successive substrate binding to two or more binding sites within this large cleft. In this way, even though both cisplatin and ASP are transported by hOCT2, they are capable of binding slightly different domains of the transporter with different affinities and maximal inhibition of ASP uptake by cisplatin cannot be achieved. This structure of the binding site with overlapping interaction domains for different substrates may also explain the contradictory observations regarding the interaction of platin derivatives with OCT-mediated transport of tracer substances (see below). For the first time, we have investigated these transport processes also in freshly isolated human proximal tubules and hepatocyte couplets. The results of these experiments confirm what was observed with hOCT1 and hOCT2, namely that cisplatin interacts with the transport system of the fluorescent organic cation ASP in proximal tubules, but not in hepatocyte couplets (14). The platin accumulation of hOCT2-HEK293 expressing cells after a 10 min incubation with 100 µM cisplatin at 37 °C was greater than that observed in HEK293 cells at 37 °C or in hOCT2-HEK293 cells at 4 °C, again confirming the importance of hOCT2 for cisplatin uptake. Only HEK293 cells expressing hOCT2 responded to cisplatin incubation with increased apoptosis. Apoptosis was suppressed by simultaneous incubation with cisplatin and cimetidine, a typical organic cation, suggesting competition for transport at the transporter and hence a reduction of cellular cisplatin toxicity (14).

Isoform-specific cisplatin transport has also been demonstrated in rat OCTs: in this model, too, the isoform 2 of OCT mediates cisplatin uptake, while rOCT1 seems not to be involved in this process (17). In an *in-vivo* model, the same authors showed that the renal uptake clearance of cisplatin was greater in male than in female rats, while the hepatic uptake clearance was similar in males and females. Furthermore, N-acetyl-b-D-glucosaminidase activity in bladder urine and urine volume were markedly increased two days after the administration of 2 mg/kg of cisplatin in male rats. Cisplatin did not induce any elevation of urinary N-acetyl-b-D-glucosaminidase activity in castrated male rats. These findings are explained by the higher, hormone-dependent expression of rOCT2 in male animals (18).

Other investigations have shown a significantly higher sensitivity of hOCT2-transfected cells for cisplatin toxicity compared to non-transfected cells (19). However, hOCT2-expressing cells were found to be much more sensitive to oxaliplatin than to cisplatin toxicity (19). After a two-hour incubation, accumulation of oxaliplatin but not of cisplatin was markedly increased in both hOCT1- and hOCT2-expressing cells. All these effects were competed for by the organic cation cimetidine. These transporters were identified at mRNA level also in colon cancer cell lines (hOCT1 in LS180, DLD, SW620, HCT116, HT29, and RKO cell lines) and tumour samples (hOCT1 in 20/20 and hOCT2 in 11/20 samples), opening up new prospects for the expression of OCT as markers for selecting specific oxaliplatin-based therapies in individual patients (19).

However, another study investigating the influence of cisplatin, oxaliplatin and carboplatin on the uptake of the organic cation TEA by hOCT1, hOCT2 and hOCT3 transiently transfected HEK cells, demonstrated that cisplatin, but not oxaliplatin markedly decreased TEA uptake by hOCT1 and hOCT2 (20). Both the cytotoxicity and accumulation of cisplatin were enhanced by the expression of hOCT2 and weakly by hOCT1, while those of oxaliplatin were enhanced by the expression of hOCT2 and weakly by hOCT3. These results again suggested that the basolateral hOCTs are important for the renal tissue distribution of cisplatin and oxaliplatin from the circulation. Since kidney cells are polarised and, in order to guarantee a vectorial transport of substances, possess a characteristic transporter distribution between the basolateral (the interstitium-facing side) and apical (urine-facing side) membrane, the contribution of a number of apical organic cation transporters (hMATE1, hMATE2-K, hOCTN1 and hOCTN2) to the accumulation of platin derivatives in proximal tubule cells was also investigated (20). The membrane apical transporters hMATE1 and hMATE2-K mediated the transport of cisplatin and oxaliplatin. Taken together, these data indicate that cisplatin was transported by hOCT1, hOCT2, hMATE1 and hMATE2-K, and oxaliplatin by hOCT2, hOCT3, hMATE1, and hMATE2-K (20). In this way, cisplatin and oxaliplatin appear to have very similar transport pathways in the kidney. In a further study by the same group, the cellular accumulation of both cisplatin and oxaliplatin induced by the expression of hMATE1 and hMATE2-K was investigated, applying an artificial H^+-gradient to activate the MATE transporters (these are stimulated by oppositely generated H^+-gradients across the plasma membrane). On ammonium chloride-generated intracellular acidification, remarkable transport of oxaliplatin by hMATE2-K and significant transport by hMATE1 were observed, while no significant stimulation of the accumulation of platinum was found after treatment with cisplatin, carboplatin and nedaplatin (21). It was suggested that the lower nephrotoxicity of oxaliplatin as compared with cisplatin, is related to the low renal accumulation of oxaliplatin because of its transport by MATE out of proximal tubule cells.

In conclusion, these data show that hOCT2 plays an important role in the uptake of cisplatin and oxaliplatin from the blood in renal tubular cells. hMATE1 and hMATE2-K seem to be important for the secretion of oxaliplatin but not of cisplatin into the urine and consequently are implied in the lower renal toxicity of oxaliplatin. The interplay of these renal transport systems in cisplatin and oxaliplatin transport is illustrated in Fig. 1. Since hOCT2 also seems to be expressed in colon cancer cells, it could be a target for a more efficient therapy of these tumours.

In future, we need to investigate whether competition for cisplatin uptake by hOCT2 with another organic cation can effectively reduce cisplatin nephrotoxicity in vivo without compromising its anticancer action. Moreover, we should also investigate whether patients who are less sensitive to cisplatin nephrotoxicity express polymorph hOCT2.

Grant support: Innovative Medizinische Forschung IMF CI 120437 and Else Kröner- Fresenius-Stiftung (P56/06//A57/06).

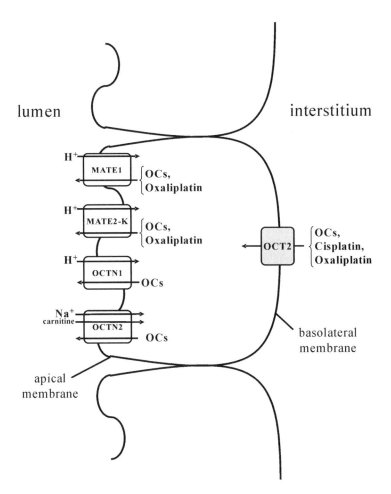

Fig. 1 Transport systems for cisplatin and oxaliplatin in human renal proximal tubules. *OCs* = organic cations

References

1. Boulikas T, Vougiouka M. Cisplatin and platinum drugs at the molecular level. Oncol Rep 2003;10:1663–82.
2. Rabik CA, Dolan ME. Molecular mechanisms of resistance and toxicity associated with platinating agents. Cancer Treat Rev 2007;33:9–23.
3. Ludwig T, Riethmuller C, Gekle M, Schwerdt G, Oberleithner H. Nephrotoxicity of platinum complexes is related to basolateral organic cation transport. Kidney Int 2004;66:196–202.
4. Wang D, Lippard SJ. Cellular processing of platinum anticancer drugs. Nat Rev Drug Discov 2005;4:307–20.
5. Reece PA, Stafford I, Russell J, Gill PG. Nonlinear renal clearance of ultrafilterable platinum in patients treated with cis-dichlorodiamineplatinum (II). Cancer Chemother Pharmacol 1985;15:295–9.
6. Endo T, Kimura O, Sakata M. Carrier-mediated uptake of cisplatin by the OK renal epithelial cell line. Toxicology 2000;146:187–95.
7. Kolb RJ, Ghazi AM, Barfuss DW. Inhibition of basolateral transport and cellular accumulation of cDDP and N-acetyl- L-cysteine-cDDP by TEA and PAH in the renal proximal tubule. Cancer Chemother Pharmacol 2003;51:132–8.
8. Pan BF, Sweet DH, Pritchard JB, Chen R, Nelson JA. A transfected cell model for the renal toxin transporter, rOCT2. Toxicol Sci 1999;47:181–6.
9. Koepsell H, Endou H. The SLC22 drug transporter family. Pflugers Arch 2004;447:666–76.
10. Koepsell H, Schmitt BM, Gorboulev V. Organic cation transporters. Rev Physiol Biochem Pharmacol 2003;150:36–90.
11. Gorboulev V, Ulzheimer JC, Akhoundova A, et al. Cloning and characterization of two human polyspecific organic cation transporters. DNA Cell Biol 1997;16:871–81.
12. Wright SH, Dantzler WH. Molecular and cellular physiology of renal organic cation and anion transport. Physiol Rev 2004;84:987–1049.
13. Motohashi H, Sakurai Y, Saito H, et al. Gene expression levels and immunolocalization of organic ion transporters in the human kidney. J Am Soc Nephrol 2002;13:866–74.
14. Ciarimboli G, Ludwig T, Lang D, et al. Cisplatin nephrotoxicity is critically mediated via the human organic cation transporter 2. Am J Pathol 2005;167:1477–84.
15. Gorboulev V, Shatskaya N, Volk C, Koepsell H. Subtype-specific affinity for corticosterone of rat organic cation transporters rOCT1 and rOCT2 depends on three amino acids within the substrate binding region. Mol Pharmacol 2005;67:1612–9.
16. Popp C, Gorboulev V, Muller TD, Gorbunov D, Shatskaya N, Koepsell H. Amino acids critical for substrate affinity of rat organic cation transporter 1 line the substrate binding region in a model derived from the tertiary structure of lactose permease. Mol Pharmacol 2005;67:1600–11.
17. Yonezawa A, Masuda S, Nishihara K, Yano I, Katsura T, Inui K. Association between tubular toxicity of cisplatin and expression of organic cation transporter rOCT2 (Slc22a2) in the rat. Biochem Pharmacol 2005;70:1823–31.
18. Urakami Y, Nakamura N, Takahashi K, et al. Gender differences in expression of organic cation transporter OCT2 in rat kidney. FEBS Lett 1999;461:339–42.
19. Zhang S, Lovejoy KS, Shima JE, et al. Organic cation transporters are determinants of oxaliplatin cytotoxicity. Cancer Res 2006;66:8847–57.
20. Yonezawa A, Masuda S, Yokoo S, Katsura T, Inui K. Cisplatin and oxaliplatin, but not carboplatin and nedaplatin, are substrates for human organic cation transporters (SLC22A1–3 and multidrug and toxin extrusion family). J Pharmacol Exp Ther 2006;319:879–86.
21. Yokoo S, Yonezawa A, Masuda S, Fukatsu A, Katsura T, Inui K. Differential contribution of organic cation transporters, OCT2 and MATE1, in platinum agent-induced nephrotoxicity. Biochem Pharmacol 2007;74:477–87.

Peripheral Neurotoxicity of Platinum Compounds

Alessandra Gilardini and Guido Cavaletti

Abstract The peripheral neuropathies induced by antineoplastic drugs are an important side effect of cancer treatment having a relevant impact on the field of research at the present time. Platinum compounds are the most widely used anti-cancer drugs and their neurotoxicity on the peripheral nervous system seems to be defined, using both *in vitro* and *in vivo* experimental models, by specific molecular pathways that involve programmed cell death. The goal of research is the under-standing of the neurotoxic mechanisms of platinum compounds in order to develop neuroprotective agents that can ameliorate the quality of life of cancer patients.

Keywords Peripheral neuropathies; Chemotherapy; Platinum compounds

Introduction

Among the several neurotoxic drugs, antineoplastic agents represent a major clinical problem given their widespread use and the potential severity of their toxicity. On clinical grounds, several classes of very effective drugs induce sensory and/or motor impairment during chemotherapy or even after treatment withdrawal, depending on the target and site of the neurotoxic action.

Platinum drugs are among the most neurotoxic antineoplastic agents. The lead platinum compounds in cancer chemotherapy are cisplatin, carboplatin, and oxaliplatin, although several other compounds are under active development and investigation. These platinum drugs share some structural similarities and, prob-ably, mechanisms of action although they have marked differences in their thera-peutic use, pharmacokinetics, and adverse effect profiles (1).

Cisplatin, carboplatin, and oxaliplatin are virtually unable to cross the blood-brain barrier which protects the central nervous system, while they have easy access

A. Gilardini and G. Cavaletti (✉)
Department of Neurosciences and Biomedical Technologies,
University of Milan "Bicocca", Monza, Italy
e-mail: guido.cavaletti@unimib.it

A. Bonetti et al. (eds.), *Platinum and Other Heavy Metal Compounds
in Cancer Chemotherapy*, DOI: 10.1007/978-1-60327-459-3_40,

to the peripheral nervous system. Besides this common feature, there are several pharmacokinetic differences among cisplatin, carboplatin, and oxaliplatin, and these differences are probably responsible for the different clinical features of their peripheral neurotoxicity. Cisplatin is the most highly protein bound (>90%), followed by oxaliplatin (85%) and carboplatin (24–50%) (1). Moreover, after intravenous administration, about 33% of the dose of oxaliplatin is bound to erythrocytes. Oxaliplatin undergoes rapid non-enzymatic biotransformation to form a variety of reactive platinum intermediates which bind rapidly and extensively to plasma proteins and erythrocytes. The antineoplastic and toxic properties appear to reside in the non-protein bound fraction, whereas oxaliplatin bound to plasma proteins or erythrocytes has been considered to be pharmacologically inactive (1).

Mechanisms of Neurotoxicity

The precise mechanism of the cytotoxic and neurotoxic actions of the platinum compounds has not yet been fully elucidated. However, some points have been clearly established regarding their mechanisms of action, particularly as far as cyto-toxicity is concerned. Several interstrand and intrastrand cross-links in DNA, particularly including two adjacent guanine or two adjacent guanine–adenine bases, can be observed following cisplatin exposure. In comparison with cisplatin- or carboplatin-induced DNA lesions, diaminocyclohexane (DACH) platinum DNA adduct formation has been associated with greater cytotoxicity and inhibition of DNA synthesis. In addition, there appears to be a significant lack of cross-resistance between oxaliplatin and cisplatin, which may be related to the bulky DACH carrier ligand of oxaliplatin, hindering DNA repair mechanisms within tumor cells (1).

Our knowledge on the mechanisms of action of platinum drugs is largely based on experimental models, and most of them are focused on cisplatin. It is clear that the antineoplastic activity of platinum drugs is primarily due to platinum-DNA inter-action, and platinum-DNA adducts have been searched and reported also in dorsal root ganglia (DRG) neurons in experimental models (1). It is generally accepted that the morphological counterpart of the occurrence of these DNA-adducts is represented by the well-known "segregation" of the nuclear components consistently reported in different experimental models (Fig. 1). However, it is very likely that other mechanisms are involved in the neurotoxicity of platinum drugs, including intracytoplasmatic protein binding, ion channel interaction and interference with intracellular signaling pathways. Regarding the intracellular events elicited by platinum drugs in neurons, particular interest is raised by the demonstration that DRG neuron apoptosis can be obtained in *in vitro* and *in vivo* models, although rather high doses of cisplatin are required to achieve this result (1). In the search for the mechanism underlying neuronal apoptosis upregulation of cyclin D1, a cell-cycle associated proteins expression is a significant observation which suggests two distinct hypotheses. One possibility is that stressed neurons express cell-cycle related proteins as a part of the death pathway. However, cell-cycle related proteins

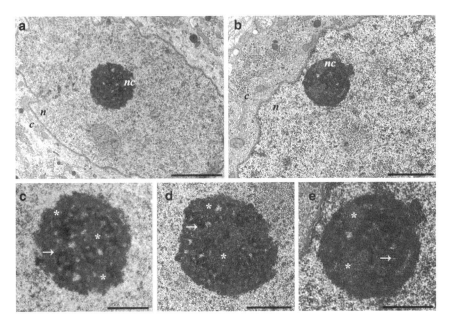

Fig. 1 Electron micrographs of dorsal root ganglia neurons of control and cisplatin-treated rats. The nucleolus (*nc*) of healthy rats has a central position (**a**) and a heterogeneous distribution of both the fibrillar (*arrows*) and granular (*asterisks*) components of the chromatin (**c**). In cisplatin-treated neurons most of the nucleolus are smaller and assume an eccentric position, while the cytoplasm (*c*) and nucleoplasm (*n*) are normal (**b**). In (**d**) and (**e**) different stages of segregation of the two different components of the chromatin are observed
Bars: **A-B,1 mm; C-D-E 500 nm**

have also been shown to be expressed in neurons, without contributing to the death pathway. Moreover, in non neuronal cells, cell-cycle related proteins are expressed in response to DNA damage, but they are involved in the repair program and not the death program. In ischemic models, upregulation of cyclins has been observed in neurons that do not undergo apoptosis. Therefore, cyclin D1 expression might simply be a response to a cisplatin-induced insult, but is not directly responsible for neuronal apoptosis (2).

A more recent hypothesis to explain cisplatin-induced apoptosis in neurons points to an alternative pathway, involving mitochondria. In fact, it has been demonstrated that the mitochondrial-cytochrome *c* pathway is activated and the fas death receptor pathway is not necessary for cisplatin-mediated death. This observation is intriguing, since the fas system has been implicated in the chemo-therapeutic effect of cisplatin at drug concentrations similar to those found in patient sera (3).

Another interesting field of investigation is represented by the interaction of platinum drugs with the Mitogen-Activated Protein Kinases (MAPK) family. Using cortical neurons treated with cisplatin as an experimental model, the activation of ERK1/2 was observed after cisplatin treatment, and this was interpreted as a protective response by neurons to injury (4). The effect of cisplatin and oxaliplatin on MAPK activation has also been studied using the human neuroblastoma cell line SH-SY5Y (5). Preliminary results demonstrate that platinum derivatives are able to affect neuronal survival and to modulate the MAPK family members, activating p38 and reducing the activation of JNK/SAPK and ERK1/2, suggesting that the stress signaling pathway induced in neuronal cells by platinum derivatives is the same as that reported by many authors in cancer cell lines (6, 7).

Clinical Highlights

From the clinical standpoint, cisplatin-induced neuropathy is sensory, predominantly characterized by symptoms of large myelinated fiber damage, such as numbness and tingling, paresthesias of the upper and lower extremities, reduced vibration and position sense perception, reduced deep tendon reflexes, and incoordination with gait disturbance. Risk factors for more severe neurotoxicity include diabetes mellitus, alcohol consumption or inherited neuropathies; all conditions which by themselves induce peripheral nerve damage. Advanced age has not been identified as an independent risk factor when there is no co-morbidity.

After completion of cisplatin chemotherapy only a part of the patients have significant neurotoxic symptoms, whereas 3–4 months later, the proportion is definitely higher. This phenomenon (called "coasting") is clinically very relevant, since it makes it difficult to assess the real severity of the DRG neuron damage during cisplatin administration. Resolution or amelioration of symptoms occurs in most of the patients over the next 12 months (despite the fact that abnormal neurological examination is frequently permanent) and, in patients with mild signs of cisplatin-related neuropathy, re-treatment with platinum drugs is generally feasible after several months.

Conventional dosages of carboplatin rather than cisplatin have been associated with a lower risk of peripheral neuropathy (e.g. mild paresthesias). Although they are generally less severe, qualitatively, the symptoms of carboplatin peripheral neuropathy are exactly the same as those observed with cisplatin.

The features of oxaliplatin neurotoxicity are rather different from those of cisplatin and carboplatin. In fact, besides chronic sensory neurotoxicity, in about 90% of patients oxaliplatin treatment has been associated with acute neurosensory toxicity, including dysesthesia and paresthesia. This peculiar type of neurosensory toxicity predominantly affects the fingers, toes, the pharyngolaryngeal tract, the perioral and oral regions, and it is generally induced or aggravated by exposure to cold. Such symptoms, which can be effectively treated with different antiepileptic agents (1), may occur within 30–60 min from the beginning or shortly after each course of oxaliplatin. Acute neurotoxicity is generally mild in severity; it disappears within a few hours or days and does not require oxaliplatin treatment withdrawal. Some patients may also develop muscle cramps or spasms. The acute neurotoxic effects of oxaliplatin result from drug-related inhibition of voltage-gated sodium currents (1). It has been suggested that oxalate ions, which are released during oxaliplatin metabolism, might be responsible for the inhibitory effects on the voltage-gated sodium channels because of their calcium chelating activity.

In addition to the acute neurotoxic symptoms caused by oxaliplatin, about 10–15% of patients treated with this agent develop a moderate neuropathy. The symptoms of chronic neuropathy include non-cold-related dysesthesia, paresthesias, superficial and deep sensory loss, and eventually sensory ataxia and functional impairment which persist between treatment cycles. Most of these symptoms usually disappear a few months after oxaliplatin withdrawal.

Neurophysiological studies in platinum drug-treated patients evidence reduction in the amplitude of the sensory potentials with minimal changes in the sensory nerve conduction velocity. Pathological examination of sural nerve biopsies has evidenced axonal degeneration, without any evidence of primary demyelination.

Models to Study Interventions

Several *in vitro* models have been used to study the neurotoxicity of platinum drugs and to investigate the possibility of protecting neurons from their toxicity (1). Moreover, animal models of the peripheral neurotoxicity of platinum drugs, which reliably reproduce most of the clinical and pathological changes observed in humans, have been developed in different laboratories and fully characterized neurophysiologically, biochemicaly, pathologicaly and analyticaly (1). The use of these models has led to increased knowledge regarding the mechanism of platinum drug peripheral neurotoxicity after chronic administration and biotransformation and, moreover, has permitted in vivo testing of the effect of putative neuroprotective agents (e.g. Org2766, reduced glutathione, nerve growth factor, vitamin E, acetyl-L-carnitine, erythropoietin,…) which have been subsequently evaluated in clinical trials or which are currently undergoing clinical investigation.

References

1. Cavaletti G, Marmiroli P. Chemotherapy-induced peripheral neurotoxicity. Expert Opin Drug Saf 2004;3:1–12.
2. Fisher SJ, McDomalds ES, Gross L, Windebank AJ. Alterations in cell cycle regulation underlie cisplatin induced apoptosis of dorsal root ganglion neurons in vivo. Neurobiol Dis 2001;8: 027–35.
3. McDonald ES, Windebank AJ. Cisplatin-induced apoptosis of DRG neurons involves bax redistribution and cytochrome c release but not Fas receptor signaling. Neurobiol Dis 2002;9: 220–33.
4. Gozdz A, Habas A, Jaworski J, et al. Role of N-methyl-D-aspartate receptors in the neuroprotective activation of extracellular signal-regulated kinase 1/2 by cisplatin. J Biol Chem 2003;278: 43663–71.

5. Donzelli E, Carfi M, Miloso M, et al. Neurotoxicity of platinum compounds: comparison of the effects of cisplatin and oxaliplatin on the human neuroblastoma cell line SH-SY5Y. J Neurooncol 2004;67:65–73.
6. Toyoshima F, Moriguchi T, Nishida E. Fas induces cytoplasmic apoptotic responses and activation of the MKK7-JNK/SAPK and MKK6-p38 pathways independent of CPP32-like proteases. J Cell Biol 1997;139:1005–15.
7. Zhuang S, Demirs JT, Kochevar IE. p38 mitogen-activated protein kinase mediates bid cleavage, mitochondrial dysfunction, and caspase-3 activation during apoptosis induced by singlet oxygen but not by hydrogen peroxide. J Biol Chem 2000;275:25939–48.

Platinum Drugs in Children with Cancer

Antonio Ruggiero and Riccardo Riccardi

Abstract Platinum compounds are very effective drugs for the treatment of childhood malignancies and their use has contributed to an increase in the long-term survival of children with cancer. Unfortunately the risk of severe disabling effects such as nephro- and ototoxicity is well known among children receiving platinum-based chemotherapy as part of their treatment. Data from literature suggest that very young children are more prone to develop cochlear damage especially when cranial radiotherapy or high cumulative doses are administered.

In view of the increasing number of children safely cured of their tumors it is fundamental that children treated with platinum drugs receive careful, continued, long-term followup.

Keywords Cisplatin; Carboplatin; Oxaliplatin; BBR3464; Ototoxicity; Children

Introduction

Chemotherapy has greatly contributed to the treatment of childhood malignancies and has led to a marked increase in the cure rate of most pediatric tumors. Platinum compounds, such as cisplatin and carboplatin, are essential components in the chemotherapeutic treatment of several pediatric tumors (Fig. 1). The use of platinum compounds has contributed to an increase in the long-term survival of children affected by cancer.

Cisplatin is an antineoplastic agent that is highly effective in the treatment of tumors in children suffering from germ cell tumors, osteosarcoma, neuroblastoma, and hepatoblastoma. However, the full clinical use of cisplatin is limited by its major toxic effects, namely, nephro- and ototoxicity. While nephrotoxicity may

A. Ruggiero and R. Riccardi (✉)
Division of Pediatric Oncology, Department of Pediatric Sciences,
Catholic University of Rome, Rome, Italy
e-mail: riccardi@rm.unicatt.it

A. Bonetti et al. (eds.), *Platinum and Other Heavy Metal Compounds in Cancer Chemotherapy*, DOI: 10.1007/978-1-60327-459-3_41,
© Humana Press, a part of Springer Science + Business Media, LLC 2009

365

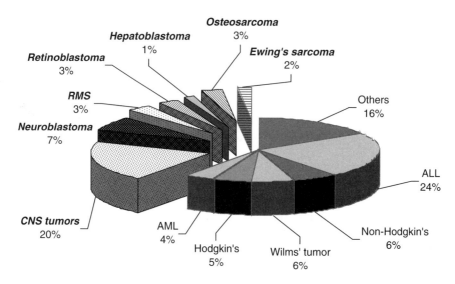

Fig. 1 Incidence of solid tumors in children less than 15 years old. Tumors *sensitive* to platinum compounds are indicated in *bold*

be significantly reduced by vigorous hydration regimens and mannitol treatment, cisplatin-related ototoxicity and associated permanent hearing loss still cause concerns. The incidence and severity of cisplatin ototoxicity appear to be greater in children than in adults. Hearing loss usually begins in the high frequency range and tends to increase in severity, spreading to the lower frequencies as ototoxicity progresses due to repeated administration and increasing cumulative doses (1).

Carboplatin is a second-generation platinum compound which was developed to obtain a less-toxic analogue which retained anticancer activity. Compared with cisplatin, carboplatin is essentially devoid of nephrotoxicity, and is less neurotoxic (Fig. 2). By contrast, haematological toxicity, principally thrombocytopenia, is the dose-limiting toxicity for carboplatin. At present carboplatin is a first-line drug for a variety of pediatric malignancies, including brain tumors, medulloblastoma, low grade gliomas, neuroblastoma, malignant mesenchymal tumors, and retinoblastoma (2). It is also active in germ cell tumors; however clinical studies have shown a lower anti-tumor effect as compared to cisplatin.

Oxaliplatin is a third-generation platinum compound which was selected for further investigation in view of its lack of cross-resistance with cisplatin and its promising antineoplastic activity in tumors with intrinsic or acquired resistance to cisplatin and carboplatin in adults. Based on preclinical reports showing synergistic effects with several anticancer agents, including irinotecan and gemcitabine, oxaliplatin is undergoing clinical evaluation in phase II trials also in children with solid tumors. Acute toxicity of oxaliplatin is relatively mild and has a transient cumulative peripheral sensory neuropathy as its dose-limiting toxicity (3, 4). However, its widespread clinical use in children will be suggested by results of ongoing phase II studies in combination with other antineoplastic compounds.

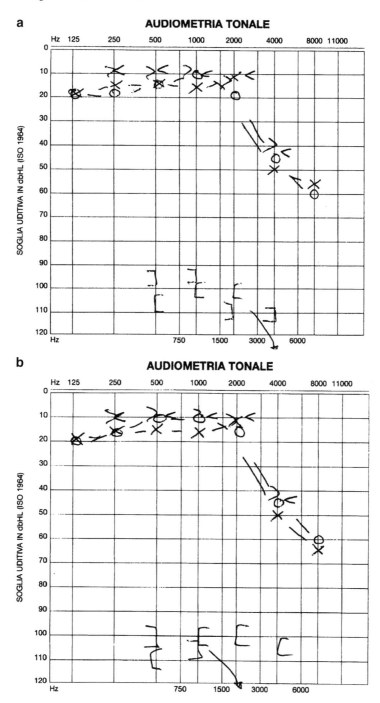

Fig. 2 Hearing loss in a child treated with cisplatin. In panel (**a**), a severe high-frequency hearing loss is noted following 8 cycles of cisplatin. In panel (**b**) no further ototoxicity following 6 additional courses of carboplatin

Pharmacodynamics and Pharmacokinetics

Platinum compounds exert their cytotoxic action by DNA platination. Reactive aquated intermediates are formed in solution after the spontaneous elimination of chloride. These cisplatin and carboplatin intermediates are rapidly bound to plasma proteins and tissues that react with nucleophilic groups to form covalent bands. After binding, the platinum intermediates are inactivated and only the free platinum products (including the parent drug) exert cytotoxic effects. Like cisplatin, carboplatin targets DNA, with the formation of DNA-interstrand crosslinks and protein-DNA crosslinks being the major toxic pathways (5).

Interestingly the adducts formed by carboplatin on DNA are essentially the same as formed by cisplatin but 20- to 40-fold higher concentrations of carboplatin are required, and the rate of adduct formation is about ten times slower (6).

The pharmacokinetic profile of bound and unbound forms of platinum differ appreciably. After administration of cisplatin, the protein-bound platinum persists in the plasma and can be detected in urine for many hours, even up to 4 days (7, 8).

By contrast, the unbound active platinum has a more rapid decline with a half-life of less than 1 h. In children, the half-lives of total and unbound cisplatin are 44 and 1.3 h, respectively (9).

The pharmacokinetic profile of carboplatin is characterized by a lower rate and degree of protein binding than cisplatin. As a consequence, the terminal half-life of unbound carboplatin is longer, ranging from 2 to 4 h. Compared with adults, pharmacokinetic parameters of carboplatin in children are similar.

Cisplatin is reported to cross the blood–brain barrier only in limited amounts. However, it can achieve significant intratumoral concentrations as a consequence of the marked blood–brain barrier disruption occurring in the vasculature of intracerebral tumors, whereas the intact blood–brain barrier in the remaining areas of the brain tissue limits protein-bound cisplatin penetration into the central nervous system. By contrast, carboplatin can achieve higher cerebrospinal fluid concentration following systemic administration as a much smaller fraction of carboplatin binds to plasma proteins due to the slower protein binding process. In our study on cerebrospinal fluid (CSF) pharmacokinetics of carboplatin in children with brain tumors, the mean AUC ratio of CSF to plasma was 0.28 (range, 0.17–0.46) suggesting a good penetration of the drug into the central nervous system (10) (Fig. 3).

Toxicity

In children, several factors have been identified as potential risk factors for cisplatin-related toxicity.

Age. A young age at the time of platinum treatment seems to increase the risk of ototoxicity. Children younger than 5 years of age have a 21-fold higher

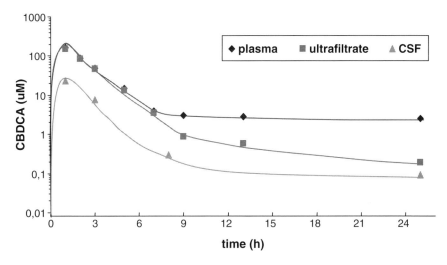

Fig. 3 Carboplatin (CBDCA) concentration vs. time curve in ventricular cerebrospinal fluid and plasma (total and ultrafiltrate) following administration (1h-infusion) of CBDCA 600 mg/m² in a patient with totally resected medulloblastoma

risk of developing moderate/severe high-frequency hearing loss compared with patients aged 15–20 years (11). This could be due to the age-related immaturity of cochlea cells or to the peculiar pharmacokinetics of cisplatin in young children.

Radiation. Hearing loss due to platinum compounds may be enhanced by prior or concomitant craniospinal radiotherapy such as in children with medulloblastoma. This deleterious effect may be present also at low cumulative doses (12).

Cumulative dose. The risk of developing ototoxicity increases with the cumulative cisplatin dose. A cumulative dose >400 mg/m² is associated with moderate to severe risk of ototoxicity (11).

Ototoxic drugs. Aminoglycosides, bleomycin, and loop-inhibiting diuretics can negatively influence the ototoxicity of cisplatin (13).

Interpatient variability. This variability may be influenced by cisplatin's degree of renal excretion and protein binding. Compared with adults, this variability is amplified in very young children due to the age-related maturation of the physiological processes responsible for drug metabolism, thus producing a large distribution volume and a slower elimination, especially in the younger age group (14–16). Recently, polymorphisms of the megalin gene have been evocated as a patient's inter-individual susceptibility factor against cisplatin-related ototoxicity (17). Megalin is a multiligand endocytotic receptor linked to the transport of cisplatin or cisplatin adducts highly expressed in renal proximal tubular cells and marginal cells of the stria vascularis of the inner ear. These studies may improve our ability to identify patients at higher risk to develop cisplatin-induced toxicity.

In addition, other factors such as renal insufficiency or intravenous bolus administration appear to enhance the cumulative risk of developing ototoxicity.

Conclusions

Platinum compounds continue to play a major role in the treatment of children with cancer. Due to its toxicity profile, carboplatin can replace cisplatin when severe cisplatin-related toxicity occurs or combined treatment with radiotherapy is planned, especially in very young children.

Children are in any case more prone to develop severe defects such as ototoxicity that have negative impact on speech, language acquisition, and educational achievement. Therefore, follow-up should focus on nephro- and ototoxicity to protect young patients from these disabling effects of potentially curative treatments.

References

1. Gilmer Knight KR, Kraemer DF, Neuwelt EA. Ototoxicity in children receiving platinum chemotherapy: underestimating a commonly occurring toxicity that may influence academic and social development. J Clin Oncol 2005;23:8588–96.
2. English MW, Skinner R, Pearson ADJ, et al. Dose-related nephrotoxicity of carboplatin in children. Br J Cancer 1999;81:336–41.
3. Di Francesco AM, Ruggiero A, Riccardi R. Cellular and molecular aspects of drugs of the future: oxaliplatin. Cell Mol Life Sci 2002;59:1914–27.
4. Kelland L. The resurgence of platinum-based cancer chemotherapy. Nat Rev Cancer 2007; 7:573–84.
5. Micetich KC, Barnes D, Erickson LC. A comparative study of the cytotoxicity and DNA-damaging effects of cis-(diammino)(1,1-cyclobutanedicarboxylato)-platinum(II) and cis-diamminedichloroplatinum(II) on L1210 cells. Cancer Res 1995;45:4043–7.
6. Knox RJ, Friedlos F, Lydall DA, et al. Mechanism of cytotoxicity of anticancer platinum drugs: evidence that cis-diamminedichloroplatinum(II) and cis-diammine-(1,1-cyclobutanedicarboxylato)platinum(II) differ only in the kinetics of their interaction with DNA. Cancer Res 1986;46:1972–9.
7. Gormley PE, Bull JM, LeRoy AF, et al. Kinetics of cis-dichlorodiammineplatinum. Clin Pharmacol Ther 1979;25:351–7.
8. DeConti RC, Toftness BR, Lange RC, et al. Clinical and pharmacological studies with cis-diamminedichloroplatinum (II). Cancer Res 1973;33:1310–5.
9. Pratt CB, Hayes A, Green AA, et al. Pharmacokinetic evaluation of cisplatin in children with malignant solid tumours: a phase II study. Cancer Treat Rep 1981;65:1021–6.
10. Riccardi R, Riccardi A, Di Rocco C, et al. Cerebrospinal fluid pharmacokinetics of carboplatin in children with brain tumors. Cancer Chemother Pharmacol 1992;30:21–4.
11. LI Y, Womer RB, Silber JH. Predicting cisplatin ototoxicity in children: the influence of age and the cumulative dose. Eur J Cancer 2004;40:2445–51.
12. Kretschmar CS, Warren MP, Lavally BL, et al. Ototoxicity of pre-radiation cisplatin for children with central nervous system tumors. J Clin Oncol 1990;8:1191–8.
13. Lanvers-Kaminsky C, Krefeld B, Dinnesen AG, et al. Continuous or repeated prolonged cisplatin infusions in children: a prospective study on ototoxicity, platinum concentrations, and standard serum parameters. Pediatr Blood Cancer 2006;47:183–93.

14. Gratton MA, Smyth BJ. Cisplatin. Continuous versus bolus. J Pediatr Hematol Oncol 2006;28:60–1.
15. Murakami T, Inoue S, Sasaki K, et al. Studies on age-dependent plasma platinum pharmacokinetics and ototoxicity of cisplatin. Sel Cancer Ther 1990;6:145–51.
16. Stöhr W, Paulides M, Bielack S, et al. Nephrotoxicity of cisplatin and carboplatin in sarcoma patients: a report from the late effects surveillance system. Pediatr Blood Cancer 2007;48:140–7.
17. Riedemann L, Lanvers C, Deuster D, et al. Megalin genetic polymorphisms and individual sensitivity to the ototoxic effect of cisplatin. Pharmacogenomics J 2008;8:23–8.

Optimising Carboplatin Dose using Patient Characteristics and Therapeutic Drug Monitoring

Aurélie Pétain, Antonin Schmitt, Fabienne Thomas, Christine Chevreau, and Etienne Chatelut

Abstract As the pharmacokinetics of carboplatin is mainly determined by renal function, AUC dosing of this drug is routinely performed. This method consists in predicting the individual carboplatin clearance and calculating the dose according to a target value of area under the plasma concentration time curve (AUC). All the equations proposed for predicting carboplatin clearance are based on body weight, age, gender, and serum creatinine level. In this way, carboplatin, which was initially contraindicated in patients with renal insufficiency, can now be administered to such patients. However, several of the assays used for serum creatinine determination are not consistent with one another. Substantial differences in carboplatin doses (even in the same patient) may be the consequence of these analytical discrepancies. A new biological parameter, cystatin C plasma level, could be an additional or even an alternative covariable for predicting carboplatin clearance. For some carboplatin regimens, such as in high-dose chemotherapy, drug monitoring of carboplatin plasma concentrations followed by Bayesian pharmacokinetically guided dosing can be implemented. In conclusion, carboplatin AUC dosing still needs to be improved in order to standardise its use in clinical practice.

Keywords Population pharmacokinetics; individual dosing; glomerular filtration rate

Introduction

Carboplatin is mainly eliminated by glomerular filtration. Initially, the drug was contraindicated in patients with poor renal function. Several formulae have been developed for individual carboplatin dosing. Calvert et al. showed a strong correlation between carboplatin clearance (CL) and glomerular filtration rate (GFR) determined by an isotopic method (1). For a decade, this methodology allowed

A. Pétain, A. Schmitt, F. Thomas, C. Chevreau, and E. Chatelut (✉)
EA3035, Institut Claudius-Regaud, Toulouse, France
chatelut.etienne@claudiusregaud.fr

A. Bonetti et al. (eds.), *Platinum and Other Heavy Metal Compounds in Cancer Chemotherapy*, DOI: 10.1007/978-1-60327-459-3_42,

physicians to prescribe carboplatin for patients with poor renal function. All the equations commonly used to predict individual carboplatin CL are based on body weight, age, gender, and serum creatinine level (Scr). However, several factors, particularly Scr, contribute to the heterogeneity observed among patients and centres. Scr levels are affected by both the muscle mass and inter-method variability of the assays. Scr can be determined by either enzymatic assay or the non-compensated Jaffé method. In order to illustrate the heterogeneity in terms of carboplatin dosing, the case of a real patient can be considered: a 63-year-old woman (82 kg, 1.8 m^2) treated with carboplatin for ovarian cancer. Her Scr, determined both by the non-compensated Jaffé method and enzymatic assay, was 126 and 91 µM, respectively. Using the first Scr value (126 µM) and the Calvert equation (with the Cockcroft-Gault formula (2) to estimate the GFR), her predicted CL would be 87 ml/min associated with a dose of 310 mg for a target area under the plasma concentration time curve (AUC) of 4 mg/ml × min. For the same patient, the second Scr value (91 µM) used in the Chatelut equation (3) (without correction for obese patients as would be required) led to a predicted CL of 108 ml/min and a dose of 540 mg for a target AUC of 5. The contributions of (1) Scr assay, (2) the equation for predicting carboplatin CL, and (3) the choice of target AUC to the overall 74%-difference in terms of dosage were 38, 10, and 25, respectively, showing the predominant impact of Scr assay. There are two possible approaches for minimizing the impact of Scr bias on carboplatin dosing. The first is to improve the method of predicting carboplatin CL by using other biological markers (*a priori* dosing method). Plasma cystatin C levels are a promising parameter. The second is to determine the actual carboplatin CL in the case of regimens based on multiple carboplatin infusion (*a posteriori* method).

Cystatin C as a New Covariate for Predicting Carboplatin Clearance

Cystatin C (CysC) is a member of the cystatin superfamily of cysteine proteinase inhibitors. It is a 120-amino-acid basic protein with a molecular weight of 13 kDa described as the product of a "housekeeping gene" that is expressed in all nucleated cells. Thus, unlike creatinine, its production is not dependent on muscle mass. Cystatin C undergoes extensive glomerular filtration and is reabsorbed by tubular epithelial cells but subsequently catabolised so that it does not return to the circulation (4). The reciprocal of CysC (1/CysC) correlates closely with the comparative GFR reference standard. Cystatin C seems to meet the criteria for an ideal GFR marker, but conflicting results have been published concerning its use in nephrology (5–7). CysC has also been studied as a marker to predict renal drug clearance and has proved superior to Scr with cefuroxime (8) and digoxin (9). Our substantial experience with carboplatin prompted us to study CysC as a marker of carboplatin elimination, which is known to be a glomerular filtration phenomenon. In a previous study (10), we showed that the best equation for predicting carboplatin clearance includes both Scr and CysC:

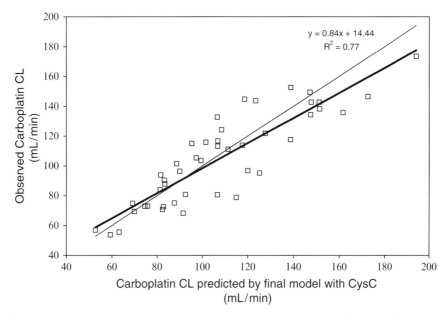

Fig. 1 Correlation between observed clearance and value calculated according to the final equation with CysC

$$CL\,(mL/min) = 110 \cdot (Scr/75)^{-0.512} \cdot (CysC/1.0)^{-0.327} \cdot (BW/65)^{0.474} \cdot (AGE/56)^{-0.387} \cdot 0.854^{SEX}$$

(with Scr in μM, CysC in mg/l, body weight in kg, age in years, and SEX = 0 if male and = 1 if female).

The correlation between observed clearance and clearance calculated with this model is shown in Fig. 1. The bias and the precision associated with the equation were 4 and 12% respectively. The deletion of either CysC or Scr from the model decreases the precision and correlation between predicted and observed clearances. We conclude that CysC as marker is at least as good as Scr in predicting carboplatin clearance. Moreover, one advantage of CysC over SCr is its low inter-laboratory variability. Two automated assays are used for most of the clinical evaluations of CysC, namely, the immunoturbidimetric (PETIA, Dako) and immunonephelemetric (PENIA, Dade-Behring) assays. When the same calibrators are used, the correlation between the two assays is extremely close (11).

Drug Monitoring of High-Dose Carboplatin

Motzer et al. (12) proposed a high-dose paclitaxel, ifosfamide, carboplatin (target AUC of 24 mg/ml × minute per cycle), and etoposide regimen (TICE) plus peripheral blood stem-cell rescue for cisplatin-resistant germ cell tumours. This treatment is used for patients who fail to respond completely to first-line chemotherapy or who present an extragonadal primary site. Three cycles of high-dose carboplatin and etoposide (400 mg/m^2/day) were administered at 14- to 21-day intervals with reinfusion of peripheral blood derived stem-cells. Each cycle consisted in three daily infusions. First, Motzer et al. determined the optimal overall AUC (3-day AUC) of carboplatin in a phase I study. The recommended AUC value was 24 mg/ml × min. The carboplatin dose was calculated according to the Calvert formula (dose = target AUC × [GFR + 25]) where GFR was initially determined by isotopic (^{99M}Tc-DTPA) determination and more recently by the Jelliffe equation. Whatever the method used to estimate GFR, the AUC values observed (for a target AUC of 24) varied considerably among patients, ranging from 12 to 48, and from 10.9 to 36.7, respectively (13). At the Institut Claudius-Regaud, we treat poor prognosis patients according to the TICE regimen, but using daily (i.e. day 1, day 2) therapeutic drug monitoring (TDM) of carboplatin ultrafiltrable plasma concentrations in order to determine the actual individual carboplatin CL. The dose is adjusted daily to effectively achieve the overall AUC of 24. Three blood samples (i.e. at the end of infusion, 1 h and 4 h after the end of infusion) are taken daily. These concentrations are analysed with a Bayesian approach using the NONMEM program and a database comprising 109 other patients. The pharmacokinetic and toxicity results of the first five patients are reported in a previous study (14). The therapeutic drug monitoring allowed us to reach the target AUC (Table 1). We retrospectively calculated the AUC that would have been obtained in these patients if we had used the Jelliffe formula: the AUC would have ranged from 15 to 41 mg/ml × min. The intra-patient variability within each cycle was very limited,

Table 1 Patients' characteristics, carboplatin pharmacokinetic parameters, and treatment

Patient	Previous cisplatin dose (mg/m^2)	Cycle	Target total AUC (mg/ml × min)	Predicted CL (ml/min)	Mean observed CL ml/min (CV%)	Observed total AUC (mg/ml × min)	Total dose (mg)	Neuro-otic common toxicity criteria
1	400	1	24	181	150 (6%)	25.0	3,750	2
		2	24	162	121 (8%)	26.5	3,210	
		3	16	130	111	NE	1,805	
2	400	1	24	226	142 (5%)	24.8	3,500	NE
		2	24	174	121 (2%)	24.1	2,940	
3	400	1	24	126	66 (26%)	24.0	1,595	3
		2	24	116	84 (15%)	25.1	2,145	
4	700	1	24	188	127 (9%)	25.0	3,230	3
		2	24	162	126 (12%)	25.7	3,180	
		3	8	179	139	7.1	990	
5	200	1	24	238	191 (3%)	24.2	4,620	3
		2	24	255	193 (8%)	24.4	4,650	
		3	16	246	174 (3%)	16.0	2,780	

CL carboplatin clearance predicted according to the Chatelut formula; *CV* coefficient of variation for interday variability; *NE* not evaluable

indicating that TDM only at day 1 would enable the overall AUC target of 24 to be achieved.

Our experience confirms the favourable clinical results (4/8 patients are in complete remission; follow-up from 1 to 7 years) in this group of patients. Besides the expected haematological toxicity, ototoxicity was the main toxic effect.

For patients treated with high-dose carboplatin, therapeutic drug monitoring is justified by the dose modifications it imposed, especially since no method of predicting carboplatin clearance appears to be good enough.

Conclusions

In addition to the prediction of carboplatin CL, physicians have to choose a target AUC for carboplatin dosing. This choice remains largely empirical. Clinical studies aimed at determining the pharmacodynamic covariates of carboplatin are required. We may suppose that demographic, biological or pharmacogenomic parameters determine carboplatin haematotoxicity. These characteristics need to be assessed and taken into account in order to achieve better individual carboplatin dosing.

References

1. Calvert AH, Newell DR, Gumbrell LA, et al. Carboplatin dosage: prospective evaluation of a simple formula based on renal function. J Clin Oncol 1989;7:1748–56.
2. Cockcroft D, Gault M. Prediction of creatinine clearance from serum creatinine. Nephron 1976;16:31–41.
3. Chatelut E, Canal P, Brunner V, et al. Prediction of carboplatin clearance from standard morphological and biological patient characteristics. J Natl Cancer Inst 1995;87:573–80.
4. Newman DJ. Cystatin C. Ann Clin Biochem 2002;39(Pt 2):89–104.
5. Dharnidharka VR, Kwon C, Stevens G. Serum cystatin C is superior to serum creatinine as a marker of kidney function: a meta-analysis. Am J Kidney Dis 2002;40:221–6.
6. Laterza OF, Price CP, Scott MG. Cystatin C: an improved estimator of glomerular filtration rate? Clin Chem 2002;48:699–707.
7. Tidman M, Sjostrom P, Jones I. A Comparison of GFR estimating formulae based upon s-cystatin C and s-creatinine and a combination of the two. Nephrol Dial Transplant 2008;23:154–60.
8. Viberg A, Lannergard A, Larsson A, Cars O, Karlsson MO, Sandstrom M. A population pharmacokinetic model for cefuroxime using cystatin C as a marker of renal function. Br J Clin Pharmacol 2006;62:297–303.
9. O'Riordan S, Ouldred E, Brice S, Jackson SH, Swift CG. Serum cystatin C is not a better marker of creatinine or digoxin clearance than serum creatinine. Br J Clin Pharmacol 2002;53:398–402.
10. Thomas F, Seronie-Vivien S, Gladieff L, et al. Cystatin C as a new covariate to predict renal elimination of drugs: application to carboplatin. Clin Pharmacokinet 2005;44:1305–16.
11. Finney H, Newman DJ, Gruber W, Merle P, Price CP. Initial evaluation of cystatin C measurement by particle-enhanced immunonephelometry on the Behring nephelometer systems (BNA, BN II). Clin Chem 1997;43(Pt 1):1016–22.

12. Motzer RJ, Mazumdar M, Sheinfeld J, Bajorin DF, Macapinlac HA, Bains M et al. Sequential dose-intensive paclitaxel, ifosfamide, carboplatin, and etoposide salvage therapy for germ cell tumor patients. J Clin Oncol 2000;18(6):1173–1180.
13. Kondagunta GV, Bacik J, Sheinfeld J, et al. Paclitaxel plus ifosfamide followed by high-dose carboplatin plus etoposide in previously treated germ cell tumors. J Clin Oncol 2007;25: 85–90.
14. Chevreau C, Thomas F, Couteau C, Dalenc F, Mourey L, Chatelut E. Ototoxicity of high-dose carboplatin. J Clin Oncol 2005;23:3649–50.

Index

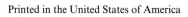

Printed in the United States of America